The Dying Patient
The Medical Management of Incurable and Terminal Illness

Edited by

Eric Wilkes OBE FRCP FRCGP FRCPsych

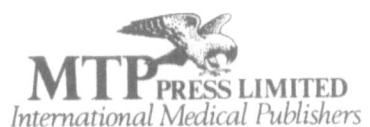

MTP PRESS LIMITED
International Medical Publishers

Published by
MTP Press Limited
Falcon House
Lancaster, England

Copyright © 1982 MTP Press Limited
Softcover reprint of the hardcover 1st edition 1982

First published 1982

The dying patient.
1. Terminal care
I. Wilkes, Eric   II. Series
362.1'9   R726.8

ISBN 978-94-011-6248-7   ISBN 978-94-011-6246-3 (eBook)
DOI 10.1007/978-94-011-6246-3

Photosetting by Swiftpages Limited, Liverpool

The
Dying Patient

Contents

List of Contributors

Sir FERGUSON ANDERSON, OBE KstJ MD FRCP
Formerly David Cargill Professor of Geriatric Medicine, University of Glasgow

TOM ARIE, FRCPsych
Professor of Health Care of the Elderly, University of Nottingham

THELMA D. BATES, FRCR
Consultant Radiotherapist and Oncologist, St Thomas's Hospital, London

JOHN R. BENNETT, MD FRCP
Consultant Gastroenterologist, Hull Royal Infirmary

IAN M. C. CLARKE, FFARCS
Director, Regional Pain Centre, and Consultant Anaesthetist, Hope Hospital, Salford

A. G. O. CROWTHER, MA MB BChir DObstRCOG
General Practitioner Sheffield; Honorary Lecturer in the Department of Community Medicine, University of Sheffield; and Medical Director, St Luke's, Sheffield

A. M. JOHNSON, MD FRCP
Consultant Cardiologist, Wessex Cardiac and Thoracic Centre, Southampton

ROB G. JONES, MB ChB MRCPsych DPM
Senior Lecturer (Psychiatry), Department of Health Care of the Elderly, University of Nottingham

E. E. LAWTON, SRN QN
Formerly Research Nurse, Department of Community Medicine, University of Sheffield

PETER W. R. LEE, MD FRCS
Consultant Surgeon, Gastrointestinal Unit, Hull Royal Infirmary

LINDA LIDDAMANT, BA
Formerly Research Assistant, St Luke's, Sheffield

G. P. MAGUIRE, FRCPsych
Senior Lecturer in Psychiatry, University Hospital of South Manchester

MARTIN G. MOTT, BSc MRCP DCH
Senior Lecturer and Consultant in Paediatric Oncology, Bristol Royal Hospital for Sick Children, Bristol

F. E. NEAL, KSG MB ChB FRCR DMRT
Consultant Radiotherapist and Oncologist, Weston Park Hospital, Sheffield; Honorary Clinical Lecturer in Radiotherapy and Oncology, University of Sheffield

MARGARET M. PLATTS, BSc MD FRCP
Reader in Medicine, University of Sheffield

MICHAEL A. SIMPSON, MB BS MRCS MRCPsych DPM
Professor of Psychiatry and Professor of Family Practice and Community Health, Temple University, Philadelphia, Pennsylvania, USA

BASIL A. STOLL, FFR FRCR DMRT
Honorary Consultant Physician to Oncology Departments, St Thomas's Hospital and Royal Free Hospital, London

SUSAN M. TEMPEST MPS
Staff Pharmacist, Yorkshire Regional Drug Information Centre, and Poisons Bureau, Leeds General Infirmary

J. M. A. WHITEHOUSE, MA MD FRCP
Professor of Medical Oncology and Director CRC and Wessex Regional Medical Oncology Unit, Southampton General Hospital, Tremona Road, Southampton

ERIC WILKES, OBE MA FRCP FRCGP FRCPsych
Professor of Community Care and General Practice, Sheffield University and Medical Director, St Luke's, Sheffield

Preface

The main purpose of this book is to bring together some description of the skills and attitudes of those working in the hospice units specializing in terminal care with those rather different but overlapping skills used daily in the palliation of chronic or incurable disease.

This varied collection of papers does not pretend to be exhaustive. Among the omissions, for example, are two major causes of death – chronic respiratory disease and stroke. This is because the treatment of the end-state of these conditions – and they are not alone in this – lies more in the gentle withdrawal of measures no longer appropriate rather than in any positive regime within the gift of the physician.

This may lead on occasion to an unjustifiable diminution of interest, but this is less likely in cases of cardiac or malignant disease.

Ischaemic heart disease remains the main killer of the western world. We may see important changes in our approach over the next decade as we document slowly and painstakingly the comparative ineffectiveness of our therapy; but in cases of progressive cardiac disease no matter how we may argue as to management or prevention, we are agreed that we must lighten the dreary burden of illness as effectively as possible.

The gradual increase of anginal pain, oedema or dyspnoea can be difficult to tolerate, yet the majority of patients accept with surprising placidity the knowledge that they have heart disease. This contrasts vividly with the horror of many who know or suspect that they have cancer. Those with chronic renal failure, in so far as any such generalization has meaning, should be placed somewhere between the two; and colleagues outside the specialty will perhaps be surprised and instructed by the blend of high technology and personal involvement that the management of such cases demands.

It is also precisely this blending of personal relationship with clinical skill that the terminal care units have re-emphasized and brought back into the centre of medical care. This is seen not only in the need for good symptom-control but in the general and time-consuming emotional support required by both patients and family when they are called on to face the problems of disseminated malignant disease.

Because of the pain, fear and mutilation experienced by a minority of these patients, most of the writings on terminal care have been concerned with cancer, and this indeed is the case here, with contributions from many different fields of medical practice and beyond.

Yet despite all this work, we still may not fully realize the scale of the need. So many of our patients are detribalized, rootless and very vulnerable. They are part of a suburban society in which so many instinctive activities atrophy that they have to be taught how to rear and play with their children, or how to make love. If they need drugs to assist in such basic functions as opening their bowels and going to sleep, how can they cope with death?

The doctors and nurses to some degree must share this common background. They have seen few dead people before their training and they too lack confidence. The dying patient may have to wait longer before the nurse answers the bell than does the less ill, but less threatening, post-operative case. Doctors who have direct clinical responsibilities have, at any rate in an American survey, a higher rate of psychiatric consultation, alcoholism and marital breakdown than non-clinicians of equivalent socioeconomic status. We are not exempt from human frailties and may be seeking in our work help with our own problems rather than effectively coping with those of others.

It is surprising that we manage so very well as often as we do, although the help may be given in spite of the system rather than because of it.

Yet we all work within the framework of a medical system that is a compound of evolution, accident and political wheeler-dealing. It has created a health service far better than the material resources of the country would lead one to expect and this, of course, leads to difficulties. It has two additional disadvantages, neither of which will be quickly or easily put right.

The first disadvantage is the routine divorcement of the general practitioner from hospital facilities, so that he can no longer care for his own straightforward cases in a local hospital bed. This is damagingly combined with a tremendous and often ill-judged demand for the practitioner's services, which averages out at nearly 10 000 consultations per practitioner per year, and which makes in the cities a 5 minute appointment system part of the doctor's survival-kit.

The second disadvantage is to some degree a corollary of the first, in that hospital consultants have to see in their outpatient clinics many cases that would not merit referral if primary care was less overwhelmed. Furthermore so far as inpatients are concerned, they have to process more and more patients through fewer beds. In a world dominated by chronic diseases, when disposal is often far more tricky than diagnosis, the whole apparatus of care is geared to speedy diagnosis and ever speedier discharge. In this situation the dying patient feels acutely the lack of an important or continuing relationship.

Most of us would admit that we are not well trained in speedily attaining trust, communication or teamwork. Just as the general practitioner may be forced to hand over to hospital a patient he has looked after for a long time, so the hospital colleague will ignore, in his important yet essentially short-term and transient role, the longer-term impact of the illness on the family or next of kin. This is not only insensitive but it is also poor preventive medicine. The impact of bereavement in physical as well as psychological terms cannot properly be left to the haphazard efforts of the other fellow. I suspect that in years to come medical historians will ponder at the inability of a reasonably good health care system to produce in major moments of crisis for the family a meeting of both the consultant and the general practitioner in joint consultation with them. This good custom has become rarer over the last two decades, and it gives a clue as to why so many terminal care units have opened since Dame Cicely Saunders started at St Christopher's Hospice less than 15 years ago. This is part of the popular indictment of our standards of medical relationships – not just for terminal cases but for the new colostomy or the recent myocardial infarct or any similar major episode affecting either the old or the young. We deliver uninvolved, convenient, sessional medicine and unhappily it is acceptable, thought not really good enough, in the eyes of dedicated high-quality colleagues in both consultant and general practice.

It is especially important, therefore, that the two psychiatric contributions should form an integral part of this book. Although psychiatry has little to offer many brave people under stress, some of their specialist knowledge and attitude should now be part of the overall competence to which all good clinicians aspire; and although the chapters of Maguire and Simpson tend to cover a little of the same ground, their subject is so crucially important and treated in such different styles that any repetition is likely to be helpful rather than tedious.

Many of us need help in handling the private fears of our patients and in the adroit use of non-verbal communication. Even more, many of us need help in handling patients who are well enough educated to require the truth but not well equipped enough to adjust to it. The senior doctors, with of course an enormous number of exceptions, do not enjoy being cross-questioned by their patients. The younger doctor is less fussed by this but is not always able to handle it as well as he would like. In this very delicate area the profession is thus manipulated often into being either inexperienced or out of date, the patient feels the doctor is either evasive or brutal, and the relative tends to feel left out. No-one can win here unless a genuine effort is made.

The book closes with a look at some of the newer administrative possibilities for terminal care, and takes a brief look at how this may be organized in future in the community, in hospital, and in the specialist unit.

It looks as if, in the short-term at any rate, the great days of British medicine are over. We need the more urgently to use our skills in a genuine attempt to compensate for the lack of resources. It is hoped that this book will be of some help in increasing our understanding of the needs of the dying patient and the family, both for the generalist and to those who are reading outside their own area of expertise; and although this book contains occasional confirmation that we are, and should remain, the most self-critical of professions, it is hoped that colleagues will find in these pages not so much new learning as relearning, not so much changing as remembering, and also much of that reassurance and support that they and their patients so richly deserve.

ERIC WILKES

1

The elderly at the end of life

Sir Ferguson Anderson

In this modern world there is going to be an increase of approximately 60 per cent in people 85 years and over before the turn of the century throughout the developed countries, and an even greater one in the under-developed countries. In the United Kingdom there will be among these very old individuals three women to every man and the great majority of these ladies will live alone. These changes will be associated with a continuing movement of population in general from rural areas into towns. There is (correctly) a general belief that older people fare best in small communities and it is known that morbidity increases markedly with age, especially in women. This background information leads to the conclusion that the care of those dying in old age is a matter worthy of thought and forward planning.

Less than 50 years ago every household in the so-called industrial nations had experience of death. The combination of high birthrates, crowded housing conditions and infectious diseases like rheumatic fever and tuberculosis, meant that at least one or two children in most families died in infancy or childhood. Before the First World War the female medical wards in hospital were approximately half-full of young girls with rheumatic fever and every week one would die with an acute myocarditis. Large sanitoria in every town were crowded with young people suffering from tuberculosis, and death was a constant companion. In spite of these hospital deaths at that time most of the total number of deaths occurred in the individual's own home and only some 5 per cent of people died in hospital. People then, especially among the poorer sections of society, were familiar with death and dying. In contrast, by 1970 66 per cent of all deaths occurred in hospital. This has had the effect of taking death-outwith the patients' homes so many young middle-aged people have never seen anybody dying nor have experienced death in the family.

Religious attitudes were different at the turn of the century too, and there was a quiet acceptance of this high deathrate, with very little recrimination against doctors, nurses or God. When death now occurs in young people it is usually regarded, rightly, as a tragedy, but in a sinister way blame is always attributed to someone, and the natural occurrence of death is much less well accepted. It seems almost macabre to state that in the years to come most people who die will certainly be old, and very many will be very elderly. Already in the United Kingdom, out of 500 000 deaths each year, half take place at over 75 years of age.

Death until recently was a taboo subject and it is only with the modern development of specialized hospices that there have been changed views and renewed interest. Diseases themselves have changed in character due to the almost complete disappearance of the great infectious diseases; and today heart disease, cancer, and diseases of the nervous system are most frequently recorded. Heart disease in old age is commonly due to coronary artery disease and cancers are predominantly found in the alimentary tract, while among afflictions of the central nervous system the most frequent is cerebrovascular disease. Studies of the pathology of old age by Howell and Piggott (1951, 1952 and 1953) showed many years ago the multiplicity of diseases in the elderly, the frequent silent onset of coronary thrombosis and the atypical presentation of some illnesses.

EDUCATION

While it is common knowledge that women live longer than men, this gift of added years is not without its drawbacks; the women who do survive longer are much less healthy than the smaller number of men who enter their 80s and 90s. These men are indeed the élite of the elderly and many of them are extremely fit. Perhaps the main problems, with elderly women in particular, are degenerative diseases associated with long-term illness, and no one can be satisfied with the progress of medicine who visits continuing-treatment hospitals for the elderly and sees the great numbers of severely disabled people who continue to live with a very poor quality of life for many years. Until new advances can be made in treatment, particularly of stroke, much skilled medical and nursing talent will need to be devoted to suitable care and maintenance of such cases. These individuals require a high amenity of accommodation, appropriately planned to suit their physical, mental and social needs, and highly skilled staff. The personnel undertaking this work must be able to relate to others and have empathy with their patients. They should be trained to reassure, guide and listen constructively. When the elderly die at home very frequently the individuals caring for them are themselves elderly; Wilkes (1965) made the important observation that 14 per cent of cancer patients dying at home were being cared for by relatives themselves over 70 years of age, while 74 per cent of caring relatives were over 50 years of age.

When dying is considered it is prudent to attempt some definition and Ackland (1974) categorized dying patients as those in whom a diagnosis of incurable disease has been made and whose doctors expect them to die within a few weeks or months. What characterizes the dying as a group is the fact that their attendants *expect* them to die.

Medical students, nurses, social workers and paramedical staff are today receiving much more instruction in the care of older people than formerly, but not yet enough in the skilled therapy of the dying. In fact, there is considerable controversy about the question of whether any instruction in the management of the dying should be given in the undergraduate or training period of the caring professions. It is argued that, for medical students particularly, this is a postgraduate subject and that understanding and appreciation of its importance will develop during routine ward work and by watching the approach of senior doctors. Often, however, newly qualified physicians find themselves suddenly faced with dying people and their relatives, without instruction of any kind; this imposes an unnecessary mental challenge. For some 7 years a seminar has been held for medical students in the third year of their instruction, by the Department of Geriatric Medicine in Glasgow. The views of young people about the care of individuals at the end of life have been varied, sometimes extremely surprising, but always interesting. The services available for dealing with the dying are described together with the problems experienced in the home care of such patients. Stress is laid on communication with relatives and on the provision of appropriate therapy. A visit is also paid to a hospice for the dying and each medical student is requested to talk to three dying patients in the hospice just as if the students were visitors and not professionals in training. The reasons for going into some detail about instruction is that, certainly in my earlier medical career, it was customary if a patient in a ward was dying to put screens around him or her, and the doctor on ward round would ask the nursing sister how that patient was keeping. On being told that the condition was worsening and that death was approaching, individuals like me very often said to the sister, 'Well carry on, you are doing a good job' and did not go and speak to the patient. This drawing back from what seemed to be a medical failure was commonplace in bygone years. Thus, there was a lack of helpful support for both the patient and also for the caring staff.

Education has improved this situation and it seems more common nowadays for young doctors to speak to their dying patients. An immense alteration in the understanding of the emotional needs of the dying has taken place in recent years as well as an increasing realization by both nurse and doctor that a death does not necessarily imply a failure in therapy. With many more people coming to the end of their lives in old age, it must be realized that this is a natural process, and one which needs to be studied in detail so that help of every possible kind is available to the individual. Elderly people do not fear death so much as the process of dying, and it must be our endeavour to make medical students and doctors consider what sort of death the patients are going to have as a consequence of the therapy prescribed for them maybe years earlier. Our knowledge in this respect is singularly lacking; for example, the treatment of hypertension without doubt reduces the incidence of cerebral haemorrhage and may cut down pathological changes in the brain arteries. This is a spectacular advance for the middle-aged and the older people up to about 75 years of age. What is going to happen to these people of 75 as they become older? What is the end result of sparing the elderly patient from a cerebral haemorrhage? Cowan and Anderson (1976) followed until death a group of elderly men and women who had reached 70 years of age when first examined. (It is essential to note that all these individuals had attained 70 years of age.) They found that it was extremely difficult to discover any factors which would give a clue as to the future length of life of these people. After the age of 70, it seems that body weight or the level of systolic or diastolic blood pressure does not influence future longevity. The most important factor was the age of the patient – the older the individual was, the more likely he was to die. Elaine Brody and her colleagues (1972) endeavoured to estimate prognosis in elderly women suffering from senile dementia. Only one medical rating predicted death significantly. When the physician and psychiatrist thought a patient needed to be watched closely was an important indicator of death. If the physician was asked, 'Who is going to die soon?', he would probably be wrong; but if the question was, 'Whom shall we have to keep close watch on?' the answer was usually correct. One subject, then, which requires much further study is the long-term follow up of elderly people and the natural history of diseases in old age.

THE ELDERLY PATIENT

Swenson (1965) makes the point that 50 years ago death came earlier in the human race and the death process was experienced mostly in a sudden or traumatic manner by those individuals gainfully employed or otherwise functioning well in society. Now, in the last quarter of the twentieth century, death commonly comes to patients who have long since been retired from active social participation and are physically or psychologically incapacitated, presumably giving them considerable time to contemplate death as an impending experience.

In caring for the older person who is dying, it is essential to place the needs of the patient first. This seems so obvious that it hardly needs stating, yet very often plans for therapy seem to be evolved without taking into effect what the end result of this or that procedure will be. Will the quality of life of the individual be improved or lessened? This not only affects the patient in a fundamental way, it has an important bearing on staff morale. It is absolutely essential to ensure that the physician tells the nursing staff in particular, and also the paramedical staff (for example physiotherapists, occupational therapists and speech therapists) what are the aims in therapy. If, for example, an elderly woman, ripe in years and with a massive stroke, who seems to be dying, is given a subcutaneous drip then the nurse may well wonder what is happening. The doctor will state that this fluid is being given in order to prevent the elderly patient, should she become conscious, from feeling a sensation of thirst; it is not being administered to prolong the act of dying but so that she may die in comfort. The fluid is being administered subcutaneously rather than intravenously, because if the needle is pulled out by the patient a vein will not be ruptured with a resultant large haematoma, and that this method of infusion has been used rather than intragastric administration so that if the elderly person withdraws the tube, fluid will simply wet the bedclothes and not go into the lungs; these explanations are worthwhile.

Misunderstanding in the direction of therapy often results in sisters and nurses losing confidence in the physician, who is with the best intention doing the right thing, but has not explained to his team what is going on. Faith in the doctor has been a tradition of British medicine, one inherited from our forefathers, but efforts must be made to maintain this faith. This means that relatives, too, must be told in simple language what is happening. It is my view that complicated explanations going into the intimate details of therapy are seldom appreciated. The old person dying is usually a loved relative and there is no doubt that a type of domestic deafness occurs in which relations do not hear even repeated explanations of what is happening. The same story may have to be told again and again until it dawns on the relatives that the end is near, and that the old person is going to die, but it is wise not to state when this event will happen.

In treating an elderly person who is presumed to be dying the first essential is to confirm the diagnosis. If this is incorrect, then subsequent therapy will obviously be totally incompetent. The doctor who sees previously unknown elderly patients must listen to them carefully. A diagnosis may already have been made and it may indicate that the illness is a fatal one. While this diagnosis may be correct, it must not be assumed to be so and the doctor must keep an open mind. On other occasions the symptoms may not fit into a previously experienced pattern of disease, and it must be borne in mind that patients have an uncanny habit of being right. Unusual symptoms should not be classified as hysterical or imaginary. With elderly people it is essential to obtain accurate information about past illnesses and previous operations and particularly about drug medication, both past and present. In old age, atypical presentation of a common illness is much more frequently seen than a rare disease.

Many physicians, especially senior doctors, seem unwittingly to consider malignancy as their first choice because the patient is elderly and on occasion seem to close their mind to alternative diagnosis. The history, full clinical examination and the investigations may indicate that the patient is indeed dying. Care then has to be taken to make certain that the complaints the patients have are due to this fatal illness and are not caused by other relatively minor pathological conditions which may make the individual's life miserable – for example, the presence of mouth ulcers or haemorrhoids. It is now recognized that side-effects of medication with drugs are not uncommon; for example, mental confusion or depression, and the possibility that symptoms such as nausea and vomiting may be due to previous physical therapy, for example radiotherapy, must be considered. If the diagnosis is in doubt, it is worth admitting the older person to hospital promptly so that a correct diagnosis may be made as soon as possible. The elderly have little time anyway, and admission should never be postponed because the individual is old. This does not mean that an elderly, emaciated person obviously in the last stages of life should be subjected to investigation in order to satisfy scientific curiosity. On the other hand, it must never be assumed because an elderly individual looks seriously ill that a fatal illness is present. Like children, old people may suddenly appear desperately unwell partly due to their severe reaction to dehydration and electrolyte imbalance. These may be aggravated by impairment of their sensation to thirst. When fluid deprivation is restored and electrolyte balance corrected, there may be a sudden dramatic improvement.

The diagnosis should be reviewed regularly: Has the diagnosis been correct? Has some change taken place? The great danger of labelling a patient with an incurable condition is that consideration is not given to the possibility that a mistake may have been made. Once it is completely evident to all that the patient is dying, then the direction of therapy, while still as active, changes. The relief of symptoms becomes the first priority and the overall purpose is to make the patient as comfortable as possible and to help him over the stile at the end of life.

It is certainly the public impression that dying now is more prolonged than it used to be and while it is not possible to make any hard and fast rules about looking after older people at the end of their life, the decisions made should be commonsense ones. Unnecessary operations should be avoided, for example a tracheotomy in a very elderly person, unconscious with a massive cerebral haemorrhage; and unpleasant manoeuvres like an intra-gastric tube in a terminally ill cancer patient. Some believe that more use should be made of euphoriants including, where appropriate, alcohol or one of the mild tranquillizing agents like thioridazine. Verzar, the eminent gerontologist, thought that the elderly at the end of their life should be permitted to chew the leaves of *Erythroxylum coca*. Consideration should be given to efforts to improve the physical and mental wellbeing of the individual according to his taste and desire. The dying have problems enough without being deprived of a favourite 'bad habit'.

PAIN

Symptoms like pain must be relieved, and Saunders (1972) has taught us that pain-relieving substances should be given regularly according to an invariable rule. Once pain has been controlled, theoretically the patient should never suffer from pain again. This requires training and teaching of medical and nursing staff. Saunders uses oral opiates for pain relief in most of her terminal patients, and the danger of drug addiction is irrelevant in dying patients. The usual dose of heroin required by mouth is 10 mg and in Saunders' (1973) series of 428 patients, only 19 per cent needed more than 20 mg at one time. It is usual to start with mild pain-relieving substances by mouth, like aspirin or paracetamol, and then proceed to codeine or drugs like dipipanone, while when the pain becomes severe, to morphine, methadone or diamorphine. Use of radiotherapy or of chemical nerve blocking can often relieve pain which cannot be relieved by any other method.

It must be borne in mind that while it is said that the pain threshold is raised in the elderly, in *everyone* including the old the pain threshold is lowered by previous discomfort, insomnia, fatigue, anxiety, fear and mental isolation. The pain threshold is raised by the easing of pain itself, sound sleep, rest, diversion and sometimes by antidepressants. Drugs of the phenothiazine group may help to dissociate the patient from his illness; for example, chlorpromazine 25 mg, three times a day by mouth, may be of use.

INSOMNIA

If drug therapy is required and pain is not the cause of the sleeplessness then chloral hydrate or chlormethiazole may be worth trying. It is always necessary to try and find out the cause of insomnia as depression, faecal impaction or a bed sore may be the real cause of the wakefulness. With insomnia, as with many other symptoms, the most important therapy is for the doctor to find time to sit down and listen to his patient talking without giving the impression that he is too busy, and that he has the desire to elicit even the most trivial-sounding complaints.

OTHER SYMPTOMS

Nausea, a most troublesome complaint, is often helped by chlorpromazine but may on occasion be caused by the associated depression, when anti-depressant drugs will be of value. Antiemetics should be tried in rotation if vomiting is a problem. If persistent vomiting occurs, and the time for any form of surgical intervention is past, it may be worthwhile passing a nasal tube and instituting intermittent or continuous suction to prevent constant retching. When dysphagia is severe, a local anaesthetic gel before food may be of value and on occasion semi-solids are most useful. The patient who has a tube inserted will require watching in case it has become blocked. Occasionally, if loss of appetite is the main symptom, small doses of prednisolone twice a day relieve symptoms and induce some euphoria. Hiccups can be overcome by having the patient breathe out and into a paper bag for a few minutes, or if carbon dioxide is available this can be used as an inhalant. If this fails chlorpromazine by injection will be effective. Persistent cough can often be relieved by pholcodine linctus in a dose of 5–10 ml, taken in hot water. Diamorphine is the strongest antitussive agent and may eventually have to be given by injection. If the sputum is purulent, a short course of an appropriate antibiotic will be helpful.

In consideration of these common symptoms it is always worthwhile performing a periodic re-examination of the dying individual to try and find out if some other cause had developed which is producing symptoms. In old people tiredness, that is, a feeling of immense fatigue, may be a very important symptom and must be investigated. Conditions like cardiac failure or very rarely potassium deficiency may be present. In the elderly, immobility may lead to stiffness and bed sores and the older patient should not be allowed to become bedridden before it is inevitable. The use of exercise with or without physiotherapy should be considered, and occupational therapy in the dying patient is often of value; if a patient has any particular ability or hobby this should be encouraged. The undertaking of minor chores in the ward or at home should be practised and praise given for work done. It is important to try and prevent apathy, boredom and despair.

MENTAL STATE

The fear of death is to be expected and the value of time spent by the doctor in reassurance cannot be overestimated. The old person if he or she desires it must be allowed to tell his or her story. The mental state is helped without doubt if the doctor will devote enough time to talking with the patient. When the inevitable question 'Am I dying?' is asked, only those who know their individual patient well can answer this question correctly. Sometimes the individual wishes reassurance. It may not even be reassurance that he will not die – it may be reassurance that there will be a minimum of pain and discomfort; and the question of when to tell a patient he is dying depends on a very accurate assessment of the whole makeup of the individual. It may be obvious that the elderly person is denying the reality of the situation and this may be a defence mechanism. Much consideration requires to be given before such denial is shattered. Crammond (1970) stated that it was easier for someone with a close personal relationship with the patient to make the decision of what to say, and my own view is that frequently the best person to be in touch with the individual at this time is his family doctor. The specialist only occasionally has this intimate relationship, but here again there is no general rule and many individuals have a very close friendship with the specialist surgeon or physician who is dealing with them at this time in their life. The general practitioner, too, needs reassurance and here the specialist in hospital has a part to play. Communication between specialist and general practitioner must always state what has been told to the patient so that no conflicting opinions may be given later, and encouragement and praise in the management of the case will do nothing but good.

It is vital to bear in mind that not only must the physical health of the patient be treated but attention must also be paid to the mental state. One important feature in regard to this is deciding when to call in the hospital padre or priest. He is an important member of the team and very frequently the person the elderly individual will want to see. Recently the father of one of my staff was dying in the medical ward, and the young house doctor telephoned the minister of the patient late at night and said 'I can do no more for this old man, I think he needs a minister'; the minister came up immediately and talked to the old man. He died later that night, and there was no doubt that this visit was very much worthwhile. The education of the medical student does pay off in that he bears in mind that he is only one of a team. Priests and padres have not been used enough in our health service, especially in our hospitals where very little provision is made for the hospital chaplain, and it is unusual for a room to be available where he can see his client in peace.

RELATIVES

Information about the diagnosis, the progress of the illness, the purpose of the therapy and the likely outcome should be given in simple language to the relatives. It is necessary to estimate their ability to understand the information given and detailed points of therapy are usually best left out of the discussion. Prognosis is difficult and it is very easy to cause great distress by stating that an old person is going to die when in fact at that time death does not occur. If, for example, a relative is told that the aged relation is definitely about to die, soon, and the old lady recovers, the relative may well be delighted but in her mind she had planned her future without her loved one and has been preparing herself for the bereavement. If, because of incorrect information, this miscalculation in prognosis is repeated then the relative is left in a state of bewilderment, having faced up to the death of her loved one several times and perhaps having made adjustments in her family life which have then to be reconsidered and replanned. Caution, therefore, is strongly advised in stating definitely that an old person is going to die, and more particularly in giving a time when this will happen. The relative is entitled to know that the loved one is seriously ill and that there is danger of death, but it is wise not to be too dogmatic in what is happening.

NURSES

The doctor in charge of the elderly dying patient has a duty to try and help his nurses as well. He must bear in mind the importance of supporting the mental health of the nursing staff and of giving explanations on each stage of treatment. In older people adequate care of the mouth is essential, and even in the terminal case it is often worthwhile reshaping ill-fitting dentures to cut down discomfort and salivation. Pain-relieving drugs may produce constipation, which may result in faecal impaction and in turn produce retention of urine, so watch must be kept on the action of the bowels. Nothing can replace good nursing in the prevention of bed sores; many people now use ripple mattresses and are aware of the danger of the phenothiazine derivatives in causing immobility.

Nutrition in terminal illness is important as there is no doubt that many people become very malnourished and unwell because of insufficient intake of, for example, protein at the end of life. Good nursing is made so much easier by ensuring that while the patient is kept free from pain, he is not made too sleepy to eat or move about the bed, as immobility is a great danger to older people. Wilkes (1973) has written about the relief of pain by inhalation of nitrous oxide and oxygen when turning a patient over with a large bed sore, and has also given advice about smell in, for example, a fungating lesion of the breast. The so-called 'death rattle' or worrying noises which may accompany the last hours of comatose patients may be due to stertorous breathing or the accumulation of mucus in the trachea or large bronchi. In stertorous breathing the noise may sometimes be relieved by placing the head in a lateral position or using an airway to prevent obstruction by the tongue. Accumulated mucus as a cause of noise may be abolished by injecting hyoscine hydrobromide 0.4 mg intravenously.

It is worth making some general points. Much more important than drugs is the establishment of a warm relationship with the doctor or nurse, and when distress or pain is the complaint, every endeavour must be made to find exactly what is causing the distress. Nurses will usually tell you that if the doctor could only find more time to speak to his dying patient, this would be of great help. The doctor also has a duty to explain to the nurse that the irritable, quarrelsome old person is in need of help. It is of little value to start an argument with such people and the doctor must be available to assist promptly in such situations.

Public reassurance is essential as many people are worried that elderly dying patients are kept alive when it would be much better for everybody's sake to allow them to die. This is usually a feeling made worse by lack of communication and understanding of what is happening, but the feeling does exist and the impression remains. It is thus important for the doctor to make certain that everyone – relatives, friends – understands what is happening and that life is not being artificially prolonged when quality has completely gone. Well-illustrated books are now available which are suitable for providing very relevant information for teenagers and upwards on dying and old age (Milne, 1977; Toomey, 1976).

THE ELDERLY AT HOME

Elderly people who die have frequently left behind an elderly relative and Wilson (1970), a health visitor in Belfast, showed that there is a withdrawal syndrome among many old people who have been bereaved and that they do not want to mix with others. They may themselves thus become ill following bereavement. Wilson's plan is that if two very elderly people are living together and one takes ill, this sort of situation should be notified to the health visitor, who should start to visit before bereavement occurs so that a friendship is built up, and if one partner dies the health visitor will keep an eye on the person remaining.

Isaacs, Livingstone, and Neville (1972) studied terminal care of the aged in Glasgow and concluded that older people who live alone and fall and those with persistent incontinence should be notified to the physician in community medicine and that dementia must be realistically handled, bearing in mind the great strain placed on relatives who keep such elderly patients at home. To my mind these suggestions become possibilities if use is made of the health care team (Anderson, 1976). Regular visiting by the health visitor of those 70 years and over, combined with a reporting-back session to the general practitioner would enable much earlier discovery of such patients. Plans could then be made for diagnosis, appropriate therapy and/or placement.

It is essential, of course, that all general practitioners should become completely aware of the facilities available for older people in terminal illness in their district. The Marie Curie night-nursing service is often of great value and in many areas there are hospices for the dying which, in properly selected cases, can be invaluable. These hospices have the additional function of providing teaching for the caring professions, and for selected volunteers too, in the management of dying people.

WHERE SHOULD AN ELDERLY PERSON DIE?

From the point of view of the family, it means care at home or care outside their own home. Most surveys have revealed that when elderly people have to come into hospital it is for nursing care because the relatives have become exhausted, and when this occurs the old, ill person must be admitted to hospital or hospice and an effort should be made to involve the relatives in the patient's further care in a limited way in this situation. The relatives will also require reassurance after admission has become unavoidable by telling them what a splendid job they have done and how they could not have managed any longer to look after the patient at home. The physician must reveal his sympathy and understanding with many caring people, who wish at all costs to keep their loved one in their own home, but a time may come when this is patently impossible and here the physician, looking at the whole situation impartially, is often the best judge.

If the patient is cared for at home the busy doctor may require help in coordinating all the services which can be procured for an old person dying at home; for example, the district nurse, night nursing, home laundry, the provision of nursing aids such as commodes, the way in which financial help can be given, and arrangements for friendly visiting if the ill old person is isolated. This coordinator may be the doctor himself, the health visitor or the social worker, but it must be ascertained that all possible services are involved, or the relatives may fail to make contact with anyone and may struggle on alone. Gibson (1971) showed the great value of elderly people dying in their own homes. If this has to be encouraged, then public reassurance is required that domiciliary services should be adequate to enable the relatives to play a full part in the care of the dying patient without being pushed over the edge into breakdown.

Visitors to Eastern countries from the West are always impressed by the short time that so many older people in these countries spend in bed before death and it seems possible that many older people in developed countries are confined to bed without any clear reasons. Perhaps the elderly individuals in the East have a greater motivation to keep active than do the single, isolated and lonely old ladies in our Western civilization. In the United Kingdom we are indeed fortunate in having an understanding legal profession who would never allow a patient to be killed, yet do not demand of us that we strive officiously to keep people alive. There seems no benefit in changing the law as long as faith in the caring physician can be preserved. The patient chooses his doctor, enjoys the privilege of friendship with him and has faith in him. He is usually completely satisfied to be advised and guided by the judgement of his physician. Any change in the law would require to be made not only by consulting the public and the doctors, but with the complete cooperation of lawyers, and would seem to me to be at the present time unnecessary. In other countries the attitudes of the legal profession are different and then doctors are placed in very difficult clinical situations where elderly people are concerned.

In contrast, nothing is more worrying to the physician than to find that a patient has been passed on to him with a diagnosis associated with certain death, when in fact the patient is not suffering from a fatal illness at all. Diagnosis in elderly people is extremely difficult and the older person may present with what appears to be a terminal neoplasm when in fact some other illness, for example acute bacterial endocarditis, is present. Even when the diagnosis has been confirmed as due to cancer, the course of many cancers in old people is different from that in the younger individual. The growth advances more slowly and the individual may die of intercurrent disease practically untouched by the cancerous growth. While unnecessary interference is always wrong, the immense advance that has been made in anaesthetics for old people and the quick, excellent surgery which is often available, can transform the outlook in many old people with cancer, and the possibility of operation for curative or palliative reason should always be kept in mind. Certainly, if a growth is obtruding a major passage, for example the oesophagus, the bowel or the urethra, then thought must be given to some sort of palliative operation. Fine judgement is required here and many general practitioners over the years have learned which surgeon to call when they want either rapid immediate action or delaying therapy which may not involve surgery at all. The doctor always has the privilege of not treating his patient with cancer in any active way, and sometimes this is the right course to take where elderly people are concerned. Chemotherapy is worthy of consideration but it is not necessary to treat every case of cancer, and on occasion masterly inactivity is the best decision.

The quality of life in the last days is of first importance. Age is in essence a secondary point. Hughes (1960) summarized the needs of dying people as being companionship, a sense of security and control of physical symptoms by medical, nursing and domestic care.

References

Ackland, Sarah (1974). Personal communication

Anderson, Sir Ferguson (1976). The effect of screening on the quality of life after seventy. *J. Roy. Coll. Phys.*, **10, No. 2,** 161

Brody, E. M., Kleban, M. H., Lawton, M. P., Levy, R. and Waldow, A. (1972). Prediction of mortality in the mentally-impaired institutionalized aged. *Jewish Chron.*, **Dec, 25,** 611

Cowan, N. and Anderson, F. (1976). Survival of healthy older people. *Br. J. Prev. Soc. Med.*, **30,** 231

Crammond, W. A. (1970). Psychotherapy of the dying patient. *Br. Med. J.*, **3,** 389

Gibson, R. (1971). Home care of terminal malignant disease. *J. Roy. Coll. Phys. London*, **5,** 135

Howell, T. H. and Piggott, A. P. (1951). Morbid anatomy of old age: Parts I and II. Pathological findings in the 9th and 10th decades. *Geriatrics*, **8,** 85

Howell, T. H. and Piggott, A. P. (1952). Morbid anatomy of old age. Parts III and IV. Findings in the late and earlier seventies. *Geriatrics*, **7,** 137, 140

Howell, T. H. and Piggott, A. P. (1953). Morbid anatomy of old age: Part V. Findings in late sixties. *Geriatrics*, **8,** 216, 267

Hughes, H. L. G. (1960). *Peace at the Last.* (London: Calouste Gulbenkian Foundation)

Isaacs, B., Livingstone, Maureen and Neville, Yvonne (1972). *Survival of the Unfittest.* (London: Routledge and Kegan Paul)

Milne, Katharine (1977). *A Time to Die.* (Hove: Wayland Publishers Ltd.)

Saunders, Cicely (1972). Care of the dying. Reprinted from the *Nursing Times* (London: Macmillan Journals)

Saunders, Cicely (1973). A death in the family; a professional view. In *Care of the Dying.* DHSS Reports, No. 5, p. 16. (London: HMSO)

Swenson, W. M. (1965). In Fulton, R. (ed.) *Death and Identity,* p. 105 (New York: John Wiley and Sons Inc.)

Toomey, Lee (1976). *Old Age.* (Hove: Wayland Publishers Ltd.)

Wilkes, E. (1965). Terminal care at home. *Lancet*, **ii,** 799

Wilkes, E. (1973). Terminal illness at home. *Mod. Geriatr.*, **3, No. 3,** 133

Wilson, F. G. (1970). Social isolation and bereavement. *Lancet*, **ii,** 1356

2

The failing mind

Rob Jones and Tom Arie

INTRODUCTION

A shark swims through the shallows. Suddenly its body rocks and its pectoral fins beat the water in the throes of a convulsion. Companion sharks swiftly appear in dangerous interest and shortly the boldest of them makes a tentative attack. Within minutes the disordered shark is destroyed by its fellows. There are few sharks in the sea with a failing and disorganized nervous system.

This dramatic anecdote serves as a reminder of a number of themes. It illustrates the devastating effect on the organism of a breakdown of the central command and control mechanisms. The more sophisticated the animal the more gentle and subtle may be the initial impairments, but beyond a certain point major effects ensue. In nature a disturbed nervous system is quite rapidly detected and ruthlessly despatched. Disease of any sort is not well tolerated. A disordered nervous system is possibly tolerated least well of all. While intraspecies cannibalism is not universally the order of the day there are plenty of predatory species around eager for a living.

Man seeks to control, ameliorate or reverse the effects of nature and to obtain a more equitable state of affairs. Human communities seem quick to label their unusual or unwell members and these include those with a failing mind, but they generally like to feel that they respond in a caring way to such problems. Yet frequently medical services are unaware of many, or even most, impaired people. It seems certain that in the past individuals afflicted with what we would now recognize as forms of dementing illness were often purged, beaten, drowned or burnt. The

17

fearful and rejecting attitudes which motivated these atrocities are now considerably muted but may still be detected.

Dementia as a word is sometimes unpopular today and some prefer other terms. The word echoes with emotive overtones of screaming irrationality and demonic deviance; however, it means literally 'out of one's mind'. We are not as intolerant as the sharks but the over-burdened family, exhausted through years of sleepless nights and heavy days, must sometimes bitterly feel that there is a covert rejecting attitude of savage effect in society's resource priorities.

The failing mind which forms the subject of this chapter is the dementing human mind. We are concerned here with the elderly but there are no vast differences in the degenerative dementias of younger people. Such a subject may seem to sit uneasily in a book of this nature because dementia, while it invariably ends in death, might not do so for many years. Most of the other sufferers described in this book frequently have considerable insight into their state and into their fate. By contrast demented individuals are characteristically unaware of the extent and nature of their disabilities. There is a sense in which this lack of insight makes dementia the most disabling condition of all. When impairments are realistically perceived there are opportunities for adaptation and the acquisition of alternative personal strategies. Where insight is missing the scope for rehabilitation is greatly reduced and dependency easily becomes massive. Dementia is unquestionably the greatest generator of dependency and makes the most expensive demand for care facing societies in the developed world.

In the vast majority of cases dementia is irreversible and incurable. Additionally it looms large in most aspects of health and social welfare services. Such services are increasingly becoming swamped by the large numbers of old people needing their attention. Population projections indicate that in this country the very old – those most prone to dementia – will be the most rapidly increasing group in coming decades, as they are already.

Community surveys indicate a prevalence of mild, moderate and severe dementia of around 10 per cent in the population of over 65 years of age (Kay, Beamish and Roth, 1969a and b); among the over 75s there is a dramatically increasing prevalence with increasing age. Thus the Newcastle Survey found that whereas about 2.3 per cent of 65–69 year olds were demented by their criteria, this figure rose to 5.5 per cent of the 75–79 year old group. In those over 80 years old the figure leapt massively to 22 per cent (Kay *et al.*, 1970).

As it is precisely this more aged section of the elderly population which is projected to increase to the greatest extent over the next two decades (Government Actuary's Department, 1975), it is clear that the failing mind will emerge even more prominently as a social problem in the closing years of the twentieth century. It has been well said that we face a 'quiet epidemic' of dementia (*British Medical Journal*, 1978).

For the individual the consequences of the failing mind are overwhelming, destructive and fatal after a variable period. For the supporters of such an individual in the community the consequences in terms of different aspects of burden, emotional suffering, family tensions and distress are nearly always similarly overwhelming and often destructive. The direct and indirect financial costs to the community of the failing mind have never been adequately measured but they are unquestionably great. If it were possible to convert intangible non-monetary aspects, such as the suffering of families, into hard currency the overall cost to the community would clearly be very great indeed.

CLINICAL FEATURES

The clinical picture of dementia reflects the deteriorating brain. Indeed some refer to 'acute brain failure', meaning confusional states, and 'chronic brain failure', meaning the dementias (Livesley, 1977). Such labels rather imply a simple mechanistic failure of the brain as an organ. In the case of dementia this is not a satisfactory analogy. The brain in its daunting complexity is associated with the essence of the individual and is not limited to any simple or single function. In the clinical course of a dementia it is not that a particular mechanical effect ceases to operate (such as the pumping of the heart in 'heart failure'), but rather that layers of sophisticated and subtle integration gradually start to become disorganized.

We favour Lishman's (1978) definition of dementia as 'an acquired global impairment of memory and personality but without impairment of consciousness'. In his view the dementia syndrome is the possible result of a number of different processes, some of which are readily detectable and may be susceptible to more than symptomatic treatment. Theoretically, the prospect exists in some cases of halting or even perhaps reversing the process of deterioration. Most doctors dealing with typical presentations in the very old do not find that they see many reversible outcomes but the attempt to seek potentially treatable causes in an individual case must never be neglected.

Apart from such cases of the dementia syndrome, two particular clinico-pathological entities exist which are accepted as diseases in their own right. These are progressive and ultimately fatal varieties of the dementing syndrome. The majority of dementias in the elderly are due to one or other of these two diseases, while in a further group the two conditions coexist. These diseases are senile dementia and arteriosclerotic dementia (or 'multi-infarct dementia (Hachinski, Lassen, and Marshall, 1974). Typically each has a somewhat different course.

To simplify, arteriosclerotic dementia may be pictured as a process in which a number of infarcts or softenings, some large but most very small, occur in the ageing brain (mainly the cortex). These infarcts tend to coalesce as time goes by, so that increasing but patchy destruction becomes evident. The appearance of such an infarcted area may be reflected in clear clinical events, particularly if the infarct is large. Often the infarcts are quite small and the symptoms which accompany them, if any, do not present to a doctor; very small infarcts may occur without revealing themselves clinically at all. By contrast the process of senile dementia encompasses a gradual generalized thinning of the cortex (though variably distributed in degree) which therefore tends towards a more steady down-ward clinical course.

Reflecting this simple account of the pathology, the clinical progression of arteriosclerotic dementia is classically patchy and proceeds in a 'stepwise' fashion. Sudden episodes, some with major deterioration and others more minor, are followed by recovery over a period to a level of functioning which is nevertheless usually poorer than previously. Further episodes are likely to occur, more or less dramatically. Again there are recovery phases but the degree of disability accumulates each time and the trend is ever downward in a zigzag manner.

The 'thinning' of senile dementia gives rise to a clinical picture of a steady gradual deterioration but it seems likely that within the overall process differing clinical progressions are distinguishable. Kral (1962) delineated 'benign senescent forgetfulness' which is clearly quite different from the process in progressive dementia of a rapid and grave illness characterized by the early appearance of parietal lobe impairment. This latter variety is often referred to as 'Alzheimer-type' or as 'Alzheimerized' dementia. All senile dementia is characterized by specific histological changes (Corsellis, 1962) and a genetic background has been established (Slater and Cowie, 1971); but it seems clear that within the overall entity are a number of different subsyndromes. As yet these are ill-understood. Relationships between varying clinical courses and possible neuropathological differences at the tissue level remain to be explored. It is increasingly evident that there is a potentially rich vein of research at the biochemical level.

Other clinical differences between arteriosclerotic dementia and senile dementia are noteworthy. Thus arteriosclerotic dementia, like vascular disease in general, tends to affect men much more than women, and specific neurological signs are much more likely to be found than in senile dementia. A history of 'strokes', hypertension in middle age or other manifestations of cardiovascular disease are common. The person with senile dementia, however, may appear to be fairly robust. Women present more commonly with the senile dementia picture and they tend to be somewhat older than men affected by arteriosclerotic dementia. A genetic background has been well established in the case of senile dementia, but with the individual case this is not likely to be a prominent distinguishing feature.

As the process of arteriosclerotic dementia or senile dementia proceeds a point is reached at which the clinical pictures converge in a severely disabled and demented state and the common outcome is death.

Turning more explicitly to the 'human face' of dementia the sort of clinical situation faced so often by general practitioners and others concerned with the elderly is pithily summarized in the following passage written by a psychogeriatrician (Baker, 1976):

... an old lady lives alone, with a neglected garden and dilapidated house. She has gradually lost her contacts with the outside world, and the circle of friends and neighbours who had helped her with shopping and visits have diminished as she has become increasingly dirty and neglected. She has discouraged home help and meals on wheels services and is now living in squalor and is perhaps incontinent. Her memory is failing and general health becoming frail. She may already be known to the police because of wandering from the house, and neighbours and others have begun to put pressure on medical and social services to have her removed. An incident such as a fall in the house, a fire, or another episode of wandering or fear of hypothermia has brought the firm request that she should be admitted to hospital.

The major clinical feature of the dementia syndrome is the memory disorder which most obviously affects recent memory. This is particularly so early on, but relatives and friends assert that long-term memory is also impaired and studies have confirmed that this is the case (Miller, 1973; Whitehead, 1978). Almost as prominent, especially in the early stages, is the increasing restriction in activity generally. Interests and hobbies are dropped. The repertoires of thought and behaviour become noticeably less rich. Those habits, interests and activities which have been followed longest tend to persist longest but the more subtle and sophisticated reflections of the previous personality and intellect fall away. The former 'queen of the kitchen' will continue to manage basic domestic activities, after some fashion, for a long time but it will also be long obvious to all, except perhaps to her, that only the simplest skills are still within her competence. A restriction of drive and initiative is evident as well as the decline in capability and it may be difficult to know which comes first. In some cases this deterioration in initiative is prominent for an appreciable period before other aspects of the dementing process become obvious.

A conversation deeper than brief social chitchat reveals impoverished ideation and a limited and circumscribed range of talk. There is difficulty in shifting from one topic to another and a tendency to return to persistent themes or well-rehearsed memories. As the deterioration continues the actual form of speech tends to degenerate so that perseveration, reiteration or more specific dysphasic difficulties appear.

Paralleling the deterioration of the failing mind, emotional response becomes coarsened and there is a tendency for the personality to become a caricature of its predominant premorbid style. Thus, those who before conspicuously displayed affection, and also aroused it, may continue conspicuously to do so, while those who were dominated by suspicion or irritability may be even more so.

Stresses and pressures which force the demented individual beyond comfortably familiar behaviour or activity will be likely to provoke 'catastrophic' reactions of primitive emotion and behavioural disturbance. Related to this, emotional lability or 'emotional incontinence', exaggerated emotional responses of either tears or laughter, are rapidly induced by minimal stimulation only to disappear again after their fleeting presence. This is particularly characteristic of arteriosclerotic dementia. A further feature of this illness is the appearance of vague or well-defined depressive states. In senile dementia insight into the increasing disability is mostly absent but the patchy nature of the arteriosclerotic dementing process frequently leads to patients having a very painful and distressing awareness of their decline; such awareness may understandably be associated with severe depression.

The dementing brain, already decreasingly in touch with the complexities of the world or able to fend off its insults, is very vulnerable to the various processes likely to lead to confusional states. Such episodes are often the presenting feature to the caring services.

Eventually the deterioration may develop to such a degree that recognizable speech is lost. Emotion and behaviour are reduced to very primitive forms and a stage of full dependence on others for all physical needs is reached. Incontinence of bowel and bladder have many causes and may be evident at any stage; when a certain level of cerebral disorganization is reached these are the rule, though skilled nursing may defer or minimize their impact.

Apart from arteriosclerotic dementia and senile dementia there are a few other recognized disease entities which give rise to the dementia syndrome. Huntingdon's chorea with its characteristic movement disorder, family history, personality change and occasional symptomatic schizophrenia is well known, though it is unlikely to present for the first time in the elderly patient. Surviving cases of Alzheimer's presenile dementia are increasingly being referred to psychogeriatricians for further care. Finally Pick's disease should be mentioned though it is very rare that it is seen, let alone reliably diagnosed. The predominantly frontal lobe nature of the process is said to lead to the change in personality which is a prominent early feature, preceding more obvious decline in memory.

Very rarely does the full clinical picture of dementia develop quite rapidly, and it is more usual for the progression to take years. It seems clear that with senile dementia at least there are a number of subtypes with varying clinical progressions. It must be admitted that we have a very limited understanding of these and of their different natural histories. Despite apparently typical patterns of presentation we are constantly being surprised.

Finally it must be appreciated that in the elderly dementia rarely appears in a pure and uncomplicated form. Social and psychological factors, both pre-existing and newly arisen, very commonly affect the picture. Even if this is not the case, one can usually expect degrees of sensory disability or frank physical illness to complicate matters, and often all these problems come together to produce a picture of great complexity.

The search for causes of dementia in social and environmental factors has not been fruitful – and at present there are few prospects for effective 'primary prevention' through modification of such factors. But the clinical picture and the pattern and extent of disability are greatly influenced by environmental factors. An environment impoverished of stimulation and permissive of apathy and inactivity will give rise to a much more disabled dementia than need be. Similarly, removal from the cues and aids of a familiar environment is likely to be associated at least temporarily with a much worse level of function; practical matters – such as accessibility of toilets – obviously bear on problems of continence. Some clinical features are particularly associated with some of the so-called treatable dementias, and these are referred to in the next section.

DIFFERENTIAL DIAGNOSIS

Exact diagnosis is crucial; but the vigour with which investigations are pursued obviously depends on the clinical picture and the history. The main questions which arise follow three lines:

(1) Could this be a confusional state rather than a dementia?
(2) Could this picture predominantly be the result of a functional disorder?
(3) Is there a potentially treatable cause or exacerbating factor for this dementia?

It is sensible to regard with the gravest suspicion any dementing state with a reported acute onset or short history. Certainly whenever the history is said to be 3 months or so, and probably whenever the history is said to be in months rather than years, it is safest to regard the condition as a confusional state until proven otherwise. Fortunately the positive features of the confusional state would usually be evident. Lishman's definition (1978) referred to dementia as being a state found in an alert patient, whereas confusional states are characterized by clouding of consciousness.

The concept of consciousness has consistently proved rather elusive of definition. The related concept of clouding of consciousness has been associated with similar difficulties. We refer to a variable degree of diminution in the normally accepted level of alert awareness of the individual. When this is severe enough to manifest as drowsiness or degrees of coma there is clearly no difficulty, but more minor and subtle impairment is frequently hard to detect. There are problems of definition but also we lack any thoroughly reliable means of detecting or measuring clouding of consciousness. Perhaps it is understandable that many clinicians do not know what is meant.

A distinctive feature of confusional states is the variation, over a short space of time, both in lucidity and in the clinical picture generally. A more telling observation is that the quantity and content of the mental life of the confused patient is much richer than that of the demented individual who displays a relatively impoverished psyche. There is nearly always some physical background to a confusional state and such patients tend to be more obviously ill. Careful physical examination and routine investigations will usually provide sufficient clues if doubt remains. Difficulties arise as confusional states commonly occur in the course of the dementias. This is particularly the case with arteriosclerotic dementia. The elderly brain is already especially prone to confusional states and the more that there is some underlying dementia the more easily and less specifically will these be provoked. Detection and treatment of confusional states may not always prove as rewarding as hoped, but neglecting this yields no reward at all.

Of the functional psychiatric syndromes depression is the commonest illness to masquerade as dementia; and it is a very common condition in the elderly. The depressive nature of psychomotor retardation and stupor may be difficult to identify but the possibility of a depressive basis must not be overlooked. Usually the nature, intensity and depth of the profound mood disturbance are betrayed in some form to the aware observer if only by a meaningful look, gesture, or occasional depressive utterance. Lishman (1978) has characterized the 'pseudo-dementias' as a 'number of conditions (with) a clinical picture resembling organic dementia ... yet physical disease proved to be little if at all responsible'. One of the main varieties is the so-called depressive pseudo-dementia. More rarely the picture may be one of an 'hysterical pseudo-dementia', with approximate and ridiculous answers to questions which betray greater underlying ability than is being displayed; thus a patient when asked the colour of milk might confidently reply 'green'.

The picture of depressive pseudo-dementia is thought to result from a combination of retardation, diminished interest, impaired attention and concentration, and perhaps intense preoccupation. The full mechanism is not understood but probably reduced cortical arousal is important and this has been demonstrated in elderly depressives, as has the reversibility of 'organic' impairment on psychometric testing.

Certain elderly depressed patients have a persistent tendency to avoid questions, and particularly questions designed to test their cognitive function, by the strategy of answering 'I don't know' to virtually every question. This is fairly characteristic; the demented patient tends by contrast to make up an answer or give some excuse for not knowing. It is almost as if the elderly depressive is refusing to take responsibility for any knowledge because of the preoccupying burden of his affect.

A careful history and mental examination will either clarify the issue or raise sufficient doubt as to make a trial of antidepressant therapy worthwhile. The dramatic effect of such treatment when appropriately applied is most gratifying; and it may be helpful even in the patient who is dementing if there is also significant depression.

Occasionally other functional psychiatric states may cause problems. A very deteriorated, ageing schizophrenic patient may at first sight appear demented. Rarely, the schizophrenic 'bufoonery syndrome' presents, as the name implies, with clowning and ridiculous behaviour amongst which may be apparent cognitive impairment. Very occasionally a hypomanic state in an elderly patient may masquerade as a dementia and sometimes difficulties arise with neurotic reactions and hysterical phenomena. As with depression, in most cases the history, examination and a period of observation will establish the correct diagnosis.

Once the diagnosis of a dementing disorder is clear, the question arises as to the possibility of a potentially treatable cause or exacerbating factor. In the very elderly with

most cases a diagnosis of dementia, senile or arteriosclerotic, can be made at home . . . [as the] history in an elderly person of progressive deterioration over months or years is so typical that when it coincides with the clinical findings, both physical and mental, the diagnosis can be regarded as conclusive. . . . It is not necessary in such patients to pursue elaborate investigations designed to find one of the rare and so-called reversible causes of dementia, when clinical evidence of them (for example, anaemia, hypothyroidism, or other abnormal neurological signs) are not in evidence (Arie, 1973a and b).

Having given this *caveat* it remains useful to have available a realistic list of the potentially treatable causes. Table 1 below lists the major causes of progressive dementia which have been regarded as potentially treatable. Most of these are within the ken of any competent physician provided that there is access to reasonable investigations to supplement and inform clinical awareness. Some are worthy of extra note.

Subdural haematoma, where treatment can be lifesaving, and can result in full recovery, is a persistent finding in studies of missed diagnoses. With its fluctuating levels of awareness, with or without papilloedema and other neurological signs, it should always be considered. A history of trauma is very commonly absent. The CAT (computerized axial tomography) scan is the most powerful investigation to exclude the possibility but it is not totally conclusive (Marsden, 1978).

Normal pressure hydrocephalus (Adams *et al.*, 1965) has been a popularly quoted cause of potentially reversible dementia, but few psychiatrists claim to have seen successful diagnosis and treatment. This may be a self-fulfilling pessimistic prophecy; and early cases probably go to neuro-

Table 1 Potentially treatable causes of the dementia syndrome

Local causes	Raised intracranial pressure	Tumours (benign or malignant) Subdural haematoma Cerebral abscess
	Normal pressure Hydrocephalus	
	Cerebral infections	Neurosyphilis Tuberculous meningitis
	Cerebral inflammations	DLE (disseminated lupus erythematosis) Cranial arteritis
Systemic causes	Endocrine disorders	Myxoedema
	Metabolic disturbances	Hypocalcaemia Hypoglycaemia Uraemia Hepatic encephalopathy Porphyria
	Vitamin deficiency	Vitamin B_{12} deficiency
	Toxic agents	Alcohol
	Prolonged anoxic states	Respiratory failure

logists rather than psychiatrists. The classical picture is one of dementia, gait disturbance, and the early appearance of urinary incontinence which is disproportionate to the degree of dementia. It is said particularly to follow subarachnoid haemorrhage, meningitis or head injury. Marsden (1978) states that RIHSA studies have been the most widely employed diagnostic techniques though he adds that none of the current techniques are entirely satisfactory. Ventriculoatrial shunting is the operative treatment of choice.

It has been written that if the history is uncertain or atypical, if there are unusual features, if there is a past psychiatric history or suggestions of depression, and if the patient is under 70 years of age without any obvious vascular cause for dementia, then there should be further investigation. Most would agree on the inclusion of a blood count and ESR, urea and electrolytes, blood sugar, liver and thyroid function tests, serum calcium, serum vitamin B_{12} and folate, and radiography of the chest and skull. An EEG is a useful non-invasive technique, though it needs careful interpretation. Given sufficient clinical justification, a radioisotope brain scan, further more sophisticated radiography or a CAT scan may be used. In contemporary practice it is sensible for the clinician to have an awareness of the financial costs as well as the limitations of the investigation. These can then be set beside the possible benefit to the patient. Money unnecessarily spent on expensive investigations detracts from what is available for decent caring services.

The rewards of work in this field rarely come from detecting 'reversible' dementias. It is common experience that though such cases may be detected, it is rare that significant reversal or benefit to the patient accrues despite the 'correct' treatment. Reports of series of patients in whom 'treatable' dementias are identified seldom report the actual results of treatment.

MANAGEMENT

This is the great challenge and there is much that can be done despite the fact that it is rare that we can arrest or reverse the progression. With the common dementias the traditional medical section on 'treatment' has, at present, to be omitted. As knowledge increases this may change and rational radical treatment become a possibility. Currently instead it is necessary to think in the wider terms of management. The individual doctor or the psychiatric services have open to them, and should explore, a number of spheres of operation. This means responding to the needs of the individual patient in a perspective which includes the family, the local community and the resources available. Management is under three headings.

(1) Specific medical measures.
(2) Practical measures and advice, and coordination of domiciliary services.
(3) Management of, or advice on, the use of institutional facilities.

It is at home that the failing mind is most frequently seen. More than 70 per cent of the elderly demented are outside institutions and though most are with their families many are actually living alone (Kay, Beamish, and Roth, 1969a and b).

Specific medical measures
The first issue is the current setting of the patient and its appropriateness for the future. The scale of the problem – the number of the demented is measured in hundreds of thousands – and ever-insufficient resources dictate that the majority of them will be cared for at home. The decision about placement for the individual patient will involve careful consideration of the attitudes and abilities of available supporters. The next section

will consider the effect of the failing mind on the family more fully.

Once it is clear where the patient will be cared for, the use of certain specific medical measures can be considered. A major concern is ensuring that the patient reliably takes any medication prescribed. This will be trickiest with a demented individual who is living alone, but sometimes it is possible to construct a rota system of frequently visiting supporters, both professional and lay. Much has been written of the dangers of drugs in the elderly (Triggs and Nation, 1975; Caird, 1977). Intolerance leading to confusion, constipation or falls, as well as many other problems, have been rightly emphasized. The demented elderly are the group most at risk from these problems and complications.

The commonest problem is restlessness, and particularly nocturnal restlessness and wandering. Often there will be paranoid ideation, repetitive nagging questioning, frank hostility or open aggression. General measures, such as diversion and activity during the day time are helpful, but the major tranquillizers are the mainstay of management. Different clinicians have their individual favourite drugs. The important thing is that a sensible and clear regime is adopted to fit the pattern of disturbance in each case. It is equally important to monitor the effectiveness of any regime to ensure that it is not, for instance, simply producing over-sedation. The aim is to eliminate or minimize excesses of behaviour while attaining the maximum compatible degree of alertness and responsiveness. As in other spheres of medicine, it is best to be familiar with a small number of drugs. In our unit we particularly favour promazine, thioridazine or haloperidol. Despite possible extrapyramidal side-effects the last-named is particularly useful when trying to avoid oversedation. Other preparations will sometimes be necessary. A tranquillizer at night combined with a suitable hypnotic will often give a night's sleep – but sometimes at the cost of a wet bed.

The choice of hypnotic is important. Some drugs with long half-lives, such as nitrazepam and flurazepam (Bond and Lader, 1973; Castleden *et al.*, 1977) may not be suitable for the elderly, and problems may be still greater in the individual with a dementing brain. A new addition to the benzodiazepine range is temazepam which is said to be particularly short-acting; but further studies in the elderly, both pharmokinetic and clinical, are needed. Benzodiazepines also tend to have a muscle-relaxant effect and theoretically might increase the risk of nocturnal falls if the patient gets up. In our unit chlormethiazole is finding favour since it has now been shown to have a short half-life and little or no 'hangover' symptoms in the elderly (Moore *et al.*, 1975; Nayal *et al.*, 1978).

Significant depression should be treated as in the non-demented patient. A fair trial of antidepressive treatment may occasionally mean giving ECT, even when there are significant indications of a dementing process, if there is also a serious possibility that a depression is the primary disorder. With drugs the same problems apply as with antidepressants in the elderly generally. Notably these include, with the tricyclics, postural hypotension, anticholinergic effects and cardiotoxicity. The newer preparations, particularly the tetracyclics, are said to give fewer such problems while still remaining effective.

Medication can also sometimes help incontinence. When this appears to be due to an unstable or neurogenic bladder with overflow, preparations which increase bladder tone have been found to be useful, particularly if this can be combined with a regime of regular aided toileting. Emepromium bromide (Cetiprin) and the new preparation flavoxate hydrochloride (Urispas) have found favour with many clinicians. Faecal incontinence usually has a treatable cause which must be sought vigorously. Frequently it is due to a buildup of constipation with leakage and overflow. Once this has been suitably treated cellulose preparations or mild laxatives often help to prevent a recurrence. However, the best prevention of constipation is sufficient exercise and adequate dietary fibre and fluid intake. It should not be forgotten that some psychotropic drugs, especially tricyclic antidepressants, may produce constipation.

Practical measures and management
The second line of management depends on the effective deployment of available domiciliary services. These will include adaptations to the home and simple safety measures which may be carried out under the auspices of the local authority social services department. The administrative separation of the health services and social services can these days pose special problems of coordination. The success with which such difficulties have been overcome varies greatly in different areas. Health service and social service staff control only the resources of their own respective agencies, but the interests of their patients and clients demand that they collaborate in the deployment of these resources. The hierarchical organization of some professions, contrasting with the professional autonomy of doctors, may add to the difficulties; but there is plenty of evidence that given goodwill and good sense collaboration can be very effective. On occasions smoothing the tangled web of ruffled interpersonal relations between caregivers may prove a more challenging task for the psychiatrist than the psychiatric problems of his patients.

The provision of domiciliary services varies a great deal from area to area and the local social services department should be approached for full details of what is available. The main social services facilities are home helps, meals on wheels, modifications to the home, some voluntary services, and social support and case work. The area health authority deploys health visitors, district nurses and community psychiatric nurses. The latter are psychiatric nurses specifically concerned with the support of patients and their families at home. Often these nurses will work from a hospital as part of the psychiatric team; alternatively they may be extra-murally based. The area health authority may provide chiropody services, home physiotherapy and occasionally home occupational therapy. Items such as commodes, walking aids, and incontinence pads should be available through the nursing services or the social worker. Incontinence home laundry services are increasingly being set up and are proving a great boon to hard-pressed relatives. In most areas there will be voluntary organizations concerned with the welfare of the elderly who will be able to provide information, liaison or actual supportive services; Age Concern and Mind are prominent examples.

Variably available are local authority day centres, perhaps with transport, and some (too few) local authorities provide a special day centre for the elderly mentally infirm. These provisions overlap with the third line of management of dementia, which is concerned with institutions. Day centres generally do not welcome and cannot cope with the elderly demented, but local authority residential homes are willing to take a few day attenders. A day hospital or a psychogeriatric unit should be able to cope with these day-patients and such support can greatly extend the coping capacity of families. How far such day hospitals do shorten the period of inpatient care or replace the need for beds (especially for the otherwise unsupported dement) is far from clear (Bergmann *et al.*, 1978). This issue requires more study.

Another mode of living which amounts to neither a wholly dependent existence in the community nor to institutional care, is sheltered accommodation. Specially designed purpose-built small living units in a single complex are linked centrally by an alarm or calling system to a warden's accommodation. These wardens are supposed to do a normal working week, but in practice many make themselves available most of the time and adopt the task of making routine checks on all their elderly. But sheltered accommodation is generally of little use to the demented unless living with a reasonably capable spouse. It does not offer the around-the-clock surveillance which they usually need. At the same time it can allow one demented individual to produce the maximum of stress and anxiety for an over-burdened warden.

Institutional facilities

In many cases the pressures are too great for relatives, or a less well-supported patient comes to require continuous supervision but fails to receive it. At this stage institutional care either in a local authority residential home or in a psychiatric unit will be appropriate. Actual provision of residential home places falls far short of official guidelines (Department of Health and Social Security, 1972) and this situation is unlikely to change rapidly. These homes were not originally intended for the demented but increasingly they find themselves caring for such individuals. Dementia *per se* is not a bar, and in general, where supervision constitutes the major need, this would be the responsibility of the social services. However, if there is significant behaviour disorder which cannot be reasonably remedied or contained, or if there is a high level of dependency requiring frequent nursing care as well as supervision, then such continuing care is best provided in a psychogeriatric unit.

Some patients in the community are already at this level but their families still cope and strongly wish to continue doing so provided they are given good support. In addition to the sorts of services already mentioned such support will generally mean regular access to 'holiday' admissions or frequent relief admissions.

Such facilities are also important for patients supported at home but not yet so severely disabled. Supporters of an individual with a failing mind need to know that they can trust the local services. In a crisis they must be assured that there will be a quick and understanding response; and ready 'therapeutic listening' is also important. Lack of resources will often mean services are unable to provide the response which relatives initially seek. Indeed the 'right answer' as perceived by relatives in a crisis may not be what either they, or the service, ultimately see as most appropriate. Provided the response is swift, honest and realistically compassionate it will usually fortify the supporters to cope further. For such support strategies to work it is vital that the service becomes involved at an early stage. Intervention is needed long before the family has become so worn down by an excessive burden and so hardened with cynicism at apparently callous buck-passing by unhelpful agencies that they are no longer prepared to provide any sort of care and their capacity to cope breaks for good. If resources allow there is a place for 'instant' relief admission (on the same day) in order to give confidence both that one appreciates the extent of pressure on the family and that the service is capable of responding promptly.

Hospital admission may be necessary for other reasons, such as brief admission to a psychogeriatric unit for assessment. Undoubtedly the limits of the failing mind and the degree of remaining function are best assessed in the patient's home surrounding, but frequently doubt about the aetiology, or the diagnosis, necessitates specialized inpatient investigation and observation. This sort of admission is quite different, and its nature must be carefully explained to the family beforehand.

Alternatively admission may be necessary to a geriatric unit. Again this may be short-term for investigation, intermittent, or long-term. The geriatric unit, rather than the psychogeriatric unit, is appropriate when the main problems are those of physical illness or frailty – this means the patient who is not mobile or who basically needs physical nursing skills.

In few parts of the country does the level of provision satisfactorily approach the recommended norms both in terms of local authority residential accommodation and in terms of hospital accommodation for the elderly demented. In this setting the psychogeriatrician, and others, are rarely able to provide all that they would wish; they are gatekeepers seeking fairly to ration access to limited resources. Thus the criteria for admission to long-stay care will vary between areas, and they are also likely to vary from time to time within the same area as the load on the service changes. Compassionate but efficient marshalling of these scarce resources is one of the major tasks for the clinician.

Another major task is to give support to those who run and work in these hospitals and homes. This medical role is shared in the case of residential homes with general practitioners and, of course, the local geriatrician. Care of the elderly demented is among the least prestigious jobs in our acquisitive society. It is all too easy for the staff in the field to become demoralized. A vicious circle of declining morale and deteriorating standards is an ever-present threat. Additionally there is these days a climate of close scrutiny and, often, ready censure when things appear amiss.

Detailed consideration of ways of maintaining morale is beyond the scope of this chapter but it is worth briefly mentioning some themes. It is important that staff see themselves as contributing and valued members of a team. It is also important that the institution should not become, or be seen as isolated, and interaction with the community should be encouraged. The work must get done but there must also be enjoyment and satisfaction in the doing. In the end there will be no 'workers' if this is not so. Regular opportunity to ventilate frustrations and problems is invaluable and unit meetings may usefully achieve this, but staff should have evidence that problems and suggestions will be taken seriously, and acted on.

The disabilities and dispositions of the patients are also important, both in themselves and for their effects on morale. An active, lively and stimulating programme helps both to maintain staff morale and esteem, and to maximize the remaining level of function of the failing mind. One approach presently much under discussion is 'reality orientation therapy' in which an organized and concerted attempt is made to confront the dementing individual with orientating reality information. Another approach might involve a more frankly behavioural slant such as the 'token economy' whereby, in simple terms, rewards are given for the desired behaviour. Other approaches have involved giving staff greater autonomy in the running of their areas. At one level it perhaps does not matter much which line is pursued as long as it is an active purposive one which manifestly engages both staff and residents in a stimulating and rewarding manner.

The clinician in this area needs a broad view, and the very breadth of the challenge provides one of the main satisfactions of the work.

LEGAL AND FINANCIAL PROBLEMS

Financial and legal complications are very likely with the demented elderly, and perhaps increasingly as we move further towards a 'property-owning democracy'. These aspects are frequently neglected by doctors and others.

A common mistake is to think that a power of attorney may be appropriately employed. This is a legal device whereby one person empowers another specified person to act for him in his affairs. The usual justification will be some sort of physical illness or limitation which makes it difficult or impossible for the patient actually to go about his business himself. It is necessary to the legitimacy of this procedure that the empowering person be fully aware of the nature and extent of his affairs and of the significance of what he is doing in this empowering process. With most demented elderly patients, by the time that the issue arises, they will be far from competently able to meet these criteria. In practice, relatives often make temporary informal arrangements with cooperative bank managers or with the family solicitor long-familiar with both the patient and the next of kin.

When there are substantial assets involved or if there is any doubt about the suitability of the arrangements it is best that the Court of Protection be approached about the management of the patient's affairs (Sim, 1968). This Court is expressly for persons incapable of managing their affairs by virtue of mental illness. Any person may set in motion referral to the Court, and usually the approach is through a solicitor or to the personal applications branch. It acts by the appointment of a receiver authorized to act as a form of statutory agent for the patient. A common problem is the long delay between application and resolution.

Another issue is that of testamentary capacity. The law requires that for a valid will a person must be of 'sound disposing mind'. It is necessary that:

(1) They should appreciate that they are making a will.
(2) They should know the nature and extent of their estate.
(3) They should know the various competing claims upon their estate in terms of family members and close friends, and should be able to make rational judgements as to their relative worth (Sim, 1968).

Retrospective assessment of these points is often difficult to make. Later problems will often be prevented if the clinician bears these issues in mind early on in his contact with the patient and records his views.

As sufferers from 'mental disorder', the elderly demented are covered by the Mental Health Act 1959. The same legal provisions apply as with younger patients when compulsory admission to hospital is felt to be necessary. Standard texts should be referred to for full details of these procedures and also for details of Section 47 of the National Assistance Act 1948, which can provide grounds for removal to a residential home. It is important that patient's wishes are only set aside when they are demonstrably the result of mental disorder. A view that they are merely 'unwise' is not enough. Similarly it is important that the doctor, when using any of these procedures, is clear in his own mind as to whose interest is being served by their use.

Implications for the family
Isaacs (Isaacs, Livingstone, and Neville, 1972) has shown in Glasgow that very few elderly patients are admitted because families do not want them. Williamson *et al.* (1964) showed that at least in the Edinburgh of the 1960s, most dementia in the community was undetected, and therefore presumably was inadequately treated. It is the experience of every worker in this field that families carry formidable burdens, often for far too long,

and often with little complaint. More recently Opit's (1977) work has strongly suggested that much need remains unmet despite the growth of domiciliary services. Sanford's (1975) study of relatives' problems highlighted states of anxiety and depression among a number of potentially remediable factors, and above all chronic lack of sleep. Families' expectations of help are growing, but there is no evidence at all that families generally are abdicating from their responsibilities for old people.

If families stopped supporting the elderly, and particularly the elderly demented, the health and social services would quickly break down. In fact, this does not happen and instead the clinician frequently encounters families under immense strain from coping with a demented relative.

Jolley (1979; 1981; Jolley and Arie, 1980) has suggested that the care provided by a spouse for an elderly dement is the model and standard at which services should aim. Spouses take on the task of caring for each other without question and tend to accept a failing mind as a natural development to be borne with compassionate fortitude.

This can continue for a long time but increasingly the physical and perhaps mental strength of the competent partner will decline. Eventually a point may be reached where home care will no longer be possible. Sometimes the clinician will need to persuade the weakening supporter to relinquish an excessive burden of care despite their wishes to the contrary.

An interesting variant of the spouse support system occurs when the couple are recently married. Usually both have had previous marriages; understandably the affective bond and sense of obligation to support each other may be less. The marriage may have been embarked upon in a spirit of looking for some new adventure in increasing old age, and caring for an elderly dement is far from the anticipated reward. As a further complication encroaching memory difficulties lead to the identity of the new spouse being forgotten. Further, the absence of the previous spouse will also slip from mind; the new spouse in attempting intimate care may then not only be misidentified but frankly rejected or even attacked for brazen behaviour.

Many more of the elderly demented are supported by other family members, usually children. All may or may not be together in the same household. Daughters rather than sons are particularly likely to be the chief supporters. There may then be problems with the competing needs and views of sons-in-law and grandchildren. A common phenomenon is that one or two family members in particular become laden with the major burden of care. Other relatives may appear to be standing on the sidelines, merely contributing wounding unhelpful criticism of the care being provided. This is often, perhaps, a defence against their own feelings of guilt and inadequacy.

Whatever the mechanism it is not uncommon that great mounds of resentment and bitterness divide the family in their stress. Sometimes it seems as if this burden of resentment is harder for the supporter to bear than is the burden of care itself. The dominant emotional themes in the dynamics of family relationships tend to become writ large under these pressures. Old rivalries and conflicts again become manifest. Fertile ground exists for the interplay of psychological factors and it is important for the clinician to be alert to them. With his expertise he can often usefully work on these factors; at the very least he must be ready to 'listen therapeutically'.

Relations between demented parents and their supporting children frequently seem strikingly reversed. Now the child is serving every physical and emotional need of a demanding dependent parent. The state may resemble that of caring for a small child or baby but this 'baby' will regress rather than progress in development. There is also a lack of the reinforcing affective qualities of the infant. At the same time the aged parent in a totally dependent state and well-cared-for may completely deny these circumstances. Instead they may hurtfully assert both that they are neglected and that they are independent. The situation is often compounded by an insistence on seeing the son or daughter still as a young child, rightfully subject to their wiser adult will.

Large numbers of old people, as a result of the two world wars, have never married or long ago became widowed. Many have been childless. In these circumstances more distant members of the family may be involved as supporters. The same kinds of problem arise as with close relatives, but usually the situation generates less heat; the sense of obligation and the burden of past relationships is likely to be less severe. For similar reasons such support is less likely to be long-lasting.

Occasionally the clinician may be seeking to persuade that the time for home care has passed; more often the family will be seeking so to persuade him. Frequently the state of resources will mean that he cannot respond to their requests as they both might wish. Viewing the situation of the family in the perspective of many similar such families, he may form a different judgement of their priority. He should be aware that he is a fairly brief visitor in their sphere as he makes his assessments. Through all these difficulties the clinician will be seeking to serve the best interests of all as humanely and justly as possible. He will treat what can be treated and try to reduce the pain of what he cannot.

THE IMPLICATIONS OF A CHANGING COMMUNITY

The full impact of the failing mind on the community has not been fully measured. Some indication can be obtained from the effect of the elderly in general. It is well known that as a group they are the greatest users of health and social welfare resources. In hospital, they occupy around half of all NHS beds, both psychiatric and general. They have the highest consultation rates in general practice and constitute the largest sector of spending of social services departments. Since 1975, the increase in services of various sorts has failed to keep pace with the increase in the numbers of the elderly (Shore, 1980). This applies across the board, from domiciliary services through to residential care places and hospital beds. Nevertheless, there are disturbing signs that soon the argument may be advanced that the elderly overconsume the 'resources cake' to the detriment of younger age groups. The elderly will not go away or cease to be disabled. The resources squeeze will be painfully felt by all groups and there is no obvious end in sight to the present era of severely constrained public expenditure. There is an unattractive prospect of differing pressure groups competing with each other for scarce funds and resources. The elderly would be unfairly and invidiously matched in such competition against appealing infants and the attractive young.

Current economic forecasts vary from dismal in the short-term to uncertain in the long-term. It is in this context that the numbers of very old people, and *pari passu* the elderly demented, will continue to rise rapidly. This trend is projected to last for at least the next two decades. Recently there have also been some signs of an increase in births. Any such sustained change would have considerable implications for the future share-out of our limited resources.

Around 95 per cent of the elderly are living at home and the vast majority of the elderly demented are also out in the community. At present, it seems fantasy to imagine an increase in institutional provision. In the 1970s the bed base for mental illness as a whole contracted considerably. The impetus towards 'community care' for all forms of psychiatric disorder has been strong. However, trends indicate a need for a major increase in all domiciliary services for the elderly merely to keep pace with the rising numbers of old people. There has already been evidence that the effectiveness of the present level of services needs improvement. It seems certain that greater rather than lesser burdens will fall on families.

In the postwar years considerable changes have taken place in the pattern of family relationships and in the expectations of the individual. It is likely that these trends will continue but their effects on the nuts and bolts of 'community care' are difficult to foresee. In view of the importance of support at home it seems worth exploring further some of these themes.

The rise of the 'nuclear family' is a well-observed phenomenon. Our society is becoming increasingly middle-class; associated trends are high geographical mobility and high expectations for a materially rich and burden-free life. Patterns of child care are changing to accommodate the large numbers of working wives and the altered expectations of women generally.

At present the largest group of working women are the middle-aged. It is this group particularly who have been called upon to aid their ageing relatives. The economic dependence of families on these women and their own aspirations towards working independence are likely to lead to increasing problems in the home care of the elderly demented.

The effect of the increasing divorce rate is unpredictable. Presumably the eventual prospect is of large numbers of divorced elderly living alone. But this would take time to work through the generations and currently there seems to be a strong counterbalancing trend towards second marriages. However the ties in a second marriage are probably less able to provide the support in old age which the failing mind demands.

More relevant perhaps is the effect of the high divorce rate on the children of the elderly. Single living divorcees may be more inclined to return to ageing parents and provide support, but this seems unlikely; second-marriage sons-in-law and daughters-in-law will probably be less tolerant of the burdens imposed by dementia. Briefer relationships and the inevitable lack of a previous background of support in the other direction will mean fewer obligations. However, as new links are formed in second marriages and the old links from first marriages are not all destroyed, we may see a new form of 'extended family'. The value of this to the elderly demented is still uncertain.

The rising divorce rate may reflect a diminishing tolerance of difficulty and stress. Whether this is true or not, it does seem clear that the expectations of the present generation of middle-aged and young are much greater than those of their predecessors. This will have a major effect on their willingness to take on supporting roles for their elderly, and on the services which they demand as they age themselves.

A clear trend in the developed world is the need for a smaller labour force and for shorter hours from those who are at work. Through earlier retirement, work-sharing and a shorter working week, large numbers of people are likely to be available for voluntary 'community work'. Imaginative new

schemes could exploit this opportunity to set up novel ways of supple-
menting the statutory services. Extra support could be organized for
families to aid with supervision, stimulation and care of the elderly
demented. Additionally, the same technological advance which is so
changing the pattern of work may also be able to make the home a safer
environment for those with failing minds.

Yet another unpredictable area is the effect on services of the large ethnic
minority groups which have become established as part of our society.
Many of these new communities have arisen in inner city areas where all
services are relatively poor. At an anecdotal level, at least, the demand of
these groups on services for the elderly has so far been disproportionately
small. Differences of culture and family custom are probably influential
factors; but most immigrants are young and we have yet to see the 'ageing'
of these ethnic communities. There may be much for us to learn from these
communities about encouraging viable family support systems.

The attitudes of the community towards the elderly are a vital factor.
They have an important effect on decision-makers' priorities for resource
allocation, and they are crucial in determining the enthusiasm and the
numbers of those who wish to work with the elderly. However, many have
to deal with the elderly and with the elderly demented whether they wish to
or not and their competence is similarly influenced by these attitudes.

IS DEMENTIA PREVENTABLE?

Senile dementia is now generally seen as a separate process from the
normal ageing of the human brain. We are quite unable to halt either.

Some potentially 'reversible dementias' have already been described. A
few may be preventable in the primary sense, but most are not. It is
probable that the incidence of arteriosclerotic dementia can be reduced by
better treatment of hypertension from middle age onwards. Possibilities
for such prevention are likely to go hand in hand with a growing understanding of the factors involved in vascular degenerative disease. No doubt
here, as in many other diseases of old age, effective prevention may be
possible only much earlier in life.

In terms of secondary prevention with arteriosclerotic dementia various
vasodilator drugs have been used, but they have not proved useful (*British
Medical Journal*, 1979). In theory they may actually make things worse by
diverting blood away from starved areas of brain supplied by non-
responding diseased blood vessels. In younger patients vascular bypass

and transplant operations have been performed, but these are unlikely to form an important part of treatment for elderly patients. Similarly, the potential for use of anticoagulants with these patients is limited. Finally, various agents said to have a stimulatory effect on neurons have been used but again without proven benefit.

In the case of senile dementia no primary preventive measures are presently available, though certain avenues are being explored. To set these in perspective it is necessary to review briefly neuropathological and other research in this area. Most authorities now see senile dementia and Alzheimer-type dementia as aspects of the same entity. The post-mortem neuropathology is similar. Macroscopically, there is a shrunken brain with enlarged ventricles and widened cortical sulci. Microscopically the major findings are neurofibrillary tangles and silver staining senile plaques. From middle age onwards these tangles and plaques may be found to a slight extent, but they are present to a very marked degree in the demented brain. Studies have shown a relationship between the mean plaque count and the level of intellectual impairment, and it has been demonstrated that such impairment is rarely marked unless the mean plaque count is above ten per low power field (Tomlinson, Blessed, and Roth, 1970).

These themes link up with possibilities for secondary prevention suggested by studies in recent years which have shown reduced levels of the enzyme choline acetyl transferase (CAT) in the brains of the senile demented (Bowen and Davison, 1978). These reduced levels have been related both to the degree of senile plaque formation and to intellectual performance as examined shortly before death (Perry *et al.*, 1978). It has been suggested, therefore, that reduced levels of the neurotransmitter acetylcholine result from lowered levels of CAT and that this state leads to the clinical picture of senile dementia.

A number of therapeutic possibilities flow from this. Thus, giving choline or lecithin could increase the level of acetylcholine but as yet this procedure has not been shown to improve memory in normal individuals. When these agents have been used with senile dements behavioural change has been reported but not any clear improvement in memory or performance. The opposite approach is to limit the breakdown of acetylcholine by administration of an anticholinesterase. Then, whatever reduced levels were present would at least be conserved. Physostigmine has been reported to improve memory and performance under laboratory conditions, but as yet there haye been no reports of similar general success with demented individuals. On a different tack, vasopressin has been reported to play a part in the facilitation of learning in normal individuals and it has also been claimed to bring about improvement in impaired individuals. Further studies are needed and awaited in this area.

It has often been speculated that some sort of toxin may be responsible for the process of senile dementia. There have been reports of increased concentrations of aluminium and of zinc in Alzheimer brains and suggestions that there may be a causative link. At present this does not seem likely. It appears that the neuron has a tendency to accumulate aluminium and this may be a general feature of the ageing nervous system (Davison, 1978).

Another interesting observation has been the link noticed between Alzheimer's disease and Down's syndrome. A state of deterioration in midlife has been noted amongst mongols and similar histological change in their brains has been observed. Additionally there have been reports of familial associations between Alzheimer's disease, mongolism and myeloproliferative disorders (Olsen and Shaw, 1969).

However, it seems likely that the researches in virology and immunology will ultimately prove of great significance. Work with scrapie and kuru was followed by the finding that a filterable agent from the brains of individuals with Creuzfeldt–Jacob disease could transmit the illness to other primates (Gajdusek and Gibbs, 1971). There have been reports of the demonstration of a transmissible agent in some instances of familial Alzheimer's disease (Gajdusek and Gibbs, 1975). A reduced immunological competence has been described in the elderly and certain immunological abnormalities have been noted in individuals with dementia. All this work leads on to a theory of dementia involving an interaction between viruses and immunological status. Viruses may enter the central nervous system earlier in life and lie dormant without causing damage for many years. With the onset of old age, a disturbed immunological status may then allow of viral activity which gives rise to a dementing process. If specific viruses were involved the process could perhaps be prevented by inoculation earlier on in life, or in old age it could perhaps be countered by agents such as Interferon.

There are other lines of research and there have been significant findings in other types of dementing state; exciting developments are taking place with both theoretical and therapeutic implications. Real prevention or cure for the majority of dementia in the elderly is not immediately in prospect, but it seems reasonable to expect substantial advances in coming years. Such hopes may help now to inspire the workers in the field; but meanwhile the community must be persuaded and cajoled into dealing more effectively with present and foreseeable problems, for these will not go away.

References

Adams, R. D. *et al.* (1965). *N. Engl. J. Med.*, **273**, 117–126

Arie, T. H. D. (1973a). *Br. Med. J.*, **4**, 540

Arie, T. H. D. (1973b). *Br. Med. J.*, **4**, 602

Baker, A. A. (1976). *Br. Med. J.*, **2**, 571

Bergmann, K., Foster, E. M., Justice, A. W. and Matthews, V. (1978). *Br. J. Psychiat.*, **132**, 441

Bond, A. J. and Lader, M. H. (1973). The residual effects of Flurazepam. *Psychopharmacologica*, **32**, 223

Bowen, D. M. and Davidson, A. N. (1978). Biochemical changes in the normal ageing brain and in dementia. In (ed: Issacs B). *Recent Advances in Geriatric Medicine* (Edinburgh: Churchill Livingstone)

British Medical Journal (1978). Dementia – the quiet epidemic, **1**, 1

British Medical Journal (1979). Vasodilators in senile dementia, **2**, 511

Caird, F. I. (1977). Prescribing for the elderly. *Br. J. Hosp. Med.*, **17**, 610

Castleden, C. M., George, C. F., Hallett, C. and Marcer, D. (1977). Increased sensitivity to nitrazepam in old age. *Br. Med. J.*, **1**, 10

Corsellis, J. A. N. (1962). *Mental illness and the Ageing Brain: The Distribution of Pathological Change in a Mental Hospital Population (Institute of Psychiatry, Maudsley Monographs, No. 9)*. (London: Oxford University Press)

Davidson, A. N. (1978). *Age Ageing*, **7**, Supplement, 4

Department of Health and Social Security (1972). *Services for Mental Illness Related to Old Age*. Circular H M (72) 71

Gajdusek, D. C. and Gibbs, C. J. (1971). *Nature*, **230**, 588

Gajdusek, D. C. and Gibbs, C. J. (1975). *Adv. Neurol.*, **10**, 291

Government Actuary's Department, (1975). *Population Projection for the United Kingdom* (London: HMSO)

Hachinski, V. C., Lassen, N. A. and Marshall, J. (1974). *Lancet*, **2**, 207

Isaacs, B., Livingstone, M. and Neville, Y. (1972). *Survival of the Unfittest: A study of Geriatric Patients in Glasgow* (London: Routledge and Kegan Paul)

Jolley, D. (1981). Dementia – misfits in need of care. In Arie, T. (ed.) *The Health Care of the Elderly*. (London: Croom Helm)

Jolley, D. (1979). Acute confusional states in the elderly. In (ed. Davies Coakley), *Establishing a Geriatric Service*

Jolley, D. and Arie, T. (1980). *Health Trends*, **12**, 1

Kay, D. W. K., Beamish, P. and Roth, M. (1964a). *Br. J. Psychiatr.*, **110**, 146

Kay, D. W. K., Beamish, P. and Roth, M. (1964b). *Br. J. Psychiatr.*, **110**, 668

Kay, D. W. K., Bergmann, K., Foster, E. M., McKechnie, A. A. and Roth, M. (1970). *Compr. Psychiatr.*, **11**, 26

Kral, V. A. (1962). Senescent forgetfulness: benign or malignant. *Can. Med. Assoc. J.*, **86**, 257

Lishman, W. A. (1978). *Organic Psychiatry*, (Oxford: Blackwell Scientific Publications)

Livesley, B. (1977). *Age Ageing*, **6**, Supplement, 9

Marsden, C. D. (1978). In (eds. A. D. Isaacs and F. D. Post) *Studies in Geriatric Psychiatry*. (Chichester: John Wiley and Sons Ltd.)

Miller, E. (1973). *Psychol. Med.*, **3**, 221

Moore, R. G., Triggs, E. J., Shanks. C. A. and Thomas, J. (1975). Pharmacokinetics of chlormethiazole in humans. *Euro. J. Clin. Pharmacol.*, **8**, 353

Nayal, S., Castleden, C. M., George, C. F. and Marcer, D. (1978). *Age Ageing*, **7**, Supplement, 50

Olsen, M. I. and Shaw, G. M. (1969). *Brain*, **92**, 147

Opit, L. J. (1977). *Br. Med. J.*, **1**, 30

Perry, E. K., Tomlinson, B. E., Blessed, G., Bergmann, K., Gibson, P. H. and Perry, R. H. (1978). *Br. Med. J.*, **2**, 1457

Sanford, J. R. A. (1975). *Br. Med. J.*, **3**, 471

Shore, E. (1980). *Unpublished lecture* at University Department of Health Care of the Elderly, Nottingham

Sim, M. (1968). *Guide to Psychiatry*, Chapter 21, pp. 885–887. (Edinburgh: E. & S. Livingstone)

Slater, E. and Cowie, V. (1971). *The Genetics of Mental Disorders*. (London: Oxford University Press)

Triggs, E. J. and Nation, R. L. (1975). Pharmacokinetics in the aged. A review. *J. Pharmacokin. Biopharmacol.* **3**, 387

Tomlinson, B. E., Blessed, G. and Roth, M. (1970). *J. Neurol. Sci.*, **11**, 205

Whitehead, A. (1978). In (eds. A. D. Isaacs and F. Post) *Studies in Geriatric Psychiatry*, (Chichester: John Wiley and Sons Ltd.)

Williamson, J., Stokoe, I. H., Gray, S., Fisher, M., Smith A., McGhee, A. and Stephenson, E. (1964). *Lancet*, **1**, 1117

3

Caring for children with cancer

Martin Mott

Look to this day for it is life,
The very life of life.
In its brief course lie all the realities and truths of existence;
The joy of growth; the splendour of action,
The glory of power.
For yesterday is but a memory and tomorrow is only a vision,
But to-day well lived makes every yesterday a memory of happiness and every
  tomorrow a vision of hope.
Look well, therefore, to this day.

Ancient Sanskrit poem

INTRODUCTION

Modern medicine has conquered many of the diseases which were causes of premature death in the past. A consequence of this success is that previously rare conditions are now assuming an increasing importance in the mortality statistics. Although there has been a dramatic improvement in the outlook for childhood cancer, it is currently the commonest disease to kill children. Despite the fact that a substantial proportion of patients now become long-term survivors, it is not usually possible to be sure whether treatment will be successful for a particular individual. In the face of an uncertain prognosis therefore, it is important for the physician to adopt a position which can help the family to deal with the outcome, whatever it may be.

The diagnosis of cancer causes a profound shock which can seriously

45

disturb the equilibrium of all the members of the family unit. The psychological environment in which treatment takes place makes a considerable difference to the wellbeing of the whole family, whatever the final outcome. Early intervention, by concentrating attention on the potential for life rather than the possibility of death and on the importance of living to the full, one day at a time, can substantially alter this psychological environment, and it is the effect of this positive approach which is the subject of this chapter.

The key to the way in which a child and his family cope with cancer lies in their understanding of the problem. Given the dramatic advances which have occurred in paediatric oncology, it is possible in most cases to indicate that *the goal of treatment is cure, and the rehabilitation of the patient to as normal a life as possible.* The fact that the illness is serious, indeed life-threatening in nature, can be accepted much more easily in that context, and it is feasible to come to terms with the possibility or actuality of death as and when it becomes inevitable. Young parents today have often not encountered death in a near relative or friend. Close involvement with other affected families is a fact of life in a paediatric oncology unit and new parents quickly learn of the reality of death as a possible conclusion, and of the difficulty of predicting the course or outcome of the disease. This is bound to be traumatic, but can be used positively in their own development if it is handled carefully by staff who are attuned to their needs. Because of this experience totally unrealistic attitudes to their own child's future are rare.

PREPARING FOR LIFE

The majority of children presenting with cancer in the 1980s can be expected to do well. Marked improvements in prognosis have occurred in the last two decades due to a variety of factors. One of the most significant improvements has been the realization that optimum treatment requires the combined efforts of a team of specialists including paediatric surgeons, radiotherapists, chemotherapists, pathologists and radiologists. The patient and his family are *key members of this team.*

Enrolment of the child and his family into the treatment team should take place on the first day. They are asked to make their essential contribution to the team objective, that is, maximum rehabilitation, with a return to as normal a life as possible. In order to do this they need to understand the actual situation that exists, the steps that are planned to change

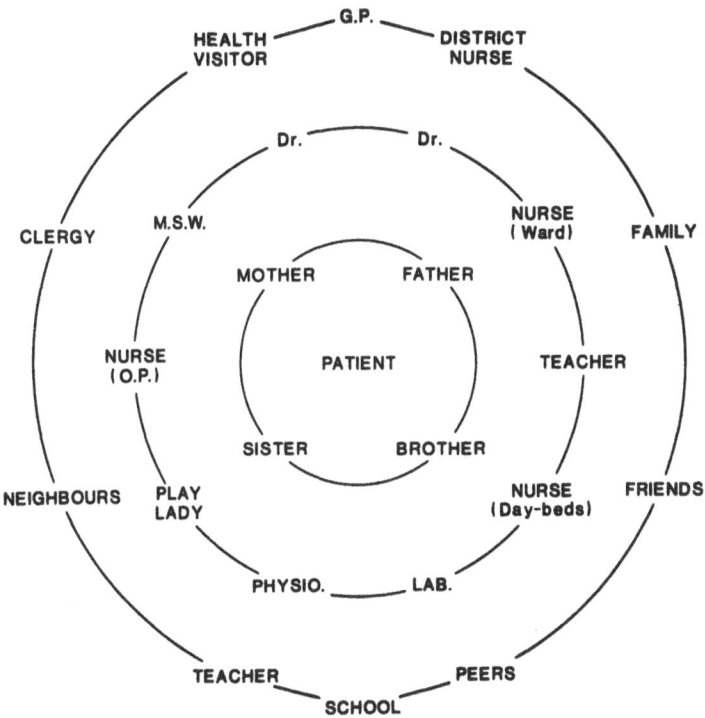

Figure 1   The treatment team

that situation and the role they are expected to play in bringing about that change. This education is a two-way process, the family being taught about the disease and its treatment, while they teach us about themselves as persons, their needs and reactions to stress.

The place of the family in the treatment team can be depicted in diagrammatic form as a central nucleus of intermediaries between the child and all other members of the team. Each member of the team can play a decisive role in the wellbeing of the family unit if care is taken to integrate their efforts. This is not the place for a detailed description of the individual role of each team member, but this does not mean that the role of any is considered less important than others (Figure 1). Active involvement of the family makes a fundamental difference which is totally convincing to anyone who remembers or still experiences the problems that occur when the parents' primary role of caring for their child is usurped or relegated by the professionals. They should be involved as much as possible in basic parental roles such as cleaning, bathing and feeding. They can also quickly be taught to take on technically 'nursing' procedures such as the recording of pulse and temperature, or fluid balance. This demands a special but very rewarding relationship with nursing staff whose aim is to enhance the parents' role rather than to replace it, working with the family rather than doing things for them. Parents and child can and should actively participate also in all physical rehabilitation, including oral and nutritional care, physiotherapy and occupational therapy.

While physical rehabilitation is important, success or failure of emotional rehabilitation is critical both for long-term survivors and for the families where a child has died. Failure can result in medical 'success' in terms of prolonged survival being ruined by the fact that life continues to be lived 'in the shadow of death'. The family will be beset by many difficulties and need to feel confident that the team are available to help them with whatever potential or actual problems arise. Feelings of guilt and inadequacy are common and it is again vital to ensure that, where possible, help for the child is channelled through the family members rather than provided from outside as a further indication that they cannot cope with the problem themselves. The problems which arise may range from the control of pain to the resolution of financial burdens occasioned by prolonged hospitalization. The impact of apparently trivial events can be devastating to the child. A common example is the major distress caused by fear of the inevitable teasing to be expected when returning to school partially or completely bald from chemotherapy. This problem has to be anticipated, acknowledged as reasonable and helped in direct proportion to the importance it has for that individual. Psychological preparation for return to school should be one of the highest priorities from the very beginning. Gentle but firm encouragement to continue schoolwork even when the child is not feeling particularly well, or is tied to an intravenous drip in hospital, strongly reinforces the idea that there is a future to be prepared for. The team may choose to use the family to educate the school personnel, and this is the ideal relationship, but it is in practice often necessary for the hospital team to develop direct contact so that there is a 'professional' reinforcement of the importance of maintaining a normal education.

Seeing a child's cancer as a family problem and encouraging the active participation of all the family helps a great deal in the rehabilitation of that family, even if death should occur. Whether or not treatment is successful, the positive approach will minimize the psychological sequelae of the disease and its treatment, and enhance the quality of life of the family.

PREPARING FOR DEATH

It is easy enough to see the value of adopting a positive approach and of involving the family when treatment is successful, but it is not so obvious when treatment fails and the child dies. A major difficulty for some is the concept of sharing 'the truth' with the dying child and his family. This difficulty arises from a simplistic notion of the nature of the truth that is shared. The facts that are presented must always be tailored to the intellectual, emotional and cultural background of the recipient, while at the same time expressing the truth. This requires an art of interpretation that depends to some extent on an understanding of the type of reaction than can be anticipated. The usual responses of the child and the family to a fatal illness have been categorized in a number of publications. There is certainly a generally recognizable pattern, but the response of every individual is unique. It sometimes helps to keep this in perspective by asking the question, 'What is an adverse reaction to death?' It is arrogant and may be dangerous to try and impose one's own theory of how, for example, grief should develop, provided it does not appear to be pathological in the sense of causing irreparable harm to the individual. There are pronounced cultural differences which may seem bizarre to the uninitiated, but which appear to play a substantial role in allowing grief to proceed naturally to a healthy conclusion.

Although the general pattern is well described in a number of standard works on death and dying, there are some points which seem worthy of further emphasis.

THE CHILD

An important factor which is frequently overlooked is that of children's exquisite sensitivity to non-verbal communication. Words are superfluous when everybody indicates by their facial expressions and by their gestures what they are so anxious to hide. Death for a young child can sometimes be quite simply thought of in terms of the fear of separation from their loved ones. Too often one sees nurses and doctors unable to share that fear and loneliness with the child because of the threat it implies to themselves – retreating from personal contact to the impersonal rituals of listening with stethoscope or counting of pulse, the academic discussion at the foot of the bed rather than playful banter and a reassuring hug or caress. Those who indulge in a conspiracy of silence often speak most eloquently by everything they do, and the message is precisely the one they are most anxious to avoid.

There is a world of difference between 2 years old, and 12, and 20, as to the form in which communication best takes place. When parents and doctors are balancing the pros and cons of preserving life or prolonging death, it is all too easy to forget that the person most concerned is the patient, and that we should listen carefully to what he tries to tell us. In the very young child particularly, this means 'listening to the child talking with his body'. After stripping away the euphemisms the question in its basic and crudest form is 'how long do you want to live?' No one believes that it should ever be asked in that direct way but there are many ways in which the answer can be obtained, if we are open to them. There is a balance between not making death a secret and not thrusting it on those who are not willing or not prepared to face it in the open at that moment, and that balance is important to the individual. The doctor must be constantly available as a friend in order to detect any change in that balance. Such availability requires the doctor's acceptance of the considerable cost of this role in emotional terms.

THE PARENT

Some degree of insight into the nature of grief may be required by parents in order to minimize its consequences on others. Grief is a natural reaction to an anticipated loss, but it cannot help the child to cope with his problems and indeed it frequently exacerbates them unless it is controlled. A common parental response is an all-embracing care of the child, which stems from the desire to protect him from the rigours of the outside world. This response frustrates any attempt to develop independence, which is an important function of childhood and is already severely hampered by his illness. Obsessional protective care can also lead to the redirection of other common feelings, such as anger and guilt, against the other parent who is barred from this exclusive relationship. Active steps may be required to encourage mutual sharing of the child and his problems by parents, so that the marital and family bonds are strengthened rather than weakened. Anger and guilt need to be turned into something constructive rather than destructive.

The reinvestment of time and energy away from the child is another common event with many potentially harmful consequences. Orchestration of the timing of this so that it does not hurt the child can be a very difficult problem, and requires early attention, since it is much easier to modify the process than it is to reverse it.

THE DOCTOR

The physician is subject to the same reactions as parents, though in a modified and diluted form, and needs to be aware of them if they are not to compromise his ability to act in the child's best interests.

The phrase, 'I can do no more for him', is common, and epitomizes what is wrong with our attitudes about death. It makes the central role of the doctor that of cure rather than care and automatically equates death with defeat. Yet if we accept the fact that all must die, and that our primary concern is with the quality and length of life, then there are always things to be done to improve a particular situation, up to and including death and the care of the bereaved relatives beyond. Such a positive approach is essential to the reasonable functioning of an oncology unit. It is the physician's proper role to plan for and orchestrate death, where it is seen to be inevitable in the foreseeable future. Situations not infrequently arise where a calculated choice can be made between different modes of death, where the impact of death will be radically different for the dying child and his family.

Treatment of cancer with cure as its goal involves surgery, radiation and chemotherapy, all of which can be unpleasant. In those whose disease is not controlled, a decision may be required at some stage to stop further attempts at curative treatment in order to alleviate unwarranted suffering. The ethical dilemma about who has the right and/or obligation to choose to stop treatment is more poignant in paediatrics because of the added complication of the doctor–patient–parent interaction. In practice, it is not often a problem if all the members of the treatment team including the child and family are in constant communication – verbal or otherwise. Children are persons with rights, and that includes the right to choose not to continue treatment when there is no prospect of cure, even though that right is customarily assumed for the very young by parents and the law.

It is important to steer parents gently away from extreme positions on the subject of stopping treatment. Capitulation too soon may lead to a perpetual concern after death that cure might have been achieved 'if only' they had persisted with treatment for longer. Persistence for too long may leave guilt that they allowed their child to be subjected to so much suffering, all to no avail. The physician must be able to reach an agreed policy with parents which is in the best interests of the child and which also fulfils their role of ensuring the very best treatment for their child. This is most easily achieved when communication is good. Such agreed policy decisions help parents to face a change of goals, for example from cure to palliation, without unnecessary stress.

THE FAMILY AS FOCUS OF THE TREATMENT TEAM

Returning the primary caring role for a sick child to parents and siblings requires considerable changes in customary practices, even in children's hospitals. Most have accepted the idea of free visiting and find that they can continue to nurse the patient despite the presence of the family. It is still common, however, to find mothers displaced while a nurse performs tasks which the mother will perform well herself as soon as the child is discharged from hospital. The professional role is jealously guarded and it requires an enlightened staff to see their job as helping the parents to perform simple nursing tasks which would normally be regarded as their province. Involvement in their child's care makes a profound difference to the family and to the way they cope with the illness. It also matters a great deal to the patient and reduces his sense of isolation and fear of separation. Comfort and security are provided by simple measures such as allowing the child to bring with him as much of his home environment as possible. The strange and frightening atmosphere of hospital is much easier to tolerate if he is dressed in his own clothes, eating his favourite food cooked by his mother, surrounded by his siblings. No one who has seen the benefits of bringing the home into the hospital in this way could doubt that the effort and trouble required are well worth it for the patient.

Just as it is important to incorporate the family and parts of the home environment into the hospital, so the reverse applies when the child leaves hospital for home. A good example is where curative treatment has been exchanged for palliative care. Where everyone has accepted that death is to be the outcome, the child will usually feel more secure and happy in his own home, provided his comfort can be guaranteed and he and his family know they can return to hospital whenever they feel the need. In this situation, part of the hospital environment may need to be transposed into the home. Close bonds of trust, affection and love develop in the weeks, months or years of active treatment between the family and staff, because they see a great deal of each other and live through many crises together. It is easy for the child and family to feel abandoned if the same staff do not continue to take an active part in management throughout the phases of terminal care and bereavement. What is required is a home-care team who are hospital-based but who continue their work within the community. The whole family (patient, parents and siblings) may have great anxieties about coping with death, for it is often their first close contact with it, and they need to feel confident that experts in dealing with the death of children are available to them night and day if required.

What is the role here of the general practitioner and his supporting staff of health visitors and district nurses in caring for children with cancer? The disease, its treatment and complications are a highly specialized field which no general practitioner can be expected to master. The GP's role is inevitably usurped by the hospital team during the period when the child may be seen several times a week or month in the hospital. Although the GP is very welcome as a participant in the treatment team, his role is implicitly supportive, and this should continue to be the case during terminal care and bereavement, with a planned and phased return of primary care into his hands as the specialized problems recede. The not-uncommon situation where a specialist rings a GP to say that he cannot cure a child and is therefore returning him to the GP's care at a time when the child and family most need specialist help is difficult to justify. Paediatric oncologists are specialists in caring for children with cancer, and that care includes death as well as curative treatment; there should be equal satisfaction in the successful management of both. The general practitioner can be a staunch ally with his specialized knowledge of the extended family, local community and available resources. Too often the family is volleyed from hospital to home as if management was an either/or option rather than a coordinated team effort.

CARE AFTER DEATH

The close ties which bind together the family and other members of the treatment team are often most needed immediately after the child's death. Senior members of the team who were not actually present at the death will usually either telephone or write a brief letter of sympathy, and this is most important to parents as a reassurance that they are not about to be abandoned. This is the worst possible time to raise the question of an autopsy, which should usually have been gently introduced at an opportune moment some days or even weeks before. Provided they are reassured that no harm or further suffering can possibly come to their child, and that the examination could yield information which might directly benefit the treatment of other children faced with the same disease in the future, there are few parents who will refuse.

Most parents are left with some doubts and uncertainties about the course and final progression of the disease and what finally caused death, and these can be very disturbing to them. A meeting a few weeks later to discuss the results of the autopsy will usually resolve many of these doubts satisfactorily, and parents often derive great comfort from the fact that the information gained has been valuable to the clinician. Such a meeting is also a good opportunity for those parents who are ready for it to return to the hospital and renew the many friendships they have developed with the staff and other parents. The presence of recently bereaved parents on the unit as an accepted part of the community may be initially threatening to new parents, but often brings a sense of reality to their own situation which is of great benefit in the long run. Bereaved parents need the warmth and reassurance of their hospital 'family', people who know what a good job they did as parents for the child who has died, and who are happy to talk about the child, because friends and relatives outside usually find the subject acutely uncomfortable and embarrassing. Parents are sometimes concerned at the speed with which siblings apparently recover, and need reassurance that this is neither true nor necessarily a bad thing. Their own ability to cope seems to be in direct proportion to the care with which they have been prepared for and helped through their bereavement, but often seems remarkably good in the first few months. Where good links have been maintained with the general practitioner, however, it is not uncommon to hear of significant problems arising maybe several years later, for the first time.

CONCLUSION

Statistics indicate that at least one out of every thousand persons reaching adult life at the turn of the century will be a survivor of childhood cancer. Yet there is a conspiracy of silence among the general public as if childhood cancer were an indecent or taboo subject. In contrast, a great deal has been written about death and dying in recent years for the professionals, so much so that in the United States thanatology has become a fashionable subject, and the dying are in real danger of being processed along theoretical pathways by people trying to come to terms with their own insecurities about death.

I have tried to describe a practical approach to dealing with childhood cancer in clinical practice, based on my own experience with many families. This approach involves a realistic facing of the situation together and an active attempt to integrate the whole family in care. Our achievements often fall short of the goals we set ourselves, but the effort expended usually seems worthwhile to all parties concerned. The virtue of learning to get the most out of each day has been known for a long time, but has been largely forgotten in our present society. It is a lesson worth relearning.

ACKNOWLEDGEMENTS

I am indebted in particular to my wife Pat and my friend and colleague Dan Wilbur for their counsel and understanding in formulating the above ideas, though responsibility for any misconceptions is entirely mine. I have learnt most from the many wonderful families with whom I have been privileged to work.

Recommended reading

Burton, Lindy (1971). Cancer children. *New Soc.*, 17 June, p. 1040
Kübler-Ross, Elizabeth (1969). *On Death and Dying.* (New York: Macmillan Publ. Co.)
Lewis, C. S. (1976). *A Grief Observed.* (London: Bantam Books Inc.)
Martinson, I. M. *et al.* (1978). Home care for children dying of cancer. *Pediatrics*, **62**, 106
Schowalter, J. E. *et al.* (1973). The adolescent patient's decision to die. *Pediatrics*, **51**, 97
Waldman, A. M. (1976). Medical ethics and the hopelessly ill child. *J. Pediatr.*, **88**, 890
Wilbur, J. R. (1975). Rehabilitation of children with cancer. *Cancer*, **36**, 809

4

Death, dying and the cardiac patient

Alan M. Johnson

In ancient Greece the heart was generally considered to be the seat of emotions and passions, and even of the intellect. At the time of Leonardo da Vinci, only 500 years ago, the soul itself was thought to reside in the heart, kindling it and through it giving life to the body. Even though these ideas have passed into history they have left, to this day, a certain mystique in matters relating to the heart. This and its very singleness arouse deep feelings when the health of the heart is called into question or actually fails. It is not surprising, therefore, that death and dying are closely linked in people's minds with the heart.

Dying, in the cardiac patient, may be considered from several points of view, as follows. Each has its own psychological and physical implications.

(1) Fear of death.
(2) Fear of not being able to die.
(3) Having 'died' and been resuscitated.
(4) The risk of sudden death.
(5) Dying, but retrieved and restored to health by surgery or by particular medical treatment.
(6) Dying from an incurable condition which may, nevertheless, be amenable to symptomatic relief by medical means which may also prolong enjoyable and useful life and greatly shorten the terminal phase of the illness.

FEAR OF DEATH

Most people, when they come to believe that they have heart disease,

57

whether or not that belief is well founded, think at once of becoming crippled and dependent, of dying by slow degrees in dreadful discomfort or pain, or of dying suddenly. The spectre of sudden death before their loved ones is often a source of special dread. The same is true of the relatives and, of course, especially the parents of children suspected or found to have an abnormal heart.

For these reasons, and because early diagnosis offers the best chance of cure or of successful palliation in most cardiac diseases, no person, whether adult or child, should be allowed to remain without a firm diagnosis once a cardiac abnormality is even mooted. Only then can the situation be managed properly and fear of the unknown be removed from patient and relatives alike. Such diagnosis may be achieved by a cardiologist using simple clinical examination, or specialized cardiac investigations may be necessary. Conviction that the doctors understand completely the condition of the heart, the immediate and long-term implications, and its management at every stage is the only possible way to peace of mind for all concerned. All this must be faithfully conveyed to the patient or relatives, or both, so creating confidence in the doctors. This is a therapeutic factor in itself.

The diagnosis may be that the heart is, after all, completely normal and healthy. For example, in children and slender adults the innocent systolic murmur that arises in the normal right ventricle often gives rise, at routine medical examinations, to suspicion of heart disease. This innocent murmur is increased by the faster circulation associated with excitement or pregnancy, or any febrile state. Similarly, in adults with innocent extrasystoles brought about by fatigue or anxiety or an intercurrent illness, the associated palpitation is liable to give rise to fear of sudden death. This fear increases the frequency of the extrasystoles, so giving rise to increasing fear and consequently a vicious circle. Once the diagnosis of normality is certain, it must be stated unequivocally. In the case of patients with innocent extrasystoles, explanation and reassurance alone often suffice to end the arrhythmia and to restore confidence, comfort and health.

From time to time doctors decline to seek specialist cardiological opinion 'for fear of frightening the patient'. It must be reiterated, therefore, that in many cases simple clinical examination by a cardiologist will suffice to establish a firm diagnosis. If, however, special investigations are required they are not of themselves frightening, painful or distressing. Many nowadays can be outpatient procedures and are completely non-invasive, such as echocardiography and phonocardiography; or are minimally 'invasive', such as nuclear cardiography which requires only a single small intravenous injection. The invasive investigations involving cardiac catheterization are performed by expert hands with a skilled team, in quiet and calm conditions, under a comfortable degree of sedation, without pain and with every preparation and precaution for the patient's safety. They require only 3 to 7 days in hospital.

FEAR OF NOT BEING ABLE TO DIE

This is an anxiety special to patients who are to be or have been provided with a permanent artificial pacemaker. They are aware that the pacemaker causes the heart to beat when it would not spontaneously do so. Such patients may think that, as life depends upon the heartbeat, death may not be possible with an artificial pacemaker in position. Of course this is not the case. The metabolic disturbances associated with terminal illness, or loss of myocardial function from ischaemic or other disease, renders the heart at last unresponsive to the pacemaker and death occurs in the normal way. Clearly, therefore, without necessarily entering into a description or discussion of these details, the patient can and must be reassured unequivocally about this.

FEAR OF HAVING 'DIED' AND BEEN RESUSCITATED

This subject merits comment because the idea of having died and been brought back from death may be deeply disturbing to an individual. The knowledge that he has suffered 'cardiac arrest' may dominate his thoughts for years with a continuing anxiety in case it happens again and if, when it does so, resuscitation might not be achieved or, worse still, might be only partially achieved with residual brain damage leading to a 'cabbage' existence. When such an event has occurred, whether following acute coronary occlusion, during unstable angina, during cardiac catheterization, coronary arteriography or cardiac surgery, or for that matter during general surgery, it is kinder to the patient, and generally to the relatives also, to avoid use of the term 'cardiac arrest' and instead to describe the event as a serious disturbance of heart rhythm which called for intensive treatment and, for a time afterwards, close observation. If the underlying cause persists and is amenable to curative or prophylactic treatment, this should of course be provided unless the initial resuscitation was itself a mistake, through error of judgement or lack of awareness of the presence of disease soon and inevitably to be fatal.

THE RISK OF SUDDEN DEATH

Certain cardiac conditions, notably ischaemic heart disease, aortic stenosis, heart block and very severe pulmonary hypertension, are particularly associated with the risk of sudden death. In these cases the question arises as to whether or not the patient or the relatives (parents in the case of children) should be informed of this. The matter arises also regarding fitness to drive.

If the cause of this risk can be eliminated, as is the case with aortic stenosis and heart block, this of course must be done.

In certain circumstances, and when the cause cannot be removed, it may be essential that the patient or relatives are made aware of such risk. It may then be possible to spare the patient the idea of sudden death while indicating that he could become ill very abruptly so as to become immediately, and for some time, unable to work or to deal with business or family affairs. In relation to fitness to drive, 'a tendency to sudden faintness' suffices to explain to the patient his unfitness to drive.

Such information will enable an individual at risk to put his affairs in order, against the time when he may suddenly and without warning 'become very ill for some time', without the spectre of sudden death clouding his every moment. Patients who know that they may die suddenly are often haunted by the mental picture of their sudden collapse and death causing at once great distress and great embarrassment to their loved ones, their friends, colleagues or workmates and to all about them. Of course the family may well be so afflicted, but they will generally prefer to accept this state of affairs in order to spare their relative from suffering constant and perhaps prolonged mental anguish in addition to other symptoms arising from his heart disease. Some patients, for particular religious or other reasons, may ask specifically whether a risk of sudden death exists in their case. A true answer should be given, gently but frankly.

In the case of children with aortic stenosis the parents cannot be spared the knowledge of this risk, for this is one of the few conditions in which avoidance of heavy physical activity must be strictly imposed in childhood, as such activity increases the risk of sudden death. Furthermore, surgery for aortic stenosis is best postponed if possible until the patient is fully grown. If surgery must be performed in childhood open aortic valvotomy will usually be advised, and some years later a further operation for aortic valve replacement will be necessary in most cases. Aortic valve replacement, once and for all, can be performed if it is possible to postpone operation until the patient is fully grown; but such postponement can only take place under close cardiological surveillance. These individuals, whether child or adult, may die suddenly before aortic stenosis has been diagnosed, when it will be discovered at the coroner's autopsy; or while the patient is on a waiting list for special cardiac investigation or surgery. For this reason they are given high priority on waiting lists. While avoidance of heavy physical effort diminishes the risk of sudden death it does not abolish it.

FEAR OF DYING, BUT RETRIEVED AND RESTORED TO HEALTH

There are several cardiac conditions that may cause severe and progressive illness, usually associated with left and right heart failure and with a falling cardiac output. The tempo of such illness may be slow, extending over months or a few years, or may be rapid, developing over weeks, days or even hours. Some of these are easily recognizable or may be strongly suspected from a simple history and clinical examination. Special cardiac investigation may, however, be needed to prove the diagnosis, to provide details required for a decision regarding suitability for cardiac surgery and, should that be advised, to show features of the condition from which the surgeon may plan the precise form that the operation should take. Among these conditions are the following.

Congenital heart disease

In the newborn and the infant, defects associated with heavy pulmonary blood flow due to left-to-right shunting of blood, such as persistent ductus arteriosus, ventricular septal defect or atrial septal defect, may cause not only a failure to thrive but lapse into progressive and fatal heart failure.

Cyanosis in the neonate or infant may pass unobserved, incredible as it often seems to the experienced observer. Severe heart failure and falling cardiac output may develop in those with heavy pulmonary blood flow or severe pulmonary hypertension, leading to death unless the true nature of the illness is recognized. In babies with reduced pulmonary blood flow severe cyanotic attacks may develop and may be fatal. Many of the babies in all of these groups are amenable to cure.

Ischaemic heart disease

Angina of effort and angina associated with emotion may become intractable to medical treatment and crippling in severity. Such patients will often have greatly limited life-expectancy. For patients found suitable following coronary arteriography, coronary artery bypass surgery now offers total relief in about 85 per cent of cases at very low risk – 1.7 per cent in our own published series (Ross *et al.* 1976). The remaining patients are partially relieved of their angina, usually to a very worthwhile degree. The benefit is long-lived and it begins to seem that life-expectancy is very significantly improved.

Myocardial infarction, in addition to causing loss of myocardial contractility and ventricular diastolic compliance, may be complicated by various mechanical problems leading to progressive illness and death.

Mitral regurgitation may result from infarction, either by such widespread loss of muscle as to cause gross left ventricular failure with dilatation of the whole ventricle and of the mitral valve ring, or by involvement of papillary muscles in the infarcted area. Mitral regurgitation resulting from papillary muscle dysfunction may develop and increase rapidly and, combined with myocardial impairment, produce overwhelming effects. Increased pulmonary venous engorgement is associated with increasing dyspnoea and leads to pulmonary oedema. This, together with overwork of the surviving myocardium, causes progressive heart failure, falling cardiac output and increasing systemic vascular resistance, setting up a vicious circle. Surgical correction of the mitral regurgitation is necessary if this circle is to be broken and the patient saved.

Ventricular septal perforation may complicate infarction of the septum. It occurs within a few days of the infarction and results in sudden development of left and right ventricular volume overload and failure, falling cardiac output and, unless corrected surgically, death.

Ventricular aneurysm, which may be anteroapical, posterior or inferior, may follow full-thickness myocardial infarction. Such aneurysmal dilatation of part of the left ventricular wall may impose a large workload upon the surviving, sound myocardium and diminish cardiac reserve, leading to progressive and intractable heart failure and to death. Life-threatening arrhythmias or unstable mural thrombus leading to recurrent systemic embolism may also complicate left ventricular aneurysm. Surgical removal of the aneurysm is indicated by any of these complications and is feasible provided that enough of the left ventricular free wall and septum is still contracting well. It can be life-saving and restores effective cardiac function. In some cases only one coronary artery is diseased, so that the remaining myocardium is normally supplied and a good result is to be expected. When other arteries are stenosed, the blood supply may be restored by coronary artery bypass grafting at the same operation. Long-term success of ventricular aneurysmectomy is dependent upon a sufficient quantity of left ventricle remaining and the adequacy of its blood supply.

Selection for surgery in any of these states depends, therefore, upon satisfactory residual left ventricular performance and assessment of this is a first requirement when surgery is considered. The non-invasive tests, echocardiography and nuclear cardiography are the first steps towards this. If these investigations show reasonably good left ventricular contractility, then left ventriculography and coronary arteriography must follow.

Valvular heart disease
Whether congenital in origin or of acquired degenerative, rheumatic or syphilitic aetiology, this may cause sudden death or the development and progression of heart failure leading to death. Surgical relief, before the heart or the lungs (or both) have suffered irreparable damage, saves life and restores health.

Hypertensive heart disease
This, unrecognized and untreated, leads eventually to progressive insidious or sudden illness and to death. Such a course of events should not occur in an age when such a range of hypotensive drugs exists and when the NHS offers so many opportunities for routine blood pressure readings.

Complete heart block
This is usually degenerative in aetiology in younger as well as older patients, but may also be a manifestation of ischaemic heart disease or of the primary cardiomyopathies. It may at first be intermittent, only later becoming permanent.

Infective endocarditis
This may present with typical development of lassitude, fever, weight loss, night sweats with rigors, anaemia, digital clubbing, petechiae including subungual splinter haemorrhages, Osler's nodes and splenomegaly; or with acute haemodynamic complications such as perforation of aortic or mitral valve cusps or chordal rupture producing severe and increasing dyspnoea progressing rapidly to life-threatening pulmonary oedema.

Spontaneous chordal rupture
This event, usually occurring in a person previously perfectly well, causes the sudden development of mitral regurgitation leading to cough and

dyspnoea that may lead to mistaken diagnosis of an acute respiratory infection. It happens most often in the fifth or sixth decade of life, but sometimes earlier or later. It appears to be increasingly common, perhaps as a result of generally greater longevity. It is, of course, associated with a mitral systolic murmur. Such a murmur may have been detected previously, even in childhood, for trivial mitral regurgitation may have pre-existed in some of these patients in association with congenital cusp redundancy, cusp prolapse or the floppy valve syndrome. The hallmark of this condition is the late systolic click, which may exist as the only evidence of the valve anomaly unless or until chordal rupture brings mitral regurgitation and the systolic murmur, or may accompany a characteristically high-pitched late mitral systolic murmur for many years before chordal rupture occurs. Measures for protection against bacterial endocarditis are of the greatest importance in such cases.

With spontaneous chordal rupture, which may occur without obvious reason or may be precipitated by heavy effort or a febrile illness, mitral regurgitation develops or increases abruptly, leading to pulmonary venous congestion and, if inadequately treated, to frank left and later right heart failure. If this state of affairs continues for too long the left ventricle may be irreparably damaged and an eminently curable condition becomes inoperable and incurable.

Acute aortic dissection
Dissection affecting the ascending aorta usually causes severe aortic regurgitation of abrupt onset. The condition presents with severe splitting or tearing anterior and posterior chest pain, often spreading or moving to the neck, arms, abdomen or legs, or to several of these sites depending upon the extent of the dissection. It leads quickly to gross dyspnoea, collapse and death unless surgical repair is undertaken urgently.

Masked conditions
In addition, some of these and other conditions may masquerade as inevitably fatal illnesses, causing misdiagnosis so that the patient is denied the opportunity of rescue and the restoration of health by way of cardiac surgery or particular medical treatment. Among those conditions already mentioned but in the event not recognized are:

Ischaemic heart disease with intractable angina
This cannot be presumed, without proof, to be beyond surgical relief, for neither clinical findings, nor electrocardiographic or chest X-ray appear-

ances, nor even all three of these together can be relied upon to distinguish between cases amenable to surgery and those not so amenable. There is also:

(1) Ischaemic heart disease with left and right heart failure due to ventricular aneurysm, but presumed without proof to be associated with generalized myocardial damage and therefore unamenable to surgical relief.

(2) Ischaemic heart disease with mitral regurgitation or ventricular septal perforation causing left and right heart failure, the murmur being mistaken for loud pericardial friction or ignored because its meaning is not understood.

Valvular heart disease

Heart failure and diminished cardiac output may have progressed so far that the murmurs arising from diseased valves are so faint that they either fail to impress the doctor with their true significance or are not detected at all. Such patients may still be retrievable and may be found in both the adult and the paediatric groups.

Heart block

This may be intermittent at first, causing Stokes–Adams attacks, and may masquerade as epilepsy and be so treated, without benefit, for some time even amounting to a few years before the correct diagnosis is made. The patient may sustain repeated and severe injuries during this time or may, of course, die in one of the attacks. The condition may also present as heart failure of which the cause seems mysterious and may be presumed incurable; or as dementia, presumed 'senile' but due in fact to impaired cerebral circulation and completely reversible by restoring a normal heart rate. Heart block may respond for a time to oral isoprenaline but, unless the patient is in the terminal stages of a mortal disease, permanent on-demand artificial pacemaking is the best and, in the long run, the least expensive form of treatment and leads to a return to a normal way of life. With Stokes–Adams attacks such treatment is mandatory. In old people one pacemaker may nowadays be expected to last a lifetime, while in the younger patient the interval between short stays in hospital for changes of the battery unit is already a few years and is still increasing.

Infective endocarditis

This may present so insidiously, with general illness, especially in the very young and the very old, that a misdiagnosis of malignant disease may be made. The true nature of the illness may not be recognized so that steps to identify the infection and to eradicate it by an effective combination of anti-biotics may not be undertaken. Death may then result from cachexia, from complicating nephritis and renal failure, or from catastrophic haemo-dynamic or intracranial complications. It must be remembered that infective endocarditis may occur in the elderly upon an aortic valve whose only abnormality is atheroma giving rise to little or nothing in the way of cardiac signs.

Spontaneous rupture of mitral chordae
This may lead to misdiagnosis of primary lung disease, from the combin-ation of dyspnoea, often with persistent cough, abnormal lung shadows in the chest X-ray, normal heart size and electrocardiogram and failure to find or to appreciate the significance of a mitral systolic murmur. The latter may, in this condition, be conducted towards the cardiac base and to the neck rather than towards the axilla.

Other conditions that may lead to apparently incurable illness by remaining unrecognized, but in which diagnosis can lead to cure, include the following.

Chronic constrictive pericarditis and chronic effusive pericarditis
In both of these intractable heart failure, presumed to be due to severe myocardial disease, or chronic incurable liver disease may be imitated. Pericardial disease must always be considered in the differential diagnosis in patients with chronic oedema or ascites without obvious explanation, and in patients with combined jaundice and oedema. Pericardectomy in either condition brings the high pulmonary and systemic venous pressures to normality by allowing the heart to fill and function normally and relieves the destructive effects of severe chronic pulmonary and systemic venous congestion.

The diagnosis of chronic constrictive pericarditis, if it is thought of, is not difficult. Anasarca, ascites, lung crepitations and pleural fluid with associated dyspnoea, and the high pressure evident in the turgid neck veins, with pulsus paradoxus and a quiet cardiac impulse all indicate the diagnosis. The electrocardiogram generally shows small voltages, often with widespread T-wave inversion, and atrial fibrillation or flutter may occur late in the condition. In the chest X-ray pericardial calcification should be sought, and it must be stressed that this may be difficult to detect in the usual posteroanterior film but very obvious in a lateral film which should therefore always be taken when the possibility of this diagnosis is entertained. Chronic effusive pericarditis, for example complicating connective tissue disease, shows similar clinical signs and, in addition, the effusion may be demonstrated by echocardiography.

Left atrial myxoma

This may lead to a chronic illness with lassitude and with weight loss sometimes progressing to cachexia. In the early stages of the illness anorexia nervosa or other psychiatric illness may be diagnosed and treatment may be directed accordingly. In the later stages malignant disease is likely to be suspected and extensive investigations may be undertaken in line with that diagnosis. Meanwhile the cardiac and pulmonary effects of the left atrial tumour develop and progress insidiously, leading to permanent damage in the pulmonary vascular bed with severe pulmonary hypertension and eventually to syncopal attacks and sometimes sudden death. A high ESR is common, the plasma proteins may be abnormal with a high globulin level and clinically a variable mitral diastolic murmur may be heard, sometimes of rather high frequency leading to suspicion of pericardial friction. A diastolic 'plop' may occasionally be heard as a pedunculated tumour drops through the mitral valve in each diastole; and the clinical signs of severe pulmonary hypertension may be evident. Systemic embolization may occur from fragments of the friable tumour breaking away; and whenever an arterial embolus is removed from a leg, histological examination should be made to exclude myxoma if the source of the embolus is not obvious. Echocardiography is a highly reliable way of showing or excluding left atrial myxoma and is an easy, quick and non-invasive outpatient investigation to be undertaken at once whenever this diagnosis is considered. Surgical removal of the tumour is a matter of urgency once it is detected.

Arteriovenous fistula

Whether in the child or the adult, congenital in a limb or in the cranium, or acquired by gunshot or other penetrating wound, this may remain undetected but may be the cause of progressive and ultimately fatal heart failure. Such fistulae should always be remembered and sought in patients dying with unexplained heart failure, for surgical obliteration of the fistula is life-saving and restores health. The author has seen just such a patient, a young man in terminal heart failure thought to be due to primary cardio-myopathy. The parents sought one last opinion before allowing him to die. He had been hit by an airgun pellet in the right thigh as a little boy, an accident that had long since been forgotten but was recalled when the boy was asked, in their presence, about the tiny scar on the thigh. An arteriovenous fistula had resulted. It was detected (indeed it was obvious once thought of), it was closed by surgery and he made a full recovery.

Aortic coarctation

Although this condition is easily diagnosed by simultaneously feeling the right radial and either femoral arterial pulse, failure to detect it remains all too common due to failure to implement this simple manoeuvre at routine medical examinations, from the initial school medical examination onwards. These pulses are normally synchronous and of equal strength. In the presence of aortic coarctation, however, the femoral pulses are diminished and delayed in comparison with the right radial pulse, or may be absent. There are, of course, several other clinical signs of coarctation and the chest X-ray after about the age of 12 years, but sometimes earlier or later, shows the characteristic rib-notching; but these are merely confirmatory of the diagnosis and will not be described here. Almost incredibly, this may not be recognized as the underlying cause of hypertension, subarachnoid haemorrhage or heart failure. The latter may occur in infancy and referral to a paediatric cardiologist will ensure correct diagnosis and early surgical relief. In the adult, however, it may still not be thought of as a cause of heart failure. An example in the author's recent experience was that of a young woman who was thought to be dying of primary cardiomyopathy but who was, mercifully and albeit in the terminal stage of her illness, referred for a cardiological opinion. The true diagnosis was immediately evident and emergency operation to resect the coarctation saved her life and restored her to health.

Thyrotoxic heart disease

This manifestation of 'masked thyrotoxicosis', is a cause of atrial fibrillation and progressive heart failure in elderly subjects, usually with toxic nodular goitre. The combination of weight loss with atrial fibrillation and heart failure, without other obvious general thyrotoxic features, may suggest cardiac cachexia secondary to an incurable form of heart disease, so that the true and curable diagnosis is missed and death results.

Congenital heart disease

When associated with heavy pulmonary blood flow in the infant, as in persistent ductus arteriosus, ventricular septal defect or occasionally atrial septal defect, this may cause respiratory symptoms leading to a misdiagnosis of pulmonary disease and to death from the effects of bronchitis and recurrent pneumonia; or, by causing feeding difficulties may lead to mis-diagnosis of gastrointestinal disease and even to death from starvation or intussusception. Such disastrous and potentially fatal mistakes in diagnosis should not occur nowadays, when there is increased awareness of the effects of congenital heart disease, and wide availability of paediatric cardiology services to assist the general practitioner or paediatrician in doubt as to the significance of abnormal cardiac or pulmonary signs. Survival of the dying baby and his subsequent progress to normality depend upon early and correct diagnosis.

FEAR OF DYING FROM AN INCURABLE CONDITION, AND THE TERMINAL PHASE

Finally, let us consider that group of patients with heart disease who are suffering from incurable and progressive conditions that shorten the life-expectancy of any age group and who truly fall within the category of the dying cardiac patient.

The conditions fall into three groups, of which only the first will receive full consideration in this chapter.

(1) Destruction of myocardium and myocardial function.
(2) Destruction of the lungs, with secondary effects upon the heart (cor pulmonale) from high pulmonary vascular resistance causing severe pulmonary hypertension, or from chronic hypoxia, or from both of these.
(3) Destruction of the kidneys, secondary to heart disease, such as bacterial endocarditis; or causing heart disease or cardiac malfunction through hypertension or progressive metabolic disturbance.

It is of course in groups (1) and (3) that organ transplant surgery enters our considerations, but this aspect will not be discussed here. We shall discuss group (1) in some depth, considering diagnosis, physical and psychological effects and management; and, more briefly, group (2). The problems of group (3) are considered in the next chapter.

Destruction of the myocardium

This occurs in ischaemic heart disease, in the primary cardiomyopathies, in some forms of chronic myocarditis following acute myocarditis and in specific heart muscle disease due, for example, to thyrotoxicosis, chronic alcoholism or amyloidosis. The commoner of these will be discussed under the pathological headings though, as all have a final common pathway to death the control of symptoms and management of the terminal state will be jointly described.

Ischaemic heart disease

Whether due to atheroma and thrombosis producing stenosis and occlusion in the coronary arteries, this may cause an insidious and progressive loss of myocardium, by microscopic degrees, leading finally to rhythm disturbances and to progressive heart failure; or it may result in abrupt destruction of areas of myocardium by acute myocardial infarction. Depending upon the extent and distribution of myocardial loss, there is a loss of contractility and impairment of ventricular diastolic compliance. With severe impairment of contractility cardiac output tends to fall and, in order that the arterial pressure shall be maintained, systemic vascular resistance is increased by arteriolar constriction. With impairment of ventricular diastolic compliance the ventricular diastolic pressure rises, and this rise is conducted retrogradely to the left atrium and the pulmonary veins. The combination of these systolic and diastolic effects causes a fall in cardiac output; and thus is acquired, abruptly with large infarcts, more gradually with insidious myocardial loss or with recurrent smaller infarcts, the state of chronic heart failure, high systemic vascular resistance and low cardiac output. Secondary to these effects, impaired renal elimination of sodium and water causes increase of blood volume, so aggravating the state of venous hypertension. Eventually venous pressure, which is the ventricular filling pressure known also as ventricular preload, exceeds the physiological optimum for the particular state of the ventricular myocardium and cardiac output falls further (Starling's law).

The picture of a rapidly or gradually progressive deterioration towards death from widespread myocardial damage and loss may be indistinguishable by clinical criteria from that associated with left ventricular aneurysm, which is sometimes a surgically amenable condition. In that condition the chest X-ray may show the typical shelf-and-prominence appearance if the aneurysm is apical and anterolateral, but rarely otherwise. The electrocardiogram usually shows persistent elevation of the ST segment in leads 'facing' the aneurysm, but this may occasionally be minimal in degree or absent and it may sometimes be seen over part of a more extensively destroyed left ventricle.

It follows, then, that one cannot say with certainty from clinical examination, even with the help of the electrocardiogram and chest X-ray, whether a particular individual has diffuse ventricular loss and cannot survive, or whether there may be a surgically remediable ventricular aneurysm. Unless, therefore, advanced age or coexisting disease gives a clear contraindication to surgical relief the matter deserves to be settled by a nuclear cardiogram and, if necessary thereafter, by left ventriculography and coronary arteriography in order to be certain that surgery cannot help before settling to the management of the terminal patient.

Primary cardiomyopathies

Congestive, or dilated, cardiomyopathy resembles that type of ischaemic heart disease associated with diffuse loss of myocardium, except that angina is not part of the clinical picture. Progressive deterioration towards death has the same pattern and general and terminal management are the same.

Hypertrophic cardiomyopathy, with or without left ventricular outflow obstruction, is associated with dyspnoea due to impaired left ventricular diastolic compliance and the resulting elevation of pulmonary venous pressure; with sudden death as in severe aortic valve stenosis previously discussed; with angina of effort and effort syncope; and with rhythm disturbances, notably heart block which calls for an artificial pacemaker. The condition may progress to the dilated form.

Restrictive cardiomyopathy is quite rare. It shows clinical features resembling those of chronic constrictive pericarditis but, unlike that condition is not, of course, amenable to surgical relief. The differential diagnosis is obviously of the greatest importance and may require angiocardiography.

Chronic myocarditis

This and the myocardial infiltrative diseases give rise to dilated or restrictive forms of left ventricular dysfunction and to the associated features of the terminal illness.

Destruction of the lungs

Chronic cor pulmonale

This leads to right ventricular failure and is the result of lung diseases associated with reduction of the pulmonary capillary bed, or impairment of gas exchange, or a combination of these. Severe pulmonary hypertension, and chronic hypoxia and hypercapnia leading to secondary polycythaemia arise from the pulmonary deficiencies and throw a heavy and increasing load upon the right heart.

Thromboembolic pulmonary hypertension
This results from continuing embolization of the lungs over months or years, usually following injuries with subsequent therapeutic immobiliz-ation, pregnancy and childbirth complicated by deep vein thrombosis, or very severe chronic varicose veins.

Primary pulmonary hypertension
This is a disease of unknown aetiology affecting most commonly girls and young women. Like the previous condition it leads to effort syncope and sudden death or to increasing right ventricular failure, tricuspid incompetence, falling cardiac output and progressive deterioration to death.

The Eisenmenger syndrome
This is associated with congenital heart disease in which there is a large communication between the atria (ostium primum defect; more rarely ostium secundum defect), the ventricles (ventricular septal defect) or the aorta and the pulmonary artery (persistent ductus, aortopulmonary septal defect, persistent truncus arteriosus). It consists of a great elevation of pulmonary vascular resistance with resulting severe pulmonary hyper-tension and right-to-left shunting of blood through the communication. This reaction in the lungs does not occur in all patients with these congenital anomalies but it does so in some and the reason is not yet known. It can develop within the first few months of life or may take a few years to develop. The pulmonary arterioles regain the thick wall and narrow lumen found in the newborn. The condition is irreversible and inoperable and is associated with a much reduced life-expectancy. Death most often occurs suddenly between the second and fourth decades, sometimes during a febrile intercurrent illness and always after years of great mental and physical distress and discomfort. Severe central cyanosis, severe cyanotic acne and severe digital clubbing produce disfigurement that neither cosmetics nor dress can disguise and combine with severe effort dyspnoea and sometimes angina and headaches to cause the distress mentioned above. Polycythaemia is always present and leads to compli-cations that include strokes from cerebral venous or arterial occlusion, or cerebral abscess, visual impairment or blindness from retinal venous or arterial thrombosis, or the nephrotic syndrome from renal vein thrombosis. Later, and sometimes heralding the end, there may be recurrent haemoptysis.
   The diagnosis of the Eisenmenger syndrome may generally be reached

by clinical examination but echocardiography and sometimes cardiac catheterization may be needed to establish beyond any doubt that surgery cannot help. In some babies the development of this awful condition may be prevented by very early diagnosis and surgery; and the existence of this syndrome reminds us always how vital may be an early cardiological opinion in babies thought or known to have congenital heart disease.

Symptoms and their control

Angina, palpitation
Dyspnoea, orthopnoea, paroxysmal nocturnal dyspnoea
Lassitude, cold extremities, 'thinness' (cachexia), decubitus ulcers
Nocturnal confusion and sleeplessness, anxiety and depression
Cheyne–Stokes respiration
Oedema

Digitalis intoxication ⎫
Prostatism ⎪
⎬ Complicating prolonged diuretic therapy
Gout ⎪
Diabetes mellitus ⎭

Good control of these symptoms calls for careful attention to detail and close surveillance, imposing a heavy load upon the doctor but, when well achieved, providing one of the most rewarding tasks in medicine. Much suffering, both for the patient and for the family, can be saved by good management of the dying patient. Indeed, a long-drawn-out and dreadful process may be transformed to a prolongation of reasonably comfortable and fulfilling life, followed either by a relatively short period of real invalidism leading to death or by sudden death while still active and 'well'.

Dyspnoea and the effects of low cardiac output

Dyspnoea on effort and the more severe degrees of the same phenomenon, orthopnoea and paroxysmal nocturnal dyspnoea, all result from a high left ventricular diastolic pressure with corresponding elevation of pulmonary venous pressure. This is the filling pressure or preload of the left ventricle. If this is lowered excessively, left ventricular output will fall according to Starling's law, unless at the same time the systemic vascular resistance (left ventricular afterload) is also reduced. Too high or too low a filling pressure reduces left ventricular output. Responses to lowered cardiac output include systemic arteriolar constriction, manifest as hypertension or skin pallor, or both. Such constriction also affects the renal arterioles and results in sodium and water retention, causing a further rise of venous pressure and further fall of cardiac output. Reduced renin excretion and increased plasma angiotensin levels cause yet more vasoconstriction, and further increase ventricular afterload.

The first attempt to break this vicious circle was by the use of digitalis and diuretics; and the introduction of potent oral diuretics some 25 years ago transformed the management of such patients. By causing a heavy diuresis the blood volume was reduced and kept reduced so long as a good diuretic response was maintained; and so left ventricular preload was reduced. This therapy was capable of controlling the situation for some time, even for several years, but eventually as myocardial disease gradually progressed the symptoms worsened again and control was lost.

Next came the means of extending control by, in addition, reducing the left ventricular afterload. This was achieved by the judicious use of drugs which cause dilatation of the systemic arterioles. If they also dilated the renal arterioles this would clearly be of considerable additional advantage, by facilitating the continuation of effective diuretic therapy.

Thirdly, drugs have been developed which produce venous dilatation, so increasing the capacity of the venous pool and contributing to a reduction of circulating blood volume, of venous pressure and of ventricular preload.

We now have, therefore, a most powerful armoury of therapeutic agents by which to control the effects of diminishing cardiac performance, due primarily to progressive myocardial disease but aggravated by excessive ventricular preload, excessive ventricular afterload and the further reduction of cardiac output that results from these. It is thus possible to eliminate paroxysmal nocturnal dyspnoea and orthopnoea and to keep effort dyspnoea to a minimum. The effects of low cardiac output, such as lassitude, cold extremities, weight loss progressing to cachexia, nocturnal confusion and excessive dreaming can also be greatly reduced or removed; and all this may be maintained for a few years in many patients who, when first seen, were *in extremis*. Diet and lifestyle are, of course, also relevant to continued control; excessive salt intake or excessive physical effort may defeat the efforts to control ventricular preload and afterload.

Angina may continue to be a distressing and limiting symptom and in controlling it further depression of myocardial function must be avoided. Generally, therefore, in these circumstances beta-blockade to assist control of angina must be used judiciously, in combination with digitalis glycosides, and with a cardioselective agent to help avoid increasing the bronchospasm that is always to some extent a feature of left ventricular failure. The dilator drugs used to reduce left ventricular preload are also coronary dilators and contribute to relief of angina.

Dependent oedema resulting from secondary right ventricular failure is generally more of a psychological than a physical problem, for no patient likes to see 'the dropsy' affecting his feet, ankles and lower legs. Some degree of this may have to be accepted and the psychological effect may be alleviated by the comment that this is water which would otherwise be in the lungs; and that one of the aims of treatment is to transfer water 'from the lungs to the ankles', so preventing shortness of breath. The ankle oedema may then be seen as a small blessing rather than acting as a source of continuing anxiety and despair.

Terminally, of course, anasarca including ascites and pleural transudates may cause distress and may even require paracentesis, though this is fortunately rare nowadays; but the object of management, as described here, is to make that terminal period as short as possible and the period of comfortable control as long as possible.

It will only be in the shorter terminal period that other distressing symptoms may need attention in their own right. Avoidance of pressure sores, at the stage of cardiac cachexia, will require the most careful preventive measures. Nocturnal sleeplessness and confusion may require help from drugs; and more terminally still, Cheyne–Stokes breathing, with the alternation of intense wakefulness during the hyperpnoeic phases and semicoma in the apnoeic phases, may cause great distress both to the patient and to any relative observing it.

Complications of prolonged diuretic therapy

Potassium depletion } Cardiac arrhythmias and further depression
Digitalis intoxication } of cardiac function

Prostatism, brought to prominence by heavy diuresis. Transurethral resection may be needed or, in the terminal state, an indwelling urethral catheter.

Precipitation or aggravation of gout

Reduced glucose tolerance, sometimes frank diabetes mellitus

Any of these may, of course, add greatly to disability and discomfort or distress and all call for prompt treatment in order to regain a perhaps fragile stability.

Drugs

Digitalis
This is used to control ventricular rate in patients with atrial fibrillation, and to assist in bringing heart failure under control even when sinus

rhythm is present. Its continued use, in the presence of sinus rhythm, to maintain freedom from heart failure in the longer term is once again under debate; but the author favours its long-term use provided adequate surveillance is continued, as it must be in these patients if the objective is to be achieved of relieving suffering in the few years, months or weeks leading to death.

For the sudden onset of atrial fibrillation in a previously undigitalized patient, if rapid control of ventricular rate is called for by a severe fall in cardiac performance, the more rapidly eliminated meslanoside (edilanid) 1–2 mg by intravenous injection may be followed by digoxin 0.25 mg twice or thrice daily for 3 days then once daily to maintain full digitalization. The dose depends upon the weight and the renal function of the particular patient. Potassium depletion must be guarded against if diuretics are concurrently used, as will be the case in most of these patients.

Diuretics

Alone or in combination with other drugs these are used to control hypertension and also, as already described, to control ventricular preload.

Depending upon the short-term or long-term objective, whether to relieve acute pulmonary oedema or to maintain already achieved stability, to take the two extreme examples, a high-potency, fast-acting or a low-potency, longer-acting drug may be chosen.

High-potency drugs include frusemide (Dryptal or Lasix), bumetanide (Burinex), mefruside (Baycaron) and ethacrynic acid (Edecrin). All of these, except mefruside which is orally administered, may be given intravenously or orally depending upon the urgency of the clinical situation. It should be remembered that the ability of the congested bowel to absorb drugs may be severely impaired, so that initially the intravenous route may have to be used.

Medium-potency diuretics include the thiazide drugs, such as chlorothiazide (Saluric), bendrofluazide (Aprinox, Centyl, Neo-Naclex), and hydroflumethiazide (Hydrenox, Naclex), the action of which is complete after 10 to 12 hours; and chlorthalidone (Hygroton) or clorexolone (Nefrolan) which may act for 48 to 72 hours. All of these are given orally.

Low-potency diuretics may usefully be combined with other diuretics of high or medium potency because they have a potassium-sparing action which may overcome or reduce the need for supplementary potassium administration. They include spironolactone (Aldactone), amiloride (Midamor) and triamterene (Dytac).

Potassium supplements

At least 24 to 36 mmol daily are needed with continuing daily diuresis, and in some cases more may be necessary. Watching the serum potassium gives a crude guide and must be employed as often as the tempo of events in a particular patient dictates. Difficulties in achieving adequate supplementation arise from the fact that the effervescent or crystalline forms of potassium supplements may cause nausea and vomiting; while the sustained release forms must not be used when oesophageal passage may be delayed as, for example, in the presence of a very large heart, for fear of causing oesophageal ulceration, haemorrhage or stricture.

Effervescent preparations include tablets of Kloref (7 mmol) and Sando-K (12 mmol), while Kloref-S is crystalline (20 mmol per sachet). Slow release preparations are Slow-K (8 mmol) and Leo-K (8 mmol).

It must always be remembered that potassium depletion potentiates the effects of digitalis, so that dangerous cardiac arrhythmias may occur if the total body potassium is not maintained.

Vasodilator drugs

These may be added to digitalis and diuretics, with potassium sparing and/or supplementation, to maintain comfortable venous pressures, pulmonary and systemic, and cardiac output while reducing left ventricular work in the presence of the progressively failing myocardium.

The long-acting nitrate isosorbide dinitrate (2 hours if chewed and swallowed, 4–6 hours if swallowed whole) acts both as an arteriolar dilator, so reducing left ventricular afterload, and as a venodilator, so reducing venous pressure and ventricular preload. The latter effect predominates. Isosorbide dinitrate (Cedocard, Sorbitrate, Vascardin) may be taken as 5 mg, 10 mg or 30 mg tablets, swallowed whole every 6 hours for this purpose, up to 120 mg daily.

Hydralazine (Apresoline) may also be used to reduce left ventricular work by causing systemic arteriolar dilatation. It should be started in small dosage, 12.5 mg twice daily, then increased by daily or two daily steps, if necessary to a maximum of 100 mg thrice daily, if it proves helpful and blood pressure, cardiac output and urine output are well maintained. This drug is appropriately used in patients who show obvious constrictive pallor of the skin, which is cool and may show some peripheral cyanosis. Such patients may complain of feeling cold, peripherally or generally, and may be hypertensive. Benefit from the drug is obvious from an improvement in colour and comfort. Its long-term use may be complicated by the lupus syndrome, pyridoxine deficiency polyneuropathy, fluid retention and weight gain.

Prazosin (Hypovase) appears to have a balanced effect in reducing both ventricular preload and afterload. For patients in whom treatment to control heart failure is expected to be prolonged, it may offer a useful alternative to the combination of nitrates and hydralazine. It is commenced with a 0.5 mg dose at evening and if well tolerated is continued in dosage 0.5 mg three times daily for 1 week and may be increased by stages thereafter to a maximum total daily dose of 20 mg.

Drugs to control gout
Allopurinol 100 mg thrice daily for 1 week, followed by 100 mg once daily permanently, combined with colchicine 0.5 mg twice daily for the first 2 months is an appropriate and effective treatment for patients in whom gout has been precipitated by diuretic therapy which must be continued.

Phenylbutazone and, to a lesser extent, indomethacin are best avoided if possible for they both cause sodium and water retention and so have a marked tendency to precipitate or aggravate heart failure. In a severe acute attack, however, indomethacin may be used for a few days for this may be less hazardous than the effects of great pain and sleeplessness in such circumstances.

Drug control of diabetes
An oral hypoglycaemic agent may be needed to control diabetes precipitated by prolonged treatment with high or medium-potency diuretics. Glibenclamide, a small tablet which is moderately short-acting and does not cause an unpleasant flush when alcohol is taken, is a suitable agent in these circumstances. A little alcohol occasionally may be pleasant, comforting and an aid to sociability in the patient much restricted in his activities.

Drugs for anxiety, depression and nocturnal restlessness and confusion
Of all the available psychotropic drugs, the most useful and suitable at the present time are diazepam (Valium), which is a good sedative round the clock, and mianserin (Bolvidon, Norval). This drug produces slight sedation in addition to its antidepressant and anxiolytic effects, has the smallest anticholinergic activity and is the least likely to cause cardiac arrhythmias even when taken in large amounts. Intravenous aminophylline may, for a time, reduce the severity of Cheyne–Stokes breathing.

Diamorphine

In the truly terminal phase of the illness in these patients, symptoms tend at last to escape from the control that was achieved over the previous weeks, months or even years, and at this stage diamorphine offers the best sedation; and even though it may increase the tendency to Cheyne–Stokes respiration this appears to impinge less upon the patient's consciousness, the struggle ceases and there is tranquillity, while awareness of relatives' presence and identity is maintained or wanes gradually to a peaceful end. During this phase, any of the previously used supportive therapy that was found difficult or unpleasant by the patient may be reduced and discontinued for, provided that the full supportive regimen that has been described above was fully and carefully applied, the stage when symptoms escape from control may, with confidence, be known to be the terminal state. Certainty in the minds of the attending doctors and nurses that their actions at this stage are the right, kind and only possible actions is a major contribution to their own confidence and peace of mind; and this calm, confidence and serenity will be transmitted through their demeanour to the patient and to the relatives. The gratitude of relatives is never greater than when a serene end has been achieved after a long illness, be it weeks, months or years. Such illness must have begun with anxiety, concern and distress. With good management the patient's and relatives' confidence will have become established, even though the relatives (and if necessary, appropriate and requested, the patient himself) will have come to understand and to accept the inevitable outcome.

Reference

Ross, J. K., Monro, J. L., Manners, J. M., Edwards, J. C., Lewis, B., Hyde, I., Conway, N. and Johnson, A. M. (1976). Cardiac surgery in Wessex; review of 1000 consecutive open-heart procedures. *Br. Med. J.*, **2**, 1485

5

Common problems in advancing chronic renal failure

Margaret M. Platts

The commonest causes of chronic renal failure – chronic glomerular nephritis, chronic pyelonephritis and polycystic disease – are incurable. Nevertheless, patients with these diseases live for many years, before their renal function deteriorates to a point at which it is insufficient to sustain life. During most of this time the patient is usually symptomless. This, indeed, is a major hazard, since the symptomless patient does not usually seek medical advice and therefore his condition may not be diagnosed until renal failure is far advanced. Symptomless hypertension may then have damaged the cardiovascular system irreversibly in addition to hastening the decline in renal function. This asymptomatic period is usually followed by a shorter period of symptomatic renal failure which begins when the glomerular filtration rate has fallen to less than 20 per cent of normal and the blood urea has reached a concentration of about 30 mmol/l. Eventually death supervenes unless the patient can be treated by haemodialysis, peritoneal dialysis or renal transplantation (renal replacement therapy).

DIAGNOSIS OF IRREVERSIBLE CHRONIC RENAL DISEASE IN THE PRESYMPTOMATIC STAGE – WHY IT IS WORTHWHILE

It may seem a cruel and pointless exercise to subject patients to investigation for the early diagnosis of an incurable condition. However, in the case of chronic renal disease the advantages of early diagnosis outweigh the disadvantage of the initial anxiety aroused. Complications may be antici-

The Dying Patient

pated and therefore prevented or alleviated by early supervision. The most obvious example is the early detection and treatment of hypertension. Normotensive patients with chronic renal disease should have their blood pressure checked at approximately annual intervals. As soon as any rise is detected it should be treated by a beta-blocking drug, with the addition of a diuretic if necessary. If the patient's blood urea is above normal any diuretic less potent than frusemide will be ineffective and 80 mg frusemide is the lowest dose worth giving. Potassium supplements should *not* be given unless there is demonstrated hypokalaemia. Blood pressure usually responds to treatment easily at this stage but if it does not methyldopa and later hydralazine should be added to the regime.

The knowledge that a patient has some impairment of renal function

Table 1 Modifications of dosage of some commonly used drugs in patients with impaired renal function

1.	*Drugs which should never be administered to patients with reduced renal function*
	Tetracycline Causes increased blood urea concentration
	Nitrofurantoin Accumulation causes peripheral neuropathy
	Clofibrate Accumulation causes muscle necrosis
2.	*Drugs requiring reduced dosage with monitoring of blood levels in all patients with reduced renal function*
	Digoxin
	Cephaloridine
	Gentamicin
	Streptomycin
	Potassium salts
3.	*Additional drugs which should not be given to patients treated by regular haemodialysis*
	Aspirin Danger of bleeding in association with heparin used for haemodialysis
	Soap or sodium phosphate enemas Absorption of sodium, potassium and water from gut
	Magnesium salts
4.	*Drugs which may be used in normal or only slightly reduced dosage in patients with severely impaired renal function*
	Penicillins Corticosteroids Heparin
	Co-trimoxazole Opiates Warfarin
	Erythromycin Paracetamol All hypotensive drugs
	Codeine phosphate
	Aluminium hydroxide
	Senna
	Progesterone contraceptive pill
5.	*Drugs which are required in larger than normal doses to produce a therapeutic effect in renal failure*
	Diuretics
	Vitamin D – except 1 α hydroxylated derivatives

helps to prevent complications due to the administration of inappropriate doses of drugs for intercurrent illnesses (Table 1). Tetracycline should never be given to patients with impaired renal function. It induces a catabolic state and the blood urea rises rapidly so that symptoms of uraemia may be precipitated for the first time. Cephaloridine, gentamicin and digoxin are drugs which should only be used in patients with impaired renal function when facilities for monitoring of blood levels are available.

Any damaged kidney is more prone to infection than the normal and, of course, a superimposed pyelonephritis will accelerate the decline in function produced by other renal diseases. Urine from these patients should therefore be cultured on the slightest suspicion of infection and treatment instituted. Ampicillin or co-trimoxazole may be used in normal doses but nitrofurantoin is best avoided because it accumulates in renal disease and may give rise to peripheral neuropathy. Patients with recurrent or persistent urinary tract infections should receive continuous medication with a sulphonamide, co-trimoxazole or ampicillin unless they have a neurogenic bladder, an indwelling catheter or calculus disease.

Patients with these conditions frequently have persistent urinary tract infections with organisms resistant to most antibiotics and probably only sensitive to colistin and gentamicin. They should not be given courses of these toxic antibiotics just because a positive culture is obtained from the urine. Antibiotic treatment in these circumstances should be reserved for occasions when the urinary infection is producing systemic symptoms such as fever and general malaise, because it is impossible to produce long-term sterilization of the urine.

Recurrent attacks of acute glomerulonephritis due to streptococci are extremely rare. Routine prophylaxis with penicillin in patients who have had a previous attack of acute nephritis or who are suffering from chronic glomerulonephritis is not required.

Young women who know that they have renal disease will usually seek advice before embarking on a pregnancy, but if they are unaware of their renal problem it may only be discovered at antenatal examination. Prior knowledge of renal disease is obviously important from the point of view of the mother's health but also because of the possibility of inheritance of polycystic disease or rare types of nephritis. Most patients with polycystic disease are only too well acquainted with their family history and the prognosis of the disease. One advantage of early diagnosis and screening of members of polycystic families is that the 50 per cent of children who do not inherit the disease may be reassured and told that they will not transmit the disease to their children. Intending parents with polycystic disease should have the dominant nature of the hereditary mechanism explained to them so that they may make their own decision on the desirability of having children. I take the opportunity of explaining to them that, although it is now usual for renal failure due to polycystic kidneys to develop in middle life, this is not inevitable. I have seen symptomless patients with polycystic kidneys in their 70s. It is explained that early diagnosis and treatment of hypertension will probably improve prognosis in the next generation and that dialysis and transplant techniques are improving so that children with polycystic disease born now will probably live to enjoy greatly improved methods of renal replacement therapy.

The matter of maternal health in pregnancy should also be discussed explicitly with the young woman with symptomless renal disease. If her blood urea concentration is stable and under about 12 mmol/l and her blood pressure is normal or well controlled with small doses of drugs, there is little or no increased maternal mortality but the incidence of toxaemia of pregnancy may be increased. Women with hypertension or higher blood urea concentrations should be advised against pregnancy. I impress on women with renal disease who are about to start a pregnancy that they must be 'model' antenatal patients and rest in hospital during pregnancy if this is advised and also accept the necessity for a therapeutic abortion if their blood pressure should get out of control. They should have their children sooner rather than later because their renal function will not improve and when their family is complete they should be sterilized thus avoiding the problem of the contraceptive pill and hypertension. With this advice I have seen one catastrophe due to pregnancy. This woman had quiescent disseminated lupus erythematosus (DLE) with normal renal function and had not taken corticosteroids for 5 years. Within 2 weeks of missing her menstrual period her lupus flared up and in spite of a therapeutic abortion and immunosuppression she died in renal failure a few weeks later.

HOW SHOULD EARLY DIAGNOSIS OF CHRONIC RENAL DISEASE BE MADE?

At an asymptomatic stage the diagnosis will usually be made as a result of investigation of proteinuria or hypertension found at a routine or antenatal medical examination or as a result of a family screen for hereditary disease.

When a person is found to have symptomless proteinuria he should have his blood pressure taken and if this is normal and the proteinuria is slight he should be asked to bring an early morning specimen for testing, to exclude postural proteinuria. However, if there is heavy proteinuria or hypertension the patient probably has renal disease and should be investigated straight away by means of blood urea and renal X-rays.

The young normotensive patient with slight proteinuria is unlikely to have renal disease particularly if an early morning specimen is negative. If the proteinuria is persistent and present in an early morning specimen but the blood pressure is normal, I usually wait 6 months. During this period the proteinuria often disappears. If it is still present after 6 months then I think full investigation including a renal biopsy is justified. There is no place for cystoscopy in the investigation of symptomless proteinuria.

The finding of small kidneys on intravenous urogram always indicates chronic disease but normal-sized or large kidneys do not exclude it. A rise in blood urea or creatinine concentration will be absent or very slight at first, but it must be remembered that the upper limits of concentration quoted on laboratory forms and in textbooks are for all ages. Renal function normally deteriorates with age and in a person under the age of 30 a blood urea over 7 mmol/l would be suspect, whereas a level of 10 mmol/l in a person of 75 years would *not* be a cause for alarm. The serum creatinine concentration is not affected by diet and is therefore a better measurement for following changes in renal function when the diet may be changed. There is an inverse relationship between the plasma creatinine concentration and the creatinine clearance so that actual measurements of clearance need rarely be made.

MANAGEMENT OF THE PATIENT WITH SYMPTOMLESS RENAL FAILURE

This is largely a matter of supervision with as little interference with normal living as possible. Supervision of blood pressure continues and urinary tract infections are treated. Dietary protein should not be restricted before there are uraemic symptoms. It is only necessary to restrict fluid and sodium intake if the patient is oedematous or hypertensive and to restrict potassium intake if the serum potassium concentration is increased (unusual). Some patients will begin to have attacks of gout due to renal retention of uric acid. Acute attacks should be treated in the usual way with colchicine or indomethacin, and then long-term therapy with allopurinol should be initiated to inhibit the formation of uric acid and prevent future attacks of gout.

Before there are uraemic symptoms there may be other biochemical

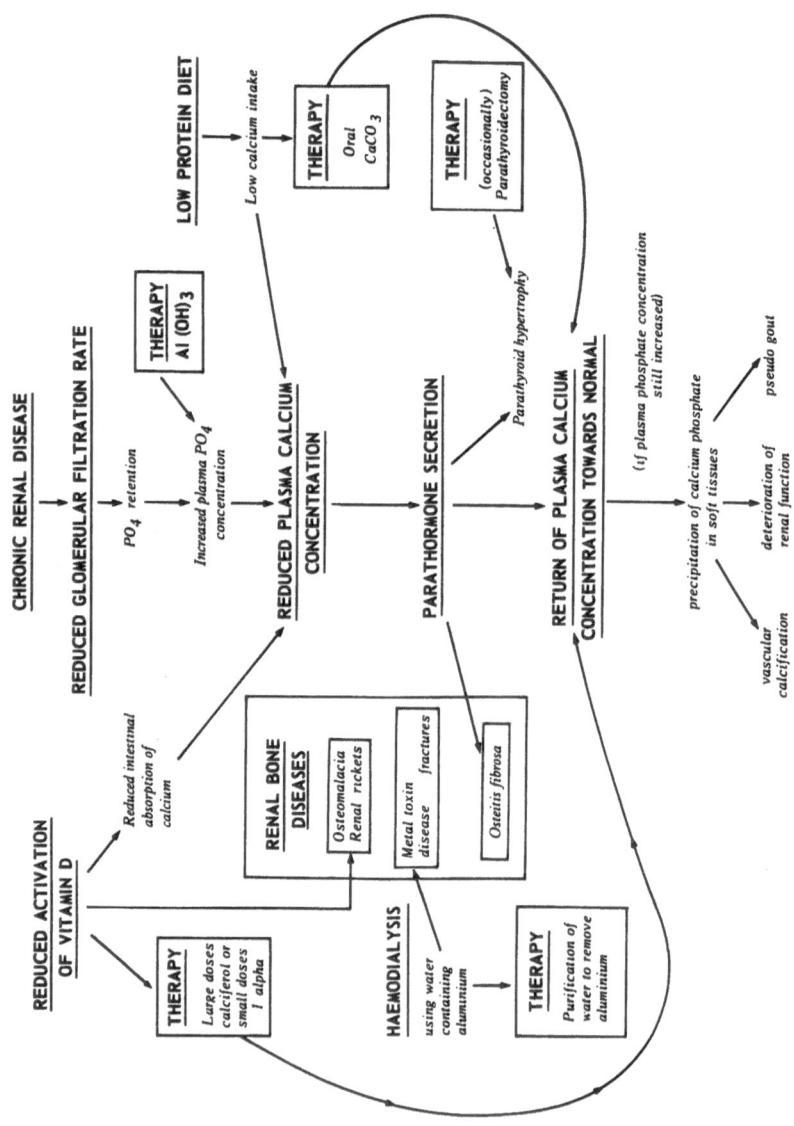

Figure 1   The mechanisms for development of renal bone diseases and the methods by which they may be prevented or treated

abnormalities which do require correction if the patient is eventually to receive some form of renal replacement therapy. As the glomerular filtration rate diminishes the plasma phosphate concentration increases. Since plasma is a supersaturated solution of calcium phosphate the plasma calcium concentration falls as the phosphate increases (Figure 1). The reduced calcium concentration stimulates the parathyroids to secrete more hormone and secondary hyperparathyroid disease ensues. In addition the kidneys are also responsible for the activation of vitamin D by hydroxylation in the 'one' position. As renal function deteriorates the patient begins to suffer from lack of vitamin D activity with poor absorption of calcium from the gut. In children and teenagers the development of clinical rickets is the commonest mode of presentation of chronic renal failure. This may be prevented by good management. The first thing is to administer oral aluminium hydroxide as soon as the plasma phosphate concentration reaches 2 mmol/l. Aluminium hydroxide combines with phosphate in the intestinal secretions and this insoluble salt is excreted in the faeces. After the plasma phosphate has been reduced to normal, vitamin D should be given if the serum calcium concentration remains below normal or if the alkaline phosphatase level in the plasma is increased. Either calciferol or one of the active 1α (one alpha) hydroxylated derivatives of vitamin D may be used. If ordinary vitamin D is used then large doses must be given such as 10 000 units daily in children and adults doubling this dose in 3 months if no improvement occurs. If 1α is used the starting dose is 1 μg daily. Whenever any form of vitamin D is given to these patients frequent measurement of serum calcium, phosphorus and alkaline phosphatase must be made. This is particularly important with 1α since it produces a more rapid increase in serum calcium than calciferol. Hypercalcaemia must be avoided even at the risk of slight undertreatment in patients with any remaining renal function since hypercalcaemia causes deposition of calcium salts in soft tissues including the kidneys and may cause rapid deterioration of renal function (Christiansen *et al.*, 1978). Hypercalcaemia may persist for several months when induced by calciferol but regresses in 1–2 weeks after 1α treatment.

When the glomerular filtration rate is reduced to about 20 per cent of normal, most patients become anaemic. This is due mainly to the failure of the kidney to secrete erythropoietin which normally stimulates the bone marrow for erythropoiesis. The anaemia rarely causes symptoms and does not respond to iron or other haematinics. Transfusion should not be performed unless the anaemia is causing symptoms which are rare with haemoglobin levels above 6 g/100 ml.

Social and psychological support in the presymptomatic stage
Young patients with early renal failure may need advice on occupation and hobbies. While the patient is asymptomatic no activity is harmful and full participation in sport and social activities should be encouraged. However, one should bear in mind the fact that the patient will eventually develop total renal failure so that an occupation not dependent on heavy manual labour is desirable. Youngsters should be encouraged to seek higher education and an occupation which depends on brain rather than brawn. Throughout the presymptomatic course the doctor should be considering whether his patient will eventually be treated by dialysis or transplantation, the criteria for which are discussed on page 92. Once the patient becomes symptomatic the further treatment will depend on whether the patient is to receive renal replacement therapy eventually or not.

MANAGEMENT OF PATIENTS NOT SUITABLE FOR DIALYSIS OR TRANSPLANTATION

When these unfortunate people develop symptomatic renal failure, treatment must be directed to the relief of symptoms and maintenance of activity for as long as possible rather than the prevention of long-term complications such as pericarditis, peripheral neuropathy and symptomatic bone disease which occur almost exclusively in patients kept alive by renal replacement therapy.

The commonest symptoms of uraemia are lethargy, nausea, vomiting, itching and breathlessness to which should be added the symptoms of uncontrolled hypertension or fluid overload.

Lethargy and intestinal symptoms are probably due directly to the unidentified nitrogenous uraemic 'toxins'. Their concentration can be reduced and these symptoms relieved by use of low-protein diets. In the first instance protein intake should be reduced to about 40 g/day, or only so far as is necessary to relieve symptoms. It is very important that a low-protein diet is not a low-calorie diet. If the patient has to break down his own tissues to provide calories no symptomatic improvement will result and the patient will lose flesh and weaken. For this reason intake of bread and potatoes should not be restricted at this stage. When symptoms recur on a diet of about 40 g/day protein the general quality of life endured by the patient must be considered. If this is reasonably good and the patient is a stalwart 'trier' then it is worth instituting a modified Giovanetti diet (Shaw *et al.*, 1965). In this, vegetable protein is largely excluded by the use

of protein-free flour for baking (Rite Diet protein-free flour) and by ration-
ing potatoes, peas and beans. Animal protein intake is then confined to
one-third of a pint of milk per day and one egg or its equivalent in meat.
Baking acceptable items with this flour is difficult but not impossible.
Calorie intake is difficult to maintain and supplements of cream,
concentrated glucose drinks (Hycal) and glucose polymer powder (renal
Caloreen) must be used. Rite Diet, Hycal and Caloreen are obtainable on
prescription in Britain.

Breathlessness in these patients is usually due to pulmonary oedema,
metabolic acidosis or, rarely, anaemia. Diuretics are relatively ineffective
because of the very low glomerular filtration rate and if used need to be
given in large doses such as 80 mg of frusemide, doubling the dose every 2
days until a diuresis is induced or a maximum daily dose of 2 g is reached.

Potassium supplements or potassium-sparing diuretics must not be
used. Cardiac arrest due to hyperkalaemia is a real hazard. Simultaneously
fluid intake must be restricted to a volume less than the urine output. In
severe cases a fluid intake of zero for 1 or 2 days is the best way of relieving
breathlessness due to pulmonary oedema. Severe hypertension causing
pulmonary oedema is nearly always associated with obvious generalized
fluid retention and will not respond to hypotensive drugs until the patient
is 'dried out'. In fact dehydration is the best treatment for hypertension at
this stage and drugs are often not necessary. Breathlessness associated with
a plasma bicarbonate concentration of less than 15 mmol/l is likely to be
due, at least in part, to acidosis and will be helped by correction with
sodium bicarbonate. This should be given orally in a dose of 1 or 2 g three
times daily. If there is also a tendency to fluid overload then a large dose of
frusemide should be given at the same time to eliminate the extra sodium
load.

Severe itching is very distressing and is difficult to relieve. Antihistamines, unfortunately, do not help. It is sometimes due to precipitation
of calcium phosphate in the skin which occurs when the plasma phosphate
concentration is very high. If this is the case then oral aluminium
hydroxide will reduce the plasma phosphate level and the itching.

Uraemic fits are rare in the well-managed patient. If they occur they are
usually associated with cerebral oedema due to severe hypertension or
fluid overload or acidosis. The tendency to fits will be reduced if these
other complications are treated. Individual fits are relieved by intravenous
diazepam.

Eventually all these measures will not prevent the patient becoming
miserable with uraemic symptoms. When this happens the kindest thing is

to give chlorpromazine and diazepam in large doses to produce a pleasant drowsy state and control nausea. If resonium A was being used to keep the serum potassium concentration down it should be stopped since cardiac arrest due to hyperkalaemia is a swift and painless way to die.

MANAGEMENT OF THE PATIENT WHO WILL EVENTUALLY RECEIVE RENAL REPLACEMENT THERAPY

The aim in these patients is to maintain comfort and activity for as long as possible before instituting renal replacement therapy without permitting the development of irreversible or disabling complications. Severe uraemic symptoms should not be allowed to develop and referral to a renal unit should occur soon after it is realized that dialysis or transplantation will eventually be required. Before referral it should be ascertained that the patient is not a carrier of serum hepatitis antigens. The reasons for early referral are as follows:

(1) The character and intellectual capacity of the patient can only be assessed accurately while he is reasonably well.
(2) A rapport between the patient and the staff of the renal unit has to be developed.
(3) Patients need time to adjust psychologically to the concept of permanent dialysis or transplantation.
(4) Most renal units have difficulty in fitting patients in and the patient may perish because facilities are not available if he is only referred when treatment is required urgently.
(5) Preparations for home dialysis such as conversion of the home or finding new accommodation take time.
(6) The arteriovenous fistula, which must be constructed for vascular access, improves with time and is best fashioned months or years before it is required for dialysis (Figure 2).
(7) The renal physician is usually best able to judge the right time to start renal replacement therapy.

Much can be done to avoid complications during conservative management of these patients. Failure to grow in children or significant weight loss in adults may be minimized by ensuring a good calorie intake at all times. Adults destined for replacement therapy should not receive diets containing less than 40 g/day of protein and children should not receive low-protein diets at all. Particular care should be taken in children to

Needles

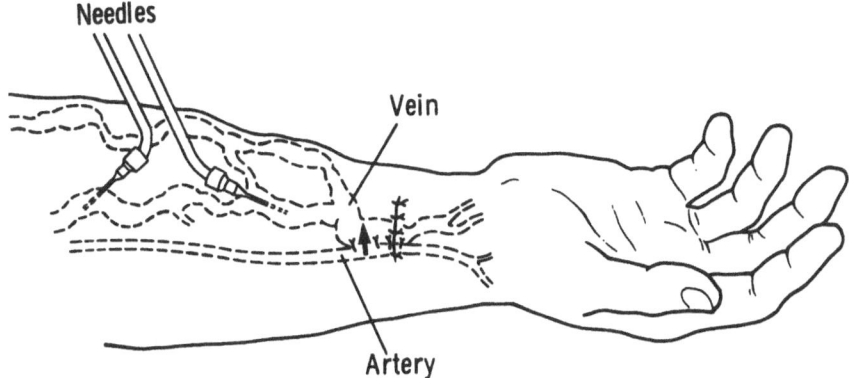

Vein

Artery

Figure 2 The forearm arteriovenous fistula used for haemodialysis. The patient inserts two needles into the distended veins for each dialysis

prevent functional vitamin D deficiency and hyperphosphataemia.

Vascular and retinal damage due to hypertension may be reduced by rigorous treatment of hypertension. Arteries and veins in the arms must be carefully preserved for vascular access. Small hand veins should be used for venepuncture or finger pricks in children.

Significant osteomalacia or hyperparathyroid bone disease can be prevented by attention to phosphorus and calcium homeostasis as described on page 87. Blood transfusion should be avoided except for very severe anaemia. This prevents formation of antibodies which may be detrimental to future transplantation or the cross-matching of blood. There has, however, been some recent evidence that blood transfusion may actually help transplant survival but transfusions should not be given specifically for this purpose at this stage. Development of serum hepatitis as a result of transfusion is a major tragedy because most dialysis units will not accept patients carrying the hepatitis antigen. Uraemic patients who get serum hepatitis usually become permanent carriers. Outbreaks of serum hepatitis on dialysis units are still common in Europe and have caused deaths of patients and staff in this country. Retinopathy in diabetic patients should receive expert attention; 50 per cent of diabetic patients become blind after starting haemodialysis. Intercurrent illnesses should be treated as they arise. In particular conditions requiring surgical treatment should be attended to. Preoperative management must not include withholding of fluids. Patients with precarious renal function are unable to concentrate their urine and easily become dehydrated. If this occurs the glomerular filtration rate drops further and if the rise in blood urea which results causes vomiting then a vicious spiral is started in which more dehydration causes more vomiting and further deterioration in renal function. Patients with reduced renal function are also unable to deal with excess fluid efficiently. So if a patient requires surgery no attempt should be made to raise his habitually low haemoglobin to normal preoperatively by a large blood transfusion. This will only cause pulmonary oedema. These patients rarely come to harm from operation while they are anaemic so long as the anaemia is not due to acute blood loss. Patients regularly receive transplants when their haemoglobin concentration is 6–7 g/100 ml. Blood transfusion during operation is limited to replacement of operative loss.

Intercurrent illness, trauma and fever increase catabolism and may raise the blood urea concentration without further irreversible impairment of renal function. Temporary dialysis is worth considering to tide patients over this type of crisis.

WHICH PATIENTS ARE SUITABLE FOR REPLACEMENT THERAPY? WHY DO WE HAVE TO 'CHOOSE'?

In theory dialysis and transplantation have rendered death from uraemia almost entirely preventable. However, most of us would agree that uraemia accompanying other distressing or fatal diseases such as severe heart disease, stroke and cancer should not be treated in this way. Nevertheless of about 40 people per million population in Great Britain who develop permanent renal failure each year and who might be expected to benefit from dialysis or transplantation only about 20 receive such treatment. The rest die. As may be seen from Table 2, 11 countries in Europe treat more patients per million population than we do. There is no reason to suppose that renal failure occurs more frequently in these countries. The only reason for the inadequacy of facilities for treatment here is the lack of sufficient funds provided by the national health service. Nevertheless, although most units are usually nearly full, most physicians in charge of renal units admit virtually all patients with permanent renal failure actually referred to them within certain age-limits. These age-limits differ in various parts of the country; in Sheffield, for example, we rarely accept patients for dialysis or transplantation over the age of 60 years. Some other regions have lower age-limits than this. In most other European countries and North America up to *50 per cent* of renal patients receiving replacement treatment are *over 60 years of age* and many of them enjoy reasonably

Table 2 Patients receiving renal replacement therapy per million population in some European countries (31 December 1978) (Combined Report, 1978)

Switzerland	198.3
Israel	170.0
Belgium	167.6
Denmark	167.6
France	154.9
Sweden	131.9
Italy	131.0
Netherlands	130.7
Federal Republic of Germany	126.8
Finland	106.0
Norway	104.4
United Kingdom	94.2
Austria	92.6
Spain	83.5
Cyprus	81.7

comfortable and pleasant lives, although the prognosis is naturally not so good as in the younger patients.

There will be insufficient facilities to treat everyone with renal failure in Britain for the foreseeable future and it seems that most of the selection of patients is occurring before referral to renal units. I think it is probable that some patients are not referred either because referring doctors believe that the quality of life of dialysed or transplanted patients is not acceptable or because they believe that the selection criteria are even more stringent than they actually are. I therefore propose to describe the various types of treatment, the quality of life to be expected and the prognosis so that doctors without much experience in nephrology may judge whether their patient with renal failure might benefit from and be accepted for dialysis or transplantation. It is also helpful to be able to answer questions from the patient or his relatives about the nature and availability of these forms of treatment. There is a natural reluctance to raise false hopes in a patient or his family by referring him for a treatment which is either not available or is unsuccessful. Renal physicians always welcome enquiries from colleagues about possibilities of treatment for particular patients. If in doubt, ask!

In 1979 most units in this country would consider the following to be contraindications to renal replacement therapy.

(1) Age over 60 or 65 years or younger than 3 years
(2) Carrier of hepatitis

(3)   Not a British taxpayer
(4)   Gross psychological derangement particularly depression or addiction to drugs or alcohol
(5)   Gross previous non-compliance with therapy
(6)   Other disease likely to be fatal in the short term or making the quality of life unacceptable
(7)   Gross mental subnormality.

The following are *not* usually absolute contraindications to replacement therapy.

(1)   Hypertension
(2)   Illiteracy
(3)   Blindness
(4)   Confinement to wheelchair
(5)   No suitable home
(6)   No caring relative
(7)   Diabetes mellitus.

Psychological preparation of the patient for replacement therapy

The young patient with slowly developing chronic renal failure is almost certainly aware that his condition is incurable and that a kidney machine or a transplant may save his life. I have found that patients usually welcome a frank approach. When some suitable opportunity arises, such as an enquiry about the probability of being accepted for life insurance, the nature of the disease, or its natural outcome, then the possibility of a kidney machine or a kidney transplant should be discussed. After this I always arrange for the patient and his spouse or parents to visit the home of another of my patients who is established on home haemodialysis. I emphasize that dialysis and renal transplantation are no longer experimental and that their sole purpose is to make the patient feel better and able to continue to be a useful member of society. A visit from our home dialysis administrator who organizes the adaptation of the home for dialysis is arranged and an appointment made for the construction of an arteriovenous fistula.

The types of treatment available for renal replacement therapy and their interrelationships are shown in Figure 3.

The mechanics of haemodialysis

Haemodialysis (Figures 4, 5, and 6) involves the passage of the patient's blood through an artificial kidney usually for three periods of about 6

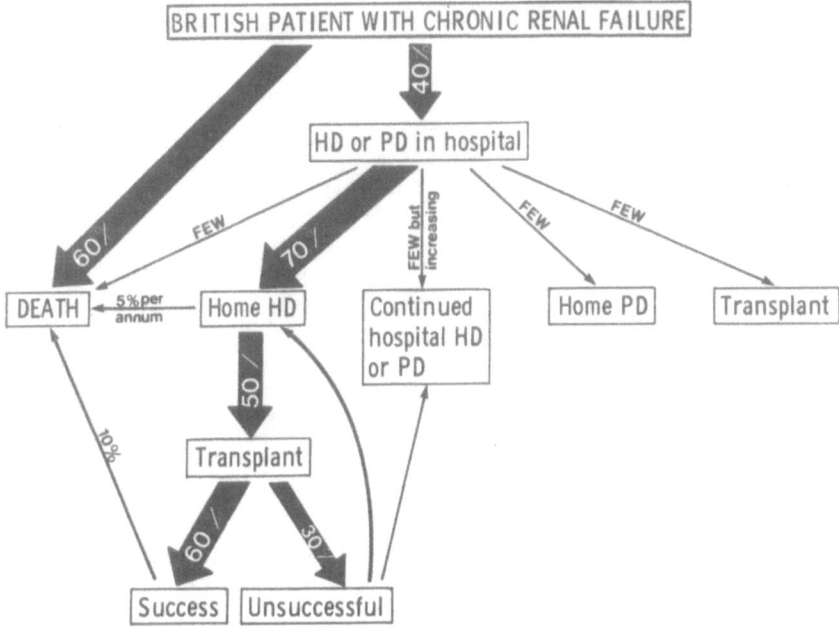

Figure 3 The pattern of treatment received by British patients with end-stage renal failure. PD = peritoneal dialysis; HD = haemodialysis

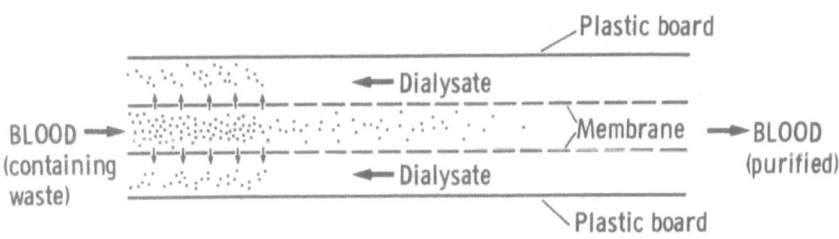

Figure 4 The artificial kidney consists of cellophane membranes supported by a rigid plastic frame. Blood passes between two layers of membrane through which uraemic toxins diffuse into the surrounding dialysate which is a physiological electrolyte solution which eventually goes to waste

hours each week. The patient attaches himself to his machine by means of two needles placed in the dilated veins of his fistula. The needles are removed after each treatment. Blood is circulated through the machine at 200 or 300 ml/min. Although complicated, the apparatus is relatively easy

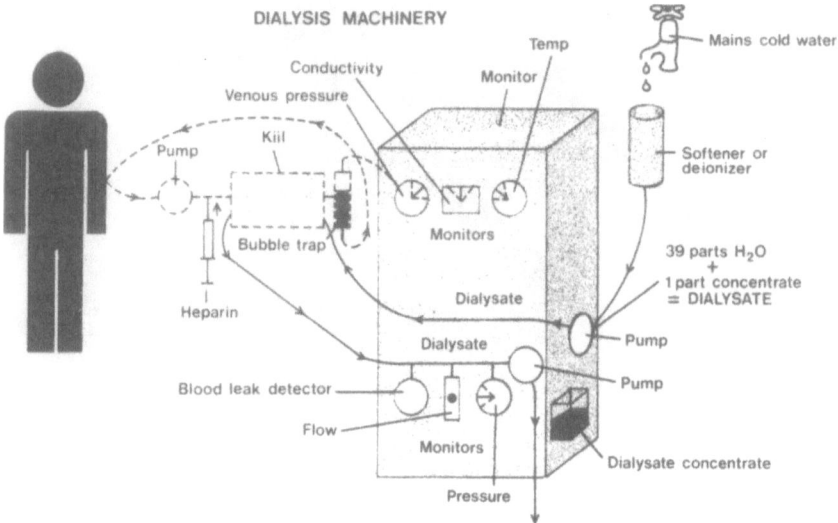

Figure 5 The general set-up for haemodialysis. Patient's blood follows the dotted line through the Kiil (artificial kidney). The monitor prepares the dialysate and checks its composition, temperature, pressure and flow rate.

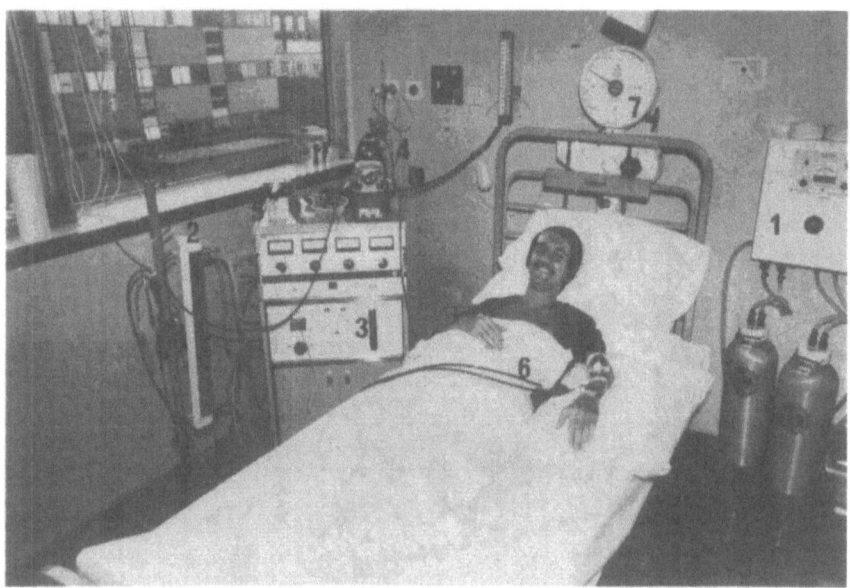

Figure 6 A patient undergoing haemodialysis. 1. Deionizer; 2. artificial kidney; 3. monitor; 4. blood pump; 5. heparin pump; 6. blood in plastic tubes between artificial kidney and needles in arm fistula; 7. bed weighing machine

to use and knowledge of electronics is not required. The difficulty in learning to use the apparatus safely is approximately equivalent to that of learning to drive a car. Virtually all people of less than 60 years of age, including older children, can learn the process in about 3 months. Patients are trained to haemodialyse in a renal unit but after this, in Great Britain, about 80 per cent of patients carry out the treatment at home. In North America and Europe only about 25 per cent of patients dialyse at home because many more beds are available in dialysis units. At home the treatments are carried out at times convenient to the patient and his family. Most patients dialyse during the evening but the apparatus is safe enough for treatment to proceed during sleep. The machine is fail-safe and breakdowns and routine servicing are dealt with by hospital technicians. Breakdown during treatment or power failure is a nuisance, but not life-threatening, because each patient dialyses often enough to ensure that he has at least 48 hours 'reserve' even if he has no residual renal function of his own. During treatment it is desirable, but not essential, for a member of the family who is familiar with dialysis to be in the house but he need not be present continuously in the dialysis room. Elderly people have more difficulty in learning new techniques and are more likely to be widowed or to have an infirm spouse who is unable to help with home dialysis, and this is perhaps the main reason why they are seldom accepted for dialysis in this country. Home dialysis requires a room reserved for that purpose. If no spare room is available a cabin is erected in the garden or the patient is found alternative accommodation. All the equipment and plumbing alterations required are paid for by the health service as is the installation of a telephone by the bedside. In Britain the patient receives financial allowances for the electricity used by the machine, telephone rental as well as the attendance allowance.

Home haemodialysis – quality of life
During the actual dialysis some patients suffer from headaches, vomiting and cramps but on most occasions the dialysis is comfortable but boring. One of the main hardships of a dialysis life is simply the time it takes. Preparation and cleaning of the equipment takes about an hour for each treatment. About 70 per cent of men on dialysis go to work and most women do their housework. Intervals between dialyses must not exceed 4 days and holidays longer than this are impracticable except in places where dialysis equipment is installed. Most units in Britain are too full to accept more than occasional holiday patients. Continental units are willing to take visitors but the cost is about £100 per dialysis and there is the ever-present

risk of acquiring hepatitis which is still prevalent in dialysis units outside
Britain. Most units have a holiday home with dialysis equipment to which
their own patients may go but this restricts patients to the same place year
after year. A few holiday portable machines are available and new ones are
being developed. At the moment these are not too reliable but it seems
likely that, in the near future, patients will be able to use equipment which
will fit in the boot of a car and can be connected to any normal tap and
electrical outlet.

Between treatments most patients feel reasonably well. Many say they
have never felt so well before in their lives but this is probably because as
chronic invalids they have forgotten the feeling of robust health. Most are
capable of sedentary occupation but heavy manual labour is rarely
possible. Walking, swimming, dancing and family games are enjoyed but
competitive sports are not possible. The main disability arises from the
anaemia with haemoglobin concentrations averaging 8 g/100 ml in females
and 9 g/100 ml in men. A few patients are dependent on regular transfusions. Severe hypertension is rare. Fluid intake is severely restricted but
the urine output is correspondingly low so that distressing thirst is not a
problem. The main dietary restrictions are of sodium and potassium.
Surreptitious consumption of potato crisps, chips and beer is an occasional
cause of death from hyperkalaemia.

Table 3   Marital status of home dialysis patients in Sheffield

	Married	*Single*	*Separated*	*Divorced*	*Widowed*
At start of home dialysis	188	52	2	3	0
Changes which occurred during dialysis life	6			9	3
13 other patients have had serious marital discord					
(Average duration of home dialysis – 2 years and 8 months)					

The marital state of Sheffield patients starting dialysis is shown in
Table 3. Divorce is common but was almost balanced by the six new
marriages which occurred during the same period. Many dialysis patients
are either impotent or frigid and have a reduced libido (Table 4). The exact
reason for this is not known but the difficulties seem to be organic rather
than psychogenic in origin. Nevertheless, some patients are helped by
treatment of common gynaecological complaints or by counselling.

Female patients must not become pregnant while being supported by
dialysis. The chances of successful conclusion of a pregnancy are remote

Table 4 Sexual activity of married home dialysis patients living in Sheffield in 1977

	Normal potency	Totally or partially impotent	No answer
Males	21	28	6
	Not frigid	Totally or partially frigid	No answer
Females	3	19	8
	Normal libido	Reduced or absent libido	No answer
Both sexes	39	31	15

Table 5 Replies of 20 widow(er)s of home dialysis patients to the question – 'While your spouse was dialysing at home did your relationship become . . .'

	Closer	*More distant*	*No reply*
Sexually	7	9	4
In other ways	14	3	3

and the hazards of an abortion in a patient who receives anticoagulants three times per week are considerable. Sterilization should be recommended to women who already have children. Young nulliparous women, however, will hope to have children when they have a successful transplant. Contraception is best by means of a sheath but the progesterone pill or progesterone intrauterine device (IUD) may be used. An ordinary IUD is not usually satisfactory because of its tendency to increase menstrual loss. Indeed menorrhagia is a troublesome, common complaint of dialysis women and aggravates their anaemia. It may need control by hysterectomy or depôt progesterone.

Widows and widowers of home dialysis patients who had died at least a year before were asked for their opinion of home dialysis and its effect on their marriage (Table 5). Although the sexual aspects of marriage were impaired a large majority felt that their marriage had been strengthened in other ways by the experience of dialysis. Living couples have also often remarked on this to me. The widow(er)s were also asked for free comments on the effect of home dialysis on family life and some of these are quoted below.

Effect on children – 'They had to grow up very quickly and, because I had very little time to spend with them, I felt that they grew away from me.'

'A bad effect in that they were shattered by worry when their father was very ill, such as when he vomited a lot and had a new shunt in, had broken bones, etc. Good effect inasmuch as they had to take responsibility in the home and in connection with each other that normally they would not have done.'

'They were not afraid of hospitals or dentists because they have seen needles in their dad's arm.'

'Their schoolwork did not deteriorate and they did not develop any nervous side-effects. They were concerned for him, but he had such courage that they were never frightened and he was helped by their cheerful and optimistic confidence. They have a mature understanding of life, and cheerful, well-balanced outlook. Susan is now training to be an occupational therapist.'

Was home dialysis worthwhile? Would you go through it again? – 'I don't think I would recommend dialysis at home. If they could be dialysed in hospital and come home to recover, at least the husband or wife would not be too exhausted to look after them. At home the kidney room dominates your life. On the other hand sharing the experience together widens your understanding of what they have to undergo.'

'I would hate to have to go through all that again. However, if it were either of my children, I would. It is a very big thing to have all the responsibility of dialysing at home. We are laymen who, for the sake of love and duty, go in at the deep end and do things we never thought possible.'

Was your general practitioner helpful? – 'Although we have a good general practitioner he was out of his depth when it came to the actual dialysing.'

'My GP knows little of dialysis and his locum knew less and cared less in fact.'

'There are three doctors in the practice to which I belong and only one of them showed any interest on one occasion, when he wished to film me putting my husband on the machine.'

General comments – 'I look back on it with horror and I do not know how I managed to cope. I had absolutely no leisure.'

'Everyone told us to lead a normal life but that was impossible because your life was almost completely full of illness.'

'I could cope with nursing but dialysing is a situation in which being emotionally involved with patient makes it very difficult and tense.'

'No regrets whatsoever about caring for my husband and the machine, it was part of our daily routine.'

About two-thirds of male patients return to work on home dialysis. We have found that there is a particular problem with young unmarried patients who were at school when they first developed renal failure and are still living with their parents (Table 6). We have had 17 such patients

Table 6   Single home haemodialysis patients less than 20 years of age

		Working	*Never worked*
No job before dialysis – no training	1	(father's shop)	5 (one unfit)
Job before dialysis	4	1 father's business 1 shop assistant 2 laboratory technicians	1 (redundant)
No job before dialysis – trained during dialysis life	6	1 jeweller 1 accountant 1 orthoptist 1 typist 1 computer operator 1 solicitor's clerk	none

under the age of 20. Those who underwent vocational training all have jobs whereas those with no vocational training remained unemployed. The latter group come from homes where education is not esteemed. They are a miserable bunch who sit at home with few interests and have a vested interest in ill-health so they can draw sickness benefit. This becomes a habit and they tend to remain symptomatic and fail to gain employment when they eventually receive a transplant. The physical health of the group which trained and obtained employment is no better than that which did not. However, the social rehabilitation and general air of contentment is much better in the employed group. The necessity for continuing education in children and adolescents on dialysis cannot be over-emphasized.

Prognosis and causes of death with home haemodialysis
Survival on home haemodialysis is improving and our results in Sheffield are typical. Of 201 patients who started treatment in the 6 years 1973–78 47 have died, eleven after transplantation. Eleven of these deaths occurred in the first 3 months of dialysis. Early death is particularly likely to occur in patients referred late who have lost a lot of weight before treatment is started. Causes of later deaths were as follows; dialysis encephalopathy, seven; cardiac failure including coronary thrombosis, nine; septicaemia, three; suicide, one; failure of vascular access, two; cerebral thrombosis, two. Dialysis encephalopathy is a very distressing, progressive dementia which was common in patients who dialysed in areas such as Sheffield where the water contains a high concentration of aluminium. It is thought to be due to accumulation of aluminium in the brain. Now that water purification is practised this disease should disappear. Figure 7 shows the survival rates for dialysis and transplant patients in Europe. It should be

The Dying Patient

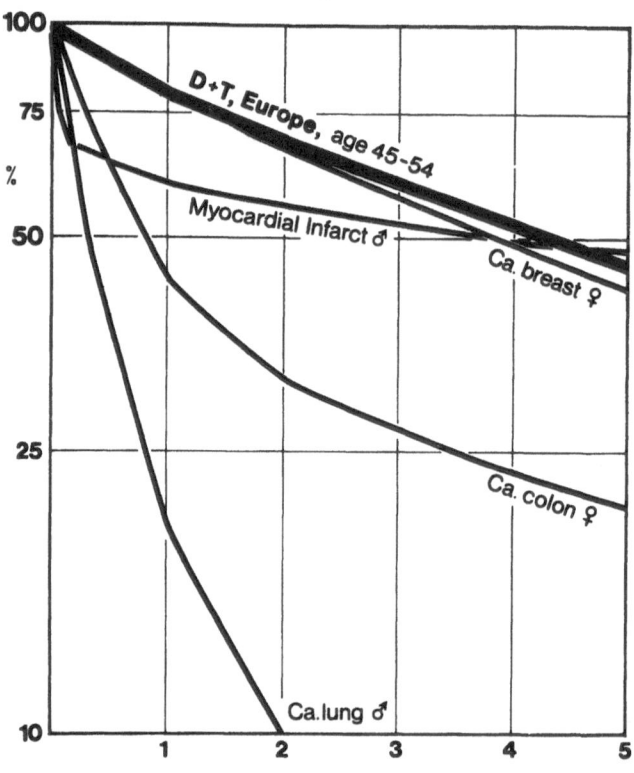

Years from Diagnosis or Starting Dialysis and Transplantation

Figure 7 Cumulative survival by dialysis and transplantation compared with some other disease (Europe, 1977) (Wing *et al.*, 1978)

noted that the prognosis is at least as good as that for carcinoma of the breast and a great deal better than the survival from various other diseases for which the treatment is not 'rationed'.

Chronic peritoneal dialysis

Until recently peritoneal dialysis was only used as a temporary measure while a patient was awaiting a place on a haemodialysis programme or the establishment of a satisfactory arteriovenous fistula. Such patients have 48 hours continuous treatment in hospital each week and the peritoneal catheter is reinserted for each treatment. More recently the advantages of peritoneal dialysis as a definitive form of treatment have become more appreciated (Oreopoulos, 1977). This stems largely from the increased expertise with the placement of 'permanent' indwelling peritoneal catheters, which are left *in situ* between treatments. These enable patients to do their own treatment at home. The procedure is relatively simple and the apparatus is cheap though the solutions used are expensive. The main requirement is that a very strict aseptic technique is practised when the bags of fluid are connected and disconnected from the cannula. At home treatment may be carried on for about 8 hours each night or as 'chronic ambulatory peritoneal dialysis'. For the latter process the patient runs 2 l of peritoneal dialysis solution into and out of his abdomen four times per day. While the fluid is in his abdomen he carries on with normal activities with the bags from which the fluid came still attached to his peritoneal dialysis catheter and carried in a pouch strapped round his waist. This technique has been used extensively in Toronto where several dozen patients have been changed to this from haemodialysis. Its practice will almost certainly increase in Britain. The biggest hazard is peritonitis but this can usually be cured while dialysis continues by the use of intra-peritoneal and systemic antibiotics. Because the technique is relatively safe and simple it is suitable for the elderly and for those who live alone. It is too early to judge the long-term prognosis with chronic peritoneal dialysis but it has been shown that patients tend to have higher haemoglobin concentrations with peritoneal than with haemodialysis. They can also enjoy unrestricted protein and fluid intake and they can travel.

RENAL TRANSPLANTATION

At best chronic dialysis is a boring nuisance and therefore most patients would prefer a successful renal transplant. A few patients such as those with a history of tuberculosis and to a lesser extent those with abnormal lower urinary tracts (spina bifida, for example) are medically unsuitable for transplant. The success rate diminishes with age and it is, therefore, not the preferred mode of treatment for most patients over 50. However, there is no doubt that the quality of life is usually improved by successful trans-plantation and the success rate is reasonable.

Donor kidneys
At the moment the main cause of a waiting list for renal transplantation is the shortage of donor kidneys. It is appropriate that in a book concerned with the care of the dying patient this matter should be discussed in some detail. It is in patients who are about to die that the matter of donation of kidneys and possibly other organs should be considered, firstly by the doctor caring for the dying patient and later by the next of kin. The greatest obstacle to the acquisition of sufficient kidneys for transplantation is

forgetfulness, ignorance and occasionally frank antagonism on the part of doctors caring for the dying. These attitudes are understandable. The doctors concerned may never have seen a person with a successful transplant and may be under the impression that transplantation is still experimental with a low success rate. Taking kidneys for transplantation does involve some extra work and trouble on the part of the people caring for the donors. Few people now would argue with the acceptability of the ethics of organ donation but it is still distressing to have to request it from relatives. However, refusal on the part of relatives is rare. Indeed when they know that death is inevitable they are often relieved to know that some benefit may be derived by others from their own bereavement.

The use of kidney donor cards has ensured that many people have thought about this matter and have told their next of kin of their wish to donate their kidneys. Even if a donor card is found on the deceased it is usual to get permission from the next of kin. In this country approximately 90 per cent of renal transplant operations are performed using cadaver kidneys. There are currently about 1000 people in Great Britain waiting for transplants and something like 3000 transplants would be required annually if most renal failure patients were to be treated in this way as is done in Australia.

In order to have a good tissue-type match it is desirable to have an even larger number of kidneys available to choose from. There are enough people dying in this country under suitable circumstances to provide this number of kidneys, and it should now be regarded as normal, good medical practice to attempt to obtain these for transplantation. Failure to do so should be considered negligent.

The best potential donor is a young person whose respiration is maintained by a respirator after irreversible brain damage. Actual age-limits are wide, approximately 5 to 60 years. Brain death should be proven in the usual ways as recommended by the College of Physicians (Luksza, 1979) and agreed by two doctors who are not members of the transplant team. An electroencephalogram is not essential. Renal disease in the donor should be excluded by history, examination of the urine and blood urea. Patients dying of malignant neoplasms, except primary cerebral tumours, which do not metastasize, as well as patients dying with significant sepsis, are not suitable donors. Because kidneys must be removed within half an hour of death under aseptic conditions, in an operating theatre, people dying outside hospital are not suitable.

If you think you have a patient who might be a suitable donor please telephone your local transplant unit before death occurs and discuss the matter. You will be advised on how best to preserve renal function in the donor. Blood will be required for tissue typing so that the best recipients for the donor's two kidneys may be selected from the computerized records in Bristol. A member of the transplant team will arrange for the removal and transport of the kidneys.

Living donors

In this country between 5 and 10 per cent of transplant patients receive their kidney from a living, related donor. The advantages of this are firstly, that the kidney is there and a long waiting period is avoided. This may be very important in patients who are doing badly on dialysis or in those in whom it is impossible to obtain satisfactory vascular access for haemodialysis. In most young children with permanent renal failure renal transplantation is the treatment of choice allowing more normal activity, diet and education. Parents are usually eager to give a kidney particularly when there is no sibling sufficiently old to give legal consent for one of his kidneys to be used.

A complete match of tissue types is only rarely obtained from a necessarily unrelated cadaver donor but there is a 25 per cent chance that a sibling will have identical tissue types. Parents are usually a half-match (A B O blood groups of donor and recipient must always be compatible). If the related donor and recipient are completely matched for tissue types as well as blood groups the chance of the transplantation being successful are over 90 per cent. With lesser degrees of match the take rate varies in different centres between 40 and 70 per cent, with good renal function after 2 years. The prognosis for a kidney from a living donor who is not a perfect tissue type match is only marginally better than a 'good' cadaver kidney. If a living donor offers a kidney he must, of course, be told of the operative risks to himself and the slight disadvantages of living the rest of his life with only one kidney. He is thoroughly investigated to ensure that he is generally healthy and has two normal kidneys (renal function tests, intravenous pyelogram and renal arteriogram).

Preparation of the recipient for renal transplantation and the operation

In Sheffield and in most other centres, patients haemodialyse at home for a considerable time before they have a transplant. This ensures that the patient is reasonably fit when he has the operation and keeps him going during the waiting time. Our waiting list is quite long and is not operated on a chronological basis. When we receive a kidney for transplantation it is given to the patient whose tissue types it best matches, not to the person who has been waiting longest. This means that patients wait from a few weeks to several years for a transplant. Before the patient's name is put on the transplant waiting list he has a cystoscopy to detect abnormalities of the lower urinary tract or ureteric reflux. If the patient has reflux, infection in his own kidneys or refractory hypertension, a bilateral nephrectomy is performed before the transplant. Some dialysis patients have large spleens and low blood white cell counts. This probably makes safe administration of azathioprine difficult, so some patients also require splenectomy before transplantation can be carried out.

When a donor kidney becomes available the dialysis patient is informed by telephone and comes into hospital for the operation immediately. Kidneys for transplantation can only be preserved for a few hours. The kidney is placed in the iliac fossa and anastomosed to internal or external iliac artery and vein and the donor ureter is implanted in the recipient's bladder. Immunosuppression is begun with azathioprine and prednisolone, initially in large doses. The first few weeks after transplantation are the most critical. It is during this period that rejection episodes are most likely to occur. These are treated by increased doses of prednisolone and therefore the patient is at risk from opportunist infections. These infections are the commonest cause of the 5 per cent of early deaths which occur after transplantation. Most rejection episodes can, however, be reversed and they are unlikely to occur after 6 months. The dose of prednisolone is then reduced to about 10 mg daily and the dose of azathioprine is about 100 mg daily. The white cell count is kept within normal limits. The modern tendency is to use smaller doses of prednisolone and not to treat rejection episodes which recur more than twice. It is better to have a live patient without a kidney than a patient who dies from an infection when his kidney is functioning.

About 40 per cent of recipients of a cadaver renal transplant are alive with good renal function after 2 years. By this time renal function is usually stable and likely to continue so. Most of the patients in whom the transplant fails are able to return to dialysis and have a second or even third or fourth transplant later.

Life with a kidney transplant

A patient with a successful renal transplant usually feels perfectly fit. His haemoglobin rises spontaneously to normal within a few weeks of the operation. About half have some degree of hypertension which requires treatment. Complications due to steroid treatment should not be great but a number of patients get ischaemic necrosis of bone, particularly of the femoral head, and require hip replacement. This complication should become less prevalent as the use of large doses of prednisolone decreases. Immunosuppression and supervision in a transplant outpatient clinic must be continued indefinitely. Dialysis, of course, is stopped and so patients can travel and enjoy virtually any hobby or occupation. Women may bear children and potency may return to men. The incidence of congenital defects in the offspring of transplant patients is only slightly above normal although immunosuppression is continued during pregnancy.

After the first 6 months the causes of death in transplant patients are predominantly those due to vascular disease. The incidence of neoplasia particularly of skin, cervix and brain is also increased. Women with a renal transplant should have regular cervical smears carried out.

Table 7   Annual cost of treatment (1979)

	£
Hospital haemodialysis	10 000
Minimal care unit haemodialysis	8000
Home haemodialysis	7000
Home peritoneal dialysis	4500
Transplantation operation (3–10 weeks in 'high dependency' hospital bed for operation)	?
Follow-up drugs annually	200
Plus cost of outpatients visits – about twelve per year	?

COST OF TREATMENT

For the foreseeable future the facilities for the treatment of end-stage renal failure in Great Britain will be restricted by cost. The approximate annual costs of maintaining patients by different methods of treatment are shown in Table 7. It is obvious that transplantation is cheaper than the other forms of treatment for most patients with end-stage renal disease under the age of 50 years. However, dialysis is needed to prepare patients for transplantation and to rescue those in whom the transplant fails. When treatment of end-stage renal failure becomes available for all who require it in Britain the proportion of older patients will increase markedly and most of these will be unsuitable for transplant, so that an expansion in dialysis services will still be required. Extension of dialysis to an older population will mean that there will be more patients who cannot dialyse at home and therefore more dialysis units will be needed, some of which may be of the 'minimal care' variety which are popular in North America and Europe. One of these units, which need not be in a hospital, should be in every town so that elderly patients without facilities for home dialysis can reach it easily. There they carry out as much of their own treatment as possible with the help of a few nurses. This kind of unit is somewhat cheaper to run than the normal British hospital-based unit. The financial restraints on treatment are not merely those for the purchase of dialysis machines. There is an embarrassment of offers from voluntary associations who wish to purchase artificial kidneys. At the moment these extra machines would not save lives. What we need are more hospital beds and in particular more nurses to staff them.

HOW IS RENAL REPLACEMENT THERAPY REFUSED TO PATIENTS?

It is perhaps a reflection of the doctors' cowardice that overt refusal of treatment is rarely made. There has been a great deal of publicity about kidney transplants and kidney machines yet patients in this country who are unsuitable for treatment rarely ask about them. It would be comforting to believe that they do not ask because they do not want these forms of treatment. I have had patients or their relatives begging for treatment on only two occasions. One was a medical student from Karachi who came here, without prior arrangement, in terminal renal failure and demanded haemodialysis under the national health service. He was of course, not entitled to this nor was he entitled to a kidney from a British cadaver. He was not rich enough to buy an artificial kidney and to pay for its running costs in Karachi. The only clinic offering private haemodialysis in Britain (National Kidney Centre in London) does treat foreign nationals but the current costs for equipment and training are approximately an initial payment of £10 000 and annual running costs at home of about £6000. The solution in this particular individual was short-term, privately funded, peritoneal dialysis in hospital followed by renal transplant from the patient's sister which fortunately was successful. The other supplicant was the daughter of a lady of 70 who had acute renal failure following a knee replacement operation. There is no age-limit for treatment of acute renal failure which is reversible and treatment is only needed for a matter of a few weeks. This daughter's anxiety about the availability of treatment for her mother was unfounded, and the old lady made a complete recovery after 2 weeks' haemodialysis.

The decision not to seek renal replacement therapy for a patient with permanent renal failure is usually made by doctors who are not renal specialists on the basis of their knowledge of the facilities available, the upper age-limit for acceptance at their local renal unit, and their beliefs about the degree of rehabilitation which is usually achieved by these methods of treatment.

I suspect that the majority of patients from whom renal replacement therapy is withheld never realize what is happening. They have the implicit faith of the British patient who believes that his 'doctor knows best.' In my experience, if a patient or his relatives raise the matter of dialysis or transplantation the patient is usually referred for an opinion. The life of a director of a renal unit would be impossible if he had to overtly refuse treatment to half of his patients. However, we shall continue to have difficulty in obtaining more facilities from the national health service unless we occasionally refuse treatment to specific patients.

Even if you have no direct experience of patients who have undergone treatment by dialysis or transplantation, you may have to deal with occasional patients with permanent renal failure. The staff of your local renal unit will be happy to arrange for you to meet patients living with renal replacement therapy so that you can form a first-hand opinion of the value of this treatment.

A louder and more concerted voice from the medical profession is needed to improve the facilities for treatment of our patients with permanent renal failure.

ACKNOWLEDGEMENT

Sister S. Smith (SRN) did most of the work involved in obtaining information on patients' marital state and difficulties. I thank her for allowing me to use the data.

References

Christiansen, C., Rodbrø, D., Christensen, M. S., Hartnack, B. and Transbol, I. (1978). Deterioration of renal function during treatment of chronic renal failure with 1,25 dihydroxycholecalciferol. *Lancet*, **2**, 700

Combined Report on Regular Dialysis and Transplantation in Europe. IX, 1978, (1979). *Proc. Eur. Dial. Transpl. Assoc.*, **16**, 6

The Dying Patient

Luksza, A. R. (1979). Brain-dead kidney donors: selection, care and administration. *Br. Med. J.*, **1**, 1316

Oreopoulos, D. G. (1977). The coming of age of home peritoneal dialysis. *Canad. Med. Assoc. J.*, **116**, 232

Shaw, A. B., Bazzard, F., Booth, E. M., Nilwarangkur, S. and Berlyne, G. M. (1965). The treatment of chronic renal failure by a modified Giovanetti diet. *Q. J. Med.*, **34**, 237

Wing, A. J., Brunner, F. P., Brynger, A., Chantler, C., Donkerwolcke, R. A., Gurland, H. J., Hathway, R. A., and Jacobs, C. (1978). Combined report on regular dialysis and transplantation in Europe, 1977 (chart). *Proc. Eur. Dial. Transpl. Assoc.*, **15**, 22

6

Management of disseminated breast cancer

Basil A. Stoll

To be conservative ... is to prefer the tried to the untried, the actual to the possible, the limited to the unbounded. ...

Michael Oakeshott

In the majority of patients with breast cancer, the disease is already disseminated even before the primary tumour is diagnosed. Evidence of this is the observation that 70 per cent of operated cases will, one by one, show evidence of metastasis over the subsequent 25 years (Brinkley and Haybittle, 1975; Mueller and Jeffries, 1975). That being so, the patient with disseminated breast cancer can be described as a dying patient only in the sense that in our present state of knowledge she is incurable. In actual fact, many of these patients require only occasional supervision and reassurance over a period of many years before reaching the stage when they need palliative care.

NATURAL HISTORY OF BREAST CANCER

The course of breast cancer is largely unpredictable. Unlike some types of cancer where recurrence manifests soon after primary treatment or not at all, in the case of breast cancer, as we noted above, evidence of overt metastasis may take many years to appear. Although 35 per cent of operated cases will show evidence of recurrence within 2 years of surgery, in 20 per cent recurrence will appear between the 2nd and the 5th years while in a further 15 per cent it will be delayed between 5 and 25 years.

...

This unpredictability extends also to the course of the disease *after* the first appearance of overt metastasis. The disease may follow a short fulminating incapacitating course, or a long indolent relatively asymptomatic course. With the recent development of effective hormonal and cytotoxic agents in the palliation of metastatic breast cancer, it has encouraged the belief that the natural growth-rate of the tumour may be slowed up by influencing both tumour and host factors. If we are successful, the patient may die *with* the disease, rather than *of* the disease.

Not only the course of breast cancer, but also the site pattern of metastasis varies widely between individuals. At each site, the tumour deposits may have their own rate of growth, carry a different prognosis and require different management. Thus, in up to 20 per cent of patients, the first clinical recurrence is local and usually asymptomatic, involving the scar, axillary or supraclavicular nodes. Bone metastasis is the presenting feature in about 35 per cent of cases, involving the ribs, spine, and pelvis most frequently. The pleura or lungs are involved in about 20 per cent of cases, and involvement of the liver, peritoneum, brain, spinal cord and opposite breast together account for about 25 per cent of all metastases (Cutler, Asire, and Taylor, 1969).

Because of this variety of patterns, about 25 to 30 per cent of patients survive more than 2 years after metastases have manifested, while 5 to 10 per cent will live for 5 years or longer. It should be emphasized that this has little to do with treatment, as even in patients with untreated disease, about 20 per cent live for 5 years or longer (Bloom, 1950). An example of the sometimes very protracted course of widespread metastatic disease is the following case history of a patient who, after 17 years is still enjoying an excellent quality of life needing only a minimum amount of treatment occasionally.

Case history

June 1963 Kathleen S., aged 39, presented with an inoperable four-quadrant tumour of the right breast. The breast and regional node areas were treated by 300 kV X-ray therapy to a maximum dose of 4000 r in 5 weeks.

June 1964 Right mastectomy and bilateral oophorectomy were carried out at the same operation. Laparotomy showed widespread peritoneal implants of cancer involving also the ovaries, and its histology was reported as similar to that of the primary breast cancer. Subsequently, the patient complained of occasional fleeting bone pains.

September 1965 Radiographs showed sclerotic metastases involving ribs, spine and pelvis. No treatment was given, but the sclerotic appearance increased over the next 10 years.

December 1974 The patient presented with ascites. This was controlled by the intermittent administration of prednisone 10–30 mg daily over the next 12 months.

September 1975 The patient complained of pain in the dorsal spine and received a course of nandrolone (Durabolin) 25 mg weekly for the next 2½ years. By June 1978, the sclerotic metastases in her skeleton had given way to a normal appearance in the X-rays, but it had taken 13 years for this (Figure 1a, b, c and d).

December 1978 Ascites recurred but was again kept under control by intermittent administration of prednisone and intra-abdominal thiotepa installation.

February 1981 When last examined the patient was still leading a normal life.

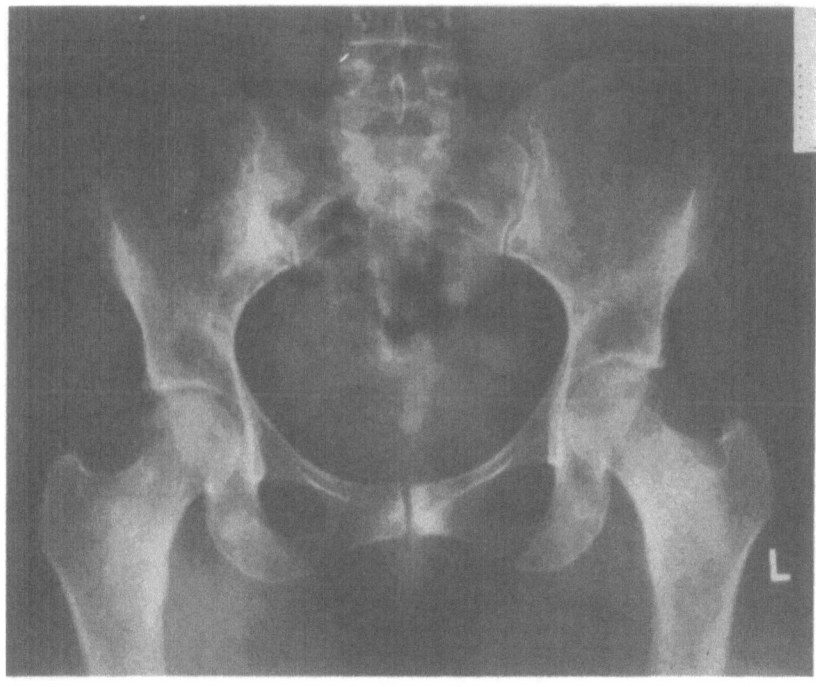

(a)

Figure 1a to d Pelvic radiographs of patient Kathleen S. showing sclerotic metastases on 28 September 1965, 15 months after oophorectomy (see text). Sclerosis increased progressively during endocrine control but a normal appearance was not seen in the bone until 13 years later (serial radiographs were taken 8 December 1972, 8 September 1975, and 19 June 1978). No radiation therapy was given to the pelvis

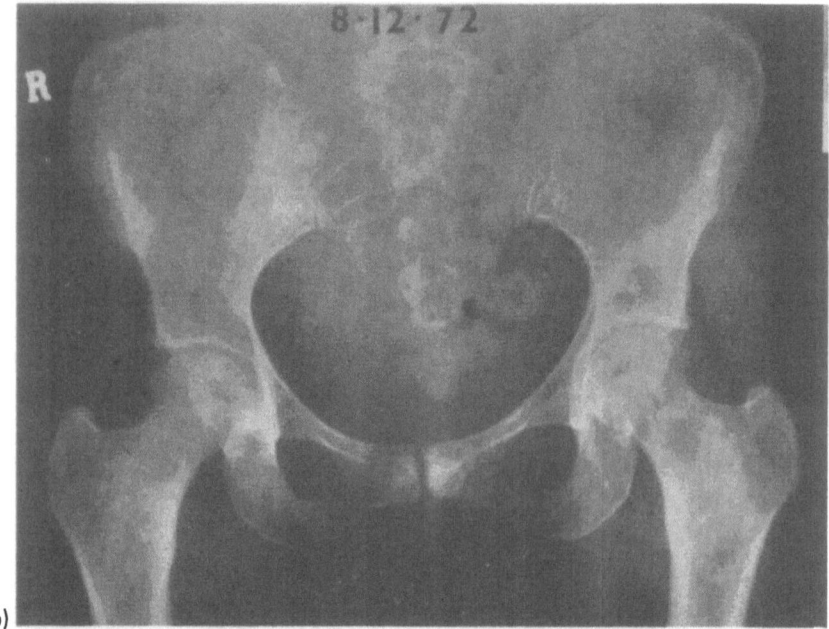

(b)

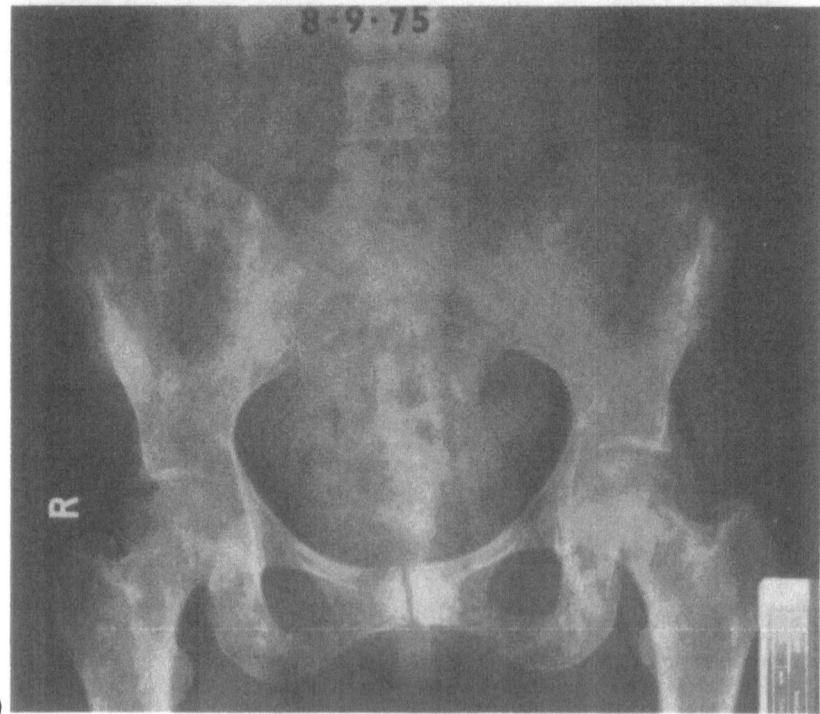

(c)

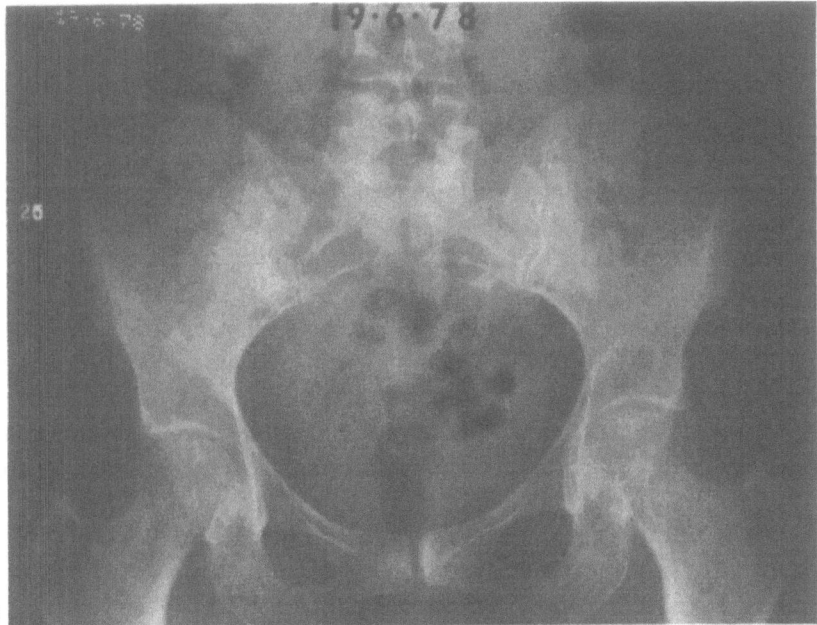

(d)

AIMS OF TREATMENT

Whether the patient presents in the first place with advanced disease, or shows recurrence after mastectomy, the first aim of treatment must be the urgent relief of symptoms. An additional aim must be the intelligent anticipation of symptoms in order to preserve the quality of the patient's remaining months or years of life. Recently, some oncologists have advocated a third aim – to embark on aggressive (and often distressing) polychemotherapy at the first clinical evidence of recurrence. It aims to delay further recurrence and thereby prolong life, but so far there is no evidence that the latter is achieved (Brunner and Cavalli, 1980; Falkson *et al.*, 1978; Stoll, 1980). As seen in the case history above, a conservative therapeutic approach is compatible not only with an excellent quality of life but also with long survival. Many types of aggressive treatment unfortunately vitiate the quality of the patient's remaining life.

The clinician needs wide experience of the diseases, considerable clinical judgement and a sense of compassion in order to steer a balanced course suited to the individual patient and her disease. Each patient is a unique problem and there can be no 'policy' for the treatment of recurrent or advanced breast cancer. There are indications for aggressive treatment but there are also others for 'masterly inactivity'.

For example, aggressive treatment in the hope of a cure can be justified as long as recurrent breast cancer can be regarded as localized. Thus, the presence of a node low down in the ipsilateral axilla after inadequate dissection, or the presence of a localized cutaneous or subcutaneous recurrence in the immediate vicinity of the mastectomy scar may justify a vigorous surgical and/or radiotherapeutic approach.

A decision of this type assumes the absence of established bloodborne metastases. It would not need to be reversed on the basis of a positive bone scan without X-ray confirmation of metastases, nor on the presence of moderate hepatomegaly without abnormal liver function tests. Widespread metastases cannot be assumed either from the presence of a solitary wedge-shaped vertebra in the presence of general osteoporosis, unless histological confirmation of tumour is obtained.

On the other hand, the presence of a bloodstained pleural effusion (especially if ipsilateral and bacteriologically negative) must be assumed malignant, even without cytological or histological confirmation. The demonstration of a space-occupying lesion in the brain or spinal cord by scan or myelogram, even without histological confirmation, must also be reported as evidence of bloodborne metastasis.

A tumour appearing in the opposite breast several years after the original mastectomy may well be a new primary growth and requires aggressive treatment in the absence of other evidence of metastases. However, in the presence of local recurrence in the scar or draining node areas, a tumour found in the contralateral breast is highly likely to be metastatic. Again, the presence of a large primary tumour widely infiltrating the breast, or large apical axillary nodes, or the presence of significant enlargement of the supraclavicular or cervical nodes on either side, or the presence of a parasternal recurrence originating in the internal mammary nodes – all are almost certain to be associated with widely disseminated disease.

ASSESSING THE TEMPO OF THE DISEASE

In order to decide the nature and extent of treatment to be given to any patient with disseminated cancer, the physician must face two questions 'How long can the patient expect to live?' and 'How can I best maintain her quality of life during that time?'. In the case of advanced cancer of the stomach or lung for example, there is no wide variation in the expected duration and quality of survival. Prognosis can be readily based on medical and treatment variables such as the microscopic type of the tumour, stage of disease, sites of spread and degree of interference with vital functions. However, in the case of advanced breast cancer, although percentage probabilities can be derived from cohorts of patients, wide variation exists between one patient and another in the tempo and pattern of the metastases.

Even in the same patient, breast cancer does not always advance irrevocably at the same rate. At different times in the natural history of the disease, growth may be rapid, slow or even imperceptible (Miller and Spratt, 1980). Because of this remarkable variability in the course of breast cancer, it has been concluded that in each individual and at any one time, there exists a biological balance between tumour factors and host factors, both local and systemic. It is these which will determine the tempo or rate of progression of the tumour.

Recognition of the tempo of the disease permits selection of a suitable form of management out of the following:

(1) Aggressive treatment associated with morbidity. This is justified only for aggressive disease, and then only if the physical and mental condition of the patient justifies it.
(2) Localized radiotherapy and conservative management. This is usually adequate to control the symptoms of most local recurrence or metastasis.
(3) No treatment at all. This is often advised for slowly growing tumours in the absence of symptoms from metastases and no danger of serious complications.

In spite of attempts to predict prognosis based on the clinical stage and histological grade of the primary tumour, the course of breast cancer in the individual is highly unpredictable until recurrence manifests following primary treatment. Even though the timing and nature of the first recurrence will provide an approximate guide, the prognosis must still be guarded. Breast cancer does not behave alike in any two patients, and not only may apparently identical types of tumour show different biological behaviour, they may also respond differently to treatment.

The following guidelines enable the clinician to judge whether the disease is more likely to have a short 'bushfire' course or a long indolent course. The clinician can then decide on the most suitable approach to treatment in the individual.

Tumour factors

Recurrence-free interval
The longer the time elapsing before the first clinical manifestation of recurrence, the greater the duration of subsequent survival. In patients whose recurrence-free interval following mastectomy is less than 2 years, the median subsequent survival period is only 6 to 12 months. For recurrence-free intervals of 2 to 5 years, the median survival is 12 to 18 months while for intervals of over 5 years, the median survival is 18 to 24 months (Cutler, Asire, and Taylor, 1969).

Site of recurrence
Deposits in the liver, peritoneum, brain or spinal cord are associated with a median survival of 6 months, while deposits in skin, lymph nodes, bone, lungs or pleura are associated with a median survival of 18 to 24 months. Lymphangitic infiltration of the lung fields predicts a worse prognosis than does the presence of discrete nodular opacities. Patients with deposits at visceral sites are much less likely to respond to hormonal or cytotoxic agents than are patients with soft tissue metastases.

Number of systems involved
The more systems involved by metastases, the shorter the subsequent survival. There is however marked variation with site, so that a combination of lymph node and lung metastases predicts a median survival of 8 months while a combination of bone and skin deposits is associated with 30 months median survival.

Delay in treatment of primary tumour
The time for which the patient has delayed treatment of the primary tumour gives few clues as to the prognosis. A large presenting tumour may be either of a rapidly growing or a slowly growing type.

Host factors

General condition
The wasted patient with gross anaemia, or the patient with a long history of severe dyspnoea from lung infiltration or pleural effusion, or a long history of uncontrolled pain – all have a poor prognosis. In such cases it is claimed that blood corticosteroid levels are high, androgen levels low, and immune reactivity defective (Mackay, 1975).

Age group
It is a generalization that breast cancer is more aggressive in the younger patient, and more slowly growing in the patient over the age of 70. Many reports witness to wide variation in the growth rate at all age groups, nevertheless, the so-called clinical 'scirrhous' cancer is more common in the older patient, and such patients may survive for many years with slowly growing skin infiltration or regional node involvement.

Endocrine status
Patients whose disease spans the menopause have a longer mean recurrence-free interval between primary treatment and the first evidence of recurrence. Bone metastases in such patients may show a mixture of sclerotic and lytic changes. On the other hand, patients whose breast cancer first presents within 5 years following the menopause tend to have a relatively more rapidly growing tumour (Stoll, 1977).

The ovarian status may be difficult to establish in women who have had a hysterectomy before the menopause. Examination of the degree of cornification in the vaginal smear or assay of the serum gonadotrophin level will be of assistance in difficult cases.

ASSESSING THE EXTENT OF THE DISEASE

The minimum information upon which an informed opinion on management can be based is a full medical and personal history, a detailed physical examination and certain selected laboratory and radiographic investigations.

The history should include details of the extent and histopathology of the primary tumour. If previous surgery has been carried out, there should be evidence as to the extent of the surgery, extent of involvement of axillary nodes and at which level, and the use of radiotherapy or cytotoxic therapy following surgery. Further important information is the duration of the free-interval before the first clinical evidence of recurrence, and its relationship to the time of the menopause.

The type and severity of the existing symptoms must be assessed and also the degree of change which has taken place in the patient's day-to-day activity. If there are multiple symptoms, it is essential to establish the *relative* importance of each symptom in the patient's disability, and also its relation to pre-existing disability such as that due to chronic arthritis, cardiac failure, diabetes, anxiety or depression.

Physical examination should look for disease in the residual breast tissue, skin flaps or regional node areas. Small areas of erythema must be regarded with suspicion and biopsied if necessary. Small subcutaneous nodules are easily missed unless the whole of the chest wall, anterior and posterior, is examined carefully with the fingertips. Nodes in the supraclavicular area, particularly in the scalene region, are also easy to overlook. The opposite breast and its draining node areas must be examined carefully and a mammogram may be necessary if there is a suspicious thickening. If any biopsy is to be carried out, a piece of the tissue should be set aside for oestrogen receptor assay.

The abdomen is examined for evidence of liver enlargement, ascites, nodes or peritoneal masses, and the pelvis and ilioinguinal areas are examined for nodes and tumour masses. Routine liver scan is not necessary unless liver function tests are abnormal, but serial assessment of liver size is recommended in patients with moderate hepatomegaly on clinical examination.

An X-ray of the chest is mandatory in every case. Slowly developing pleural or lung metastases may be asymptomatic while localized areas of fibrosis due to previous radiotherapy may cause needless anxiety unless recognized as such. Neurological abnormality is looked for in the optic discs, cranial nerves and peripheral nerves.

Skeletal pain calls for appropriate radiological investigation, and only in negative or non-symptomatic cases is a bone scan necessary for deciding on management. Tenderness to percussion is looked for over the spine and bony prominences, and severe *localized* tenderness is practically diagnostic of metastasis. If X-rays are reported negative in such a case, tomograms may be needed. Widespread symptomless osteosclerotic metastases are not uncommon, particularly in women in the perimenopausal age group.

Laboratory studies must include a full haematological investigation. Pancytopenia may suggest recent therapy by cytotoxic agents or wide-field radiation therapy. On the other hand, metastatic involvement of the marrow is suggested by thrombocytopenia, anaemia and leukocytosis associated with the presence of immature red and white cells in the peripheral blood. Liver function studies will include estimation of the alkaline phosphatase level but the latter may be abnormally raised due either to bone or liver metastases. They can be distinguished by measuring the 5-nucleotidase level in the serum which is a sensitive monitor of metastases in the liver (Van der Slik *et al.*, 1970). Serum calcium levels must always be measured in the presence of bone metastases because hypercalcaemia is not uncommonly found in such cases.

CHOOSING TREATMENT FOR THE INDIVIDUAL

Having decided the tempo of the disease and its extent, it is necessary to consider the specific characteristics of each type of treatment which make it more or less suitable for the individual patient.

The general condition or performance status of the patient

The wasted patient with anaemia, anorexia and depression will rarely respond to aggressive cytotoxic chemotherapy, and her death may even be hastened by such treatment. Psychological support and attempts to build up nutrition take precedence over aggressive antitumour therapy. Corticosteroid therapy using prednisolone 30 mg daily in association with cyclophosphamide 100 mg orally daily may sometimes cause near-miraculous improvement in the patient's condition and may enable more aggressive therapy to be started subsequently.

If metastases involve several systems, the urgency of the disability arising from each particular system will decide the priorities of treatment. Relief of pain takes priority over every other treatment.

Age and menstrual status

Treatment of the young patient will obviously be more aggressive in general than that of the older patient. In the latter, one must be guided by the patient's general health and attitude to illness before initiating distressing treatment. Patients before the menopause and also elderly patients show the highest response rate to endocrine therapy, while patients within 5 years after the menopause rarely respond to such treatment.

Aggressiveness of the disease

This is reflected by the rate of growth and extent of the tumour, and in the case of postoperative recurrence the former can be judged approximately by the recurrence-free interval. A more slowly growing tumour is more likely to be sensitive to endocrine manipulation and will usually show a positive oestrogen receptor assay on biopsy.

Predominant site of metastatic involvement

Patients with metastases in the brain or liver and those with large abdominal masses or bilateral pleural effusion are least influenced by treatment whether it is hormonal or cytotoxic. The patient with an unpinned fracture of the femoral neck, or with extensive skin infiltration and ulceration causing carcinoma-en-cuirasse, is likely to succumb from pneumonia.

Extent and type of disease

The presence of a large primary tumour and multiple large axillary deposits strongly suggests the likelihood of widespread, even if occult, disease. The choice of treatment will also be influenced by whether overt lung metastases are of the nodular or lymphangitic type and by whether bone metastases are of the sclerotic or lytic types. The former type is less aggressive in both cases and more amenable to systemic therapy whether hormonal or cytotoxic.

PLANNING SEQUENTIAL THERAPY

It was stressed above that as long as recurrent breast cancer can be regarded as localized, one can justify aggressive therapy in the hope of a cure. The converse argument applies equally. In the case of overt disseminated disease, there is so far no evidence to support the *theoretical* argument that early and aggressive treatment is more likely to prolong life because of the smaller tumour load and because it stops the development of tertiary metastases. Early aggressive cytotoxic therapy may delay the clinical appearance of the next recurrence but there is no evidence in randomized clinical trials that total survival is any longer than in the patient in whom systemic therapy is delayed until the next metastasis has become clinically overt (Brunner and Cavalli, 1980; Falkson *et al.*, 1978; Stoll, 1980).

Intensive treatment of disseminated disease, whether by surgery, radiation therapy, cytotoxic therapy or endocrine therapy must be *based on the patient's need and not on the physician's hope*. It is important to keep treatments in reserve for as long as possible and this means that a sequential plan of treatment must be projected from the outset. This involves progression from the most simple to the most complex treatment, at every step using the minimum treatment necessary for palliation. Thus, for the palliation of localized metastases or advanced local disease, the patient should first be offered localized radiation therapy even if we presume that wide subclinical spread has already occurred. Local radiation therapy will yield the highest certainty of relief with the lowest incidence of unpleasant side-effects.

Justification for the sequential approach to therapy is the acknowledgement that in our present state of knowledge the progress of the disease is inevitable and that the dominant goal of treatment is palliation. The guiding principles of sequential therapy are as follows:

(1) The most troublesome or most life-endangering manifestation will determine the most immediate form of treatment. Apart from this, one starts with the simplest and best tolerated form of treatment compatible with palliation.

(2) One does not progress to another form of therapy until adequate time has been allowed to assess the results of treatment. Whereas relief of pain from the radiation of bone metastases may take only 2 weeks, that from endocrine therapy or cytotoxic therapy may take 4 to 6 weeks. Similarly macroscopic tumour regression from the latter methods may take 3 months to show itself.

(3) Once a treatment regime has shown itself capable of controlling tumour growth, it is persisted with until response is lost.

(4) In selecting one of several possible alternative treatments, the clinician must consider not only the response rate from each method, but also the likely duration of remission, its degree of completeness and the promptness with which it occurs. Against these four conjectural benefits of treatment must be set the likely morbidity of each treatment, its effect on the patient's wellbeing and day-to-day activity and its effect on her mood and mental outlook.

(5) Mere objective regression of local tumour must not be confused with improved quality of life, and the cost to the patient in suffering must be commensurate with possible benefits from a treatment. For example, aggressive systemic therapy by combination cytotoxic therapy may achieve regression of local disease. If, however, its duration is only a matter of a few months and the disease is again recrudescent by the time the morbidity of therapy has settled, one must question whether palliation has been achieved.

(6) A mixed response to a specific therapy does not preclude its further use. For example, if localized soft tissue tumour has regressed on endocrine therapy, but in the meanwhile a painful new metastasis has appeared in bone, the hormone therapy can be continued. Radiation therapy may be used to treat the bone deposit if it is localized.

If these principles of sequential therapy are accepted:

(1) There is no advantage to be gained by a search for occult or asymptomatic metastases by tests which cause the patient inconvenience or distress. Evidence of bloodborne metastasis at one site presumes the

presence of widespread systemic disease.

(2) There is no indication to plague the patient with frequent and repeated follow-up investigations. In 90 per cent of cases, the development of new metastases is heralded by symptoms, and while chest X-rays or liver function tests may occasionally uncover occult disease, serial bone scans as a routine are not justified (Winchester *et al.*, 1979). Serial liver and brain scans are certainly not justified.

(3) A solitary metastasis calls for aggressive treatment only if it fails to respond to simpler palliative measures. The argument that a single overt metastasis in lung, bone, brain or liver may be a solitary deposit and needs aggressive therapy, is not justified either by pathological concepts or by the results of treatment. A report of long survival following intensive treatment of such a deposit by surgery or aggressive radiotherapy does not prove the effectiveness of the treatment in eradicating the disease. It merely indicates that slowly growing disease is involved.

(4) The use of anticipatory treatment for asymptomatic metastases must be discriminating and based on informed clinical experience. It may be indicated in the case of small mediastinal or cerebral metastases where their further growth may threaten life, or for lytic deposits in long bones where a pathological fracture might subsequently incapacitate the patient. It is often quite unnecessary for asymptomatic slowly growing metastases in skin or regional nodes in elderly patients, or for symptomless sclerotic bone metastases, or for discrete limited opacities in the lung fields, or for defects in the liver image visible in a scan.

(5) Sometimes a patient or her relatives may desire that aggressive treatment be carried out because of the findings of asymptomatic metastases. This may be justified on a psychological basis, but the patient must be given to understand that there is no evidence that such treatment will prolong survival. In all cases, it is better for the patient to continue as normal a life as possible, and activity should be restricted only if there is a danger that it may make symptoms appear or cause complications such as a pathological fracture.

(6) The management of advanced local disease by a combination of localized radiation therapy and systemic therapy is, in our present state of knowledge, an example of 'overkill'. Regression of the local disease often leads to the systemic therapy being continued for long periods without any evidence that it has exerted any control whatsoever on the disease. We must await the results of current randomized clinical trials in order to ascertain whether such combination therapy has any advantage over either treatment alone.

It is obvious that a decision on treatment based upon so many imponderables is not easy. That is why the physician's clinical experience and compassion are of paramount importance in selecting treatment. Where there are several apparently equally effective treatments to choose from, the difficulty is often to compare different forms of unpleasantness in the side-effects. An example of this dilemma is a decision as to the most suitable type of systemic therapy for the patient with widespread bone metastases where oestrogen receptor (ER) assay is not feasible. There are several methods of treatment all offering a one-in-three chance of relief of pain and some possibility of recalcification of bone metastases.

It is obvious that the simple, less unpleasant methods should be offered first, for example treatment by antioestrogen, androgen or amino-glutethimide. If these fail, the patient may possibly derive benefit from hypophyseal ablation or from polychemotherapy (with their attendant morbidity), but this should be an informed decision by the patient based on the knowledge that all treatments are palliative. In our present state of knowledge, no method of treatment can be presented as a possible 'cure', although that is not to say that the patient should ever be deprived of the hope of a prolonged remission.

METASTASES IN SPECIFIC CLINICAL SITUATIONS

Advanced local tumour

About 20 per cent of patients with breast cancer present with locally advanced disease but without overt evidence of distant metastases. The majority will show clinical evidence of such metastases within a year and will probably die within 3 years. Some tumours, however, such as 'scirrhous' cancer in the elderly, are compatible with many years of symptom-free survival.

As a general rule, advanced local tumour should first be treated by radiation therapy, whether or not distant metastases are present (Chu, 1977) because radiotherapy can cause regression of even the largest tumour. In advanced tumours, radiation will control growth for between 6 and 24 months. Grossly ulcerated cancer will heal in the vast majority of cases although necrosis sometimes supervenes in heavily infected rapidly growing tumours. In a patient with a relatively short expectation of life, it is important to achieve an effective dose of radiation in the smallest number of fractions and in addition megavoltage therapy should be used because it is least damaging to the surrounding normal skin.

As mentioned above, clinical trials are under way to assess the effect of concomitant systemic therapy in prolonging control of primary tumour growth, but longer follow-up is necessary before we can evaluate the results. Systemic therapy should, however, be started concomitantly if symptomatic metastases are present. If the ER assay of the primary tumour is reported positive, oophorectomy is advised in premenopausal patients and antioestrogen therapy (tamoxifen 10–20 mg b.d.) in postmenopausal patients. If, on the other hand, the tumour is reported ER negative, combination cytotoxic therapy is preferred. This is not the place to describe details of the latter treatment, but various reviews (see, for instance, Tormey and Neifeld, 1977) discuss drug dosage, toxicity and expected response rates.

In the absence of facilities for ER assay, cytotoxic therapy is generally preferred for infiltrating and rapidly growing disease in the younger patient, while tamoxifen therapy should be given a trial for localized slowly growing tumours in the older patient. Tamoxifen 10–20 mg b.d. may be tried even before radiotherapy in the case of the very old patient. Complete or partial regression of the primary tumour will occur in about 50 per cent of such cases and the hormonal therapy may have a similar controlling effect on distant metastases also, especially those in bone, lungs or pleura. Side-effects of the agent are remarkably few.

An advanced local tumour which is either ulcerated or about to ulcerate, may be managed by toilet mastectomy, particularly in the case of a slowly growing tumour in an elderly patient. Excision is, however, contraindicated if there is deep infiltration of the chest wall or if the skin is widely infiltrated and primary skin closure is unlikely. Under such conditions, surgery can precipitate wide lymphatic permeation leading to carcinoma-en-cuirasse, possibly the most distressing of all local manifestations of breast cancer. It must be remembered also that radiation therapy cannot convert an inoperable tumour into an operable tumour. Even if macroscopic shrinkage takes place, microscopic foci of viable cells will almost certainly persist following a dose of radiation which is compatible with viable skin flaps.

Local skin recurrence

Between 5 and 15 per cent of operated cases show cutaneous or sub-cutaneous lesions near the line of the scar as the first evidence of recurrence. They may be either of the nodular or infiltrating types and often closely precede or follow the appearance of distant metastases. Nodular recurrence usually starts near the line of the mastectomy scar and the nodules eventually ulcerate. The infiltrating type of local recurrence appears as diffuse thickening and reddening of the skin associated with itching or pain. The spread of the latter is usually much more rapid than that of the former.

If one or two small nodules are grouped closely together, it may be possible to excise the area successfully, particularly if they are situated in loose skin near the scar line. If, however, they are scattered at the periphery of the operation area, they are usually evidence of diffuse lymphatic permeation and are better treated by radiation therapy, preferably of the electron beam type.

Only palliative dosage of irradiation is attempted if distant metastases are present, but it should include a wide area of possible occult permeation, from the anterior midline to the posterior axillary line. Disease within the irradiated area can usually be controlled for between 6 and 24 months but when the tumour recurs, further effective radiotherapy will not usually be tolerated by the tissues.

Localized slowly growing or ER-positive tumour for which further radiation is impossible can be treated by oophorectomy in the pre-menopausal patient or by antioestrogen therapy in the postmenopausal patient. In the case of infiltrating, rapidly growing or ER-negative tumour, combination cytotoxic therapy is preferred.

Lymph node recurrence

The axillary and supraclavicular nodes are the ones most commonly involved. As they increase in size, they become fixed deeply and may eventually ulcerate through the skin. The brachial plexus may be involved either by pressure or by tumour invasion. Internal mammary node metastasis may present as a parasternal nodule growing between the upper costal cartilages, but pain and ulceration usually occur late with such metastases.

Treatment of metastatic recurrence in lymph nodes is nearly always by radiation therapy. Involved nodes show excellent regression from such treatment while they respond less well to endocrine or cytotoxic therapy. Radiation dosage is planned to a radical or palliative level depending on whether distant metastases have manifested, but in most cases the local disease can be controlled for a period which varies between 12 and 36 months.

Bone metastases

Painful and disabling metastases in bone are the most common manifest-ation of distant metastases in breast cancer. Although disseminated bone metastases require systemic therapy, irradiation of localized symptom-producing areas offers the highest likelihood of pain relief and often leads to recalcification. Some degree of pain relief is achieved almost invariably within 2 or 3 weeks, and failure to do so makes one suspect either that the diagnosis of bone metastasis is incorrect or else that an inadequate volume of tissue has been irradiated.

Some patients with bone metastases show patchy osteosclerotic metastases in the skeleton without any symptoms. These are usually associated with adenocarcinoma, or may indicate slowly growing metastases in patients whose disease straddles the menopause. They are seen also after successful endocrine therapy, and (as described in the case history at the beginning of this chapter) require no treatment as long as the patient has no pain.

In the case of a lytic metastasis in a long bone, however, localized radiotherapy is advised even it it is asymptomatic, because of the danger of pathological fracture. Pathological fracture of a long bone may lead to vascular or nerve damage and in the case of the femur, prolonged immobilization of the patient may lead to pneumonia or venous thrombosis. Such fractures are best stabilized by some form of internal fixation and this is followed by a course of irradiation. In the case of a fractured femoral neck, the femoral head may be replaced by a prosthesis. Bilateral surgical procedures on the femora or humeri are not uncommonly carried out, as patients with slowly growing lytic metastases sometimes survive for several years.

In the presence of widespread bone metastases in an elderly patient, endocrine therapy is indicated. Although recalcification of metastases will result in less than one-third of patients treated, some degree of pain relief occurs in a further third of patients for a period of some months. Response is most likely from oophorectomy in the premenopausal patient or from androgen therapy (fluoxymesterone 10 mg t.d.s.) in the postmenopausal patient. Antioestrogen therapy by tamoxifen, or hypophyseal ablation, may be tried as secondary endocrine therapy in patients showing a good response to primary endocrine manipulation.

Cytotoxic therapy by the CMF combination (cyclophosphamide, methotrexate, fluorouracil) rarely leads to recalcification in bone metastases in breast cancer, in spite of some claims to the contrary. Relief of pain for several months in however not uncommon from its use. In patients with evidence of widespread bone marrow replacement by tumour, intensive cytotoxic therapy is not feasible, but a combination of cyclophosphamide 50–100 mg daily and prednisone 15–20 mg daily is usually well tolerated. In the writer's experience, it may control the patient's symptoms for up to 2 years.

Lung metastases

These are usually of the nodular or lymphangitic types, but not uncommonly the appearance is mixed. Discrete slowly growing opacities may enlarge over a period of several years and require no treatment until they cause symptoms. At this stage they may regress under either endocrine or cytotoxic therapy, and localized radiation therapy is indicated only if haemoptysis or bronchial obstruction are major symptoms.

In the case of lymphangitis carcinomatosa involving the whole lung fields, there is often dramatic *subjective* response to the administration of 30–60 mg prednisone daily, but the radiographic picture will rarely change on this regime. A well-tolerated cytotoxic regime (such as thiotepa or cyclophosphamide) may be combined with this, and can control the disease for 9 to 12 months (Stoll, 1977).

Pleural effusion

The symptoms associated with a metastatic pleural effusion tend to vary according to the rate of its accumulation. A very large effusion which has developed slowly may barely inconvenience the patient, while a small effusion barely filling the costophrenic angle may sometimes cause severe dyspnoea. Shortness of breath may also be related to the degree of displacement of the mediastinum. Either the visceral or parietal pleura may be involved by tumour and a bloodstained effusion containing malignant cells is usually evident.

Removal of the fluid usually gives instant relief of symptoms but unless steps are taken to seal the space between visceral and parietal pleura, the fluid will reaccumulate in a few weeks. Repeated paracentesis leads not only to loss of valuable protein but also to the development of loculation in the pleural cavity which will prevent full evacuation of fluid after the first or second paracentesis. It is therefore essential that at the *first* drainage of fluid, a tube be inserted in the pleural space, and suction maintained for about 24 hours. To help pleurodesis further, a cytotoxic agent such as nitrogen mustard or thiotepa is instilled into the cavity (Anderson, Roper, and Ferguson, 1977), and after about 30 minutes suction is applied to the tube and maintained for another 24–48 hours until the X-ray shows the pleural cavity to be empty. The process can be repeated 2 weeks later if the fluid should reaccumulate and the blood count is satisfactory.

Procedures of this nature will stop further accumulation of fluid in about

75 per cent of cases and many of these patients may enjoy a comfortable life for 2 years or longer. Systemic therapy should of course be instituted if other metastases are evident – by hormones if the tumour is likely to be hormone-sensitive or by systemic cytotoxic agents if it is not.

Liver metastases

The liver is rarely the only location of metastases in the patient, but sometimes it is the major cause of symptoms. Pain and tenderness under the ribs is common. It is often relieved by prednisone 20–30 mg daily but the size of the enlarged liver is rarely decreased in such cases. Radiation therapy is not well tolerated by the liver but it may be useful for relief of jaundice due to pressure by metastatic nodes at the porta hepatis.

Endocrine therapy is rarely effective in causing regression of liver metastases even if biopsy proves them to be ER-positive. The results of cytotoxic therapy are equally disappointing although intrahepatic infusion of fluorouracil is said to be useful if other methods fail. The prognosis in the presence of rapidly growing liver metastases is very poor, but sometimes the deposits progress slowly even without treatment.

Hypercalcaemia

This is a major medical complication of breast cancer and is almost always associated with the presence of widespread bone metastases. It may occur spontaneously or it may be precipitated within a few days of initiating hormone therapy. Hypercalcaemia usually presents with nausea, vomiting, constipation and abdominal distension and may proceed to coma if untreated. Persistent hypercalcaemia inevitably leads to severe renal damage and death.

The most urgent measures are hydration by means of intravenous saline and the forcing of diuresis. Infusions of sodium sulphate or sodium citrate will increase the urinary calcium excretion (Davis, 1977). Corticosteroids at high dosage, such as 50–100 mg prednisone daily, will help to restore serum calcium levels to normal, and when this has been achieved it is often possible to continue the original hormonal therapy and even achieve regression of tumour growth.

Brain metastases

Metastases in the cerebrum usually present with symptoms of increased intracranial pressure or evidence of focal motor, sensory or eye symptoms. Personality changes as a presenting symptom are rare. Metastases involving the cerebellum usually present with ataxia or vertigo. The presence of brain metastases is usually confirmed by isotope or CAT scan and even if this shows the gross abnormality to be unilateral, it must be assumed that both sides of the brain are involved by metastases. Most cytotoxic agents fail to achieve therapeutic concentrations in the brain, although intrathecal administration of thiotepa or methotrexate is said to cause benefit in patients with meningeal involvement.

The administration of large doses of corticosteroids (such as dexamethasone 3–10 mg daily or prednisone 30–100 mg daily) will relieve the symptoms of raised intracranial pressure in most cases. The dose is subsequently titrated against the symptoms to achieve as low a level as possible. If the patient survives for 3 months and there are no other rapidly growing and life-endangering metastases, a course of radiotherapy to the brain may be considered. The whole brain is usually irradiated in such cases, but if the patient has one slowly growing metastasis, local irradiation to a high dose may be practised and will achieve as much as surgical excision.

Spinal cord compression
It is important to be alert for early signs of spinal cord compression in any patient with vertebral metastases. Bowel or bladder dysfunction, weakness of gait or sensory signs in the legs such as paraesthesia, are symptoms requiring immediate investigation and myelography. A laminectomy or deroofing operation is indicated as an emergency if a block in the spinal canal is shown.

Radiotherapy can be given later but is generally not advised as the primary measure because the neurological deficit may become permanent before the radiation has had time to relieve the pressure. As in the case of brain metastases, dexamethasone or prednisone in large doses should be given as soon as the diagnosis is made in order to reduce oedema and thus decrease the risk of permanent neurological damage.

Palliation of pain
This may be one of the most intractable problems in the patient with disseminated breast cancer. Analgesics may be adequate to relieve the pain of pleural effusion, peritonism or stretching of the liver capsule but are rarely adequate for the patient with bone metastases or infiltration of nerve roots. If the disease is too extensive for control by radiation therapy and attempts at control by endocrine or cytotoxic methods are ineffective, the use of opiates is indicated and this is discussed in Chapter 10 by Tempest and Clarke.

If the patient has a resonable life-expectancy, however, and the pain is localized, some form of surgical pain-relieving procedure may be considered. Both posterior rhizotomy and percutaneous cordotomy have their adherents but the indications are restricted. It is sometimes claimed that L-dopa can relieve pain in patients with bone metastases from breast cancer and may even predict subsequent response to endocrine ablation therapy (Minton and Dickey, 1972) but this claim has not been confirmed.

SUMMING UP

One may perhaps sum up this section on the management of the patient with disseminated breast cancer by setting out some prime examples of *inappropriate* treatment.

(1) Aggressive treatment of asymptomatic metastases.
(2) The use of two methods of treatment in combination where one would suffice.
(3) Prolonged duration of a palliative treatment, in relation to the patient's life-expectation.
(4) Severe morbidity from a treatment, in relation to the degree of palliation to be expected.

The death of a cancer patient while undergoing an aggressive treatment (whether by surgery, radiotherapy or cytotoxic agent) can be justified if the treatment is an attempt at cure and the risks have been calculated. If, however, a patient dies in the middle of a course of aggressive treatment directed at *palliation*, it indicates poor clinical judgement by the physician or surgeon.

In extenuation, it is sometimes suggested that the decision has been forced by the patient or relatives demanding that no stone be left unturned. But it needs to be emphasized that the art of medicine (as opposed to the science) requires time – time for reassurance, careful explanation, compassionate understanding and an ability to know when unnecessary suffering should be avoided. We should not feel guilty if we do not offer our technically complex treatments in this highly scientific age. But it often takes more time to explain why we do not advise it than it takes to arrange such treatment.

References

Anderson, C. B., Roper, C. L., and Ferguson, T. B. (1977). In *Breast Cancer Management – Early and Late* (ed. B. A. Stoll) (London: Heinemann Medical), p. 175

Bloom, H. J. G. (1950). *Br. J. Cancer*, **4**, 347

Brinkley, D. and Haybittle, J. L. (1975). *Lancet*, **2**, 95

Brunner, K. W. and Cavalli, F. (1980). In Stoll, B. A. (ed.) *Hormonal Management of Endocrine Related Cancer* (London: Lloyd Luke), p. 231

Chu, F. C. H. (1977). In Stoll, B. A. (ed.) *Breast Cancer Management – Early and Late* (London: Heinemann Medical), p. 101

Cutler, S. J., Asire, A. J. and Taylor, S. G. (1969). *Cancer*, **24**, 861

Davis, H. L. (1977). In Stoll, B. A. (ed.) *Breast Cancer Management – Early and Late* (London: Heinemann Medical), p. 185

Falkson, G., Falkson, H. G., Leone, L. *et al.* (1978). *Proc. Am. Soc. Clin. Oncol.*, **19**, 410

Mackay, W. D. (1975) In Stoll, B. A. (ed.) *Host Defence in Breast Cancer* (London: Heinemann Medical), p. 111

Minton, J. P. and Dickey, R. P. (1972). *Lancet*, **1**, 1069

Miller, T. and Spratt, J. S. (1980). In Stoll, B. A. (ed.) *Mind and Cancer Prognosis* (London: John Wiley and Sons), p. 31

Mueller, C. B. and Jeffries, W. (1975). *Ann. Sur.*, **182**, 334

Stoll, B. A. (1977). In Stoll, B. A. (ed.) *Breast Cancer Management – Early and Late* (London: Heinemann Medical), p. 133

Stoll, B. A. (1980). In Stoll, B. A. (ed.) *Systemic Therapy in Breast Cancer* (London: Heinemann Medical), p. 178

Tormey, D. C. and Neifeld, J. P. (1977). In Stoll, B. A. (ed.) *Breast Cancer Management – Early and Late* (London: Heinemann Medical), p. 117

Van der Slik, W., Persijn, J. P., Engelsman, E. and Riethorst, A. (1970). *Clin. Biochem.*, **3**, 59

Winchester, D. P., Sener, S. F., Khandekar, J. D. *et al.* (1979). *Cancer*, **43**, 956

7

The patient with lung cancer

F. E. Neal

Cancer of the lung is responsible for the majority of deaths from malignant disease and accounts for at least twice as many fatalities as cancer of the breast and malignant disease of the stomach. About 40 000 people die annually from this disease and there is little evidence that the mortality rate is falling. Because it is so common and usually follows a rapid and often distressing course, the disease produces situations which result in high-dependency patients who occupy much of the time of the caring professions. It is also interesting and surprising that one disease can produce such a plethora of symptoms and signs from patient to patient, even with identical primary tumours, and it is characterized by a variety of syndromes which may mimic other disease and lead to errors in diagnosis and treatment. Such a universally fatal disease will obviously present a problem for the attendant medical practitioner whether in the hospital or the community and it is a situation where, with the exception of that minority of patients who are amenable to radical treatment, the doctor is literally dealing with a dying patient from the moment of diagnosis. Progress in the treatment of cancer patients has unfortunately had little influence on the curability of lung cancer and there is little effective long-term treatment that can be offered, and often no treatment is the right treatment. In spite of this hopeless situation there is much to be done in the way of palliation, but it is fruitless to hope for more than the temporary relief of symptoms in all but a small percentage of patients. Such improvement is acceptable because the survival time is short.

The progress of this disease may be modified slightly by the histological type of tumour and by the clinical features at presentation, but generally the disease can be considered as one entity and much suffering can be

135

spared by a realistic appreciation of the problems, the natural history and the clinical peculiarities of the disease.

Although it is common, knowledge of the natural history and the survival rates is surprisingly limited, with the result that much excessive investigation and unnecessary treatment is often undertaken, unfortunately contributing to rather than alleviating patient suffering. Obviously there is an emotive problem, particularly where the younger patient is concerned, but it is important to accept that the facts are against survival and that satisfactory symptomatic control is all that is required. There are many other facets to the problem which cannot be pushed aside. Communication with the patient and family is of paramount importance, as is the frank discussion of the underlying management policy with members of the other caring professions.

GENERAL BACKGROUND

Bronchogenic carcinoma is *not* the only malignant disease which has failed to respond to modern methods of treatment, but the impact on the community is more pronounced because of its frequency and short clinical course. The 40 000 deaths from lung cancer recorded annually account for one-third of all the deaths from malignancy and 80 per cent of these sufferers are male. As with other malignancies the disease affects mainly the older age group, but there is a significant proportion of younger people who produce a particular emotional and management problem. Of all patients presenting with the disease, 20 per cent may be suitable for curative treatment by some form of surgery but the median survival time for all patients is less than 6 months, with a 5-year survival rate of 10 per cent. If the 20 per cent 'curable' group is excluded, the 5-year survival rate falls to 2 per cent.

The brunt of caring for these patients will rest with the general medical practitioner and he will need an experienced and understanding community team to help him provide the optimum care. Even allowing for the relative uncommonness of malignant disease in general practice, it is likely that there will be one or two patients requiring attention at any one time.

CLINICAL AND PATHOLOGICAL ASPECTS

There are several histological types of lung cancer, but detailed knowledge of the pathology is not essential as the clinical course is similar in the various tumour types, and although there are minor symptomatic variations the clinical course is usually determined by the anatomical position rather than histology.

The basic symptoms are those of chronic or acute respiratory disease with additional symptoms superimposed, which vary with the type and progress of the disease. The patient may present with a wide variety of problems, some of which at first sight may not suggest bronchogenic neoplasm. The anatomical site of the tumour is responsible for great variation in the symptoms, and the tumour arising centrally in the major bronchi will give rise to symptoms associated with bronchial obstruction long before the peripherally placed growth, which may reach a considerable size before making itself clinically manifest. The peripheral tumour may, however, produce early symptoms if the pleura is invaded and pain is a prominent problem. A small proportion of asymptomatic patients are discovered by routine radiography and this group may be suitable for radical treatment.

Presenting symptoms may be minimal, varying from a single episode or repeated attacks of acute respiratory infection, or the aggravation of existing symptoms of chronic bronchitis. Symptoms that are not progressive are often ignored and further delay in diagnosis results. In the older male, therefore, persistent new respiratory symptoms should always raise the suspicion of bronchogenic neoplasm, particularly if he is a heavy smoker. More disturbing symptoms like haemoptysis or hoarseness may be the initial problem, but the most dramatic presentation is that of sudden and devastating onset of superior vena caval obstruction in an otherwise fit patient. At the other extreme the unfortunate individual will present with severe respiratory symptoms or evidence of metastases and the illness will pursue a fulminating course. In all patients, whatever the stage of the primary tumour presentation, there may be widespread metastases in a variety of organs which may be obvious to the clinician but which may have been ignored or missed by the patient. There are usually chest symptoms as well but in some instances there is little evidence of local disease. It is not necessary to have a large primary tumour before metastases appear and there are sometimes bizarre and troublesome syndromes related to the ectopic hormone production without evidence of primary tumour. In spite of this variation in symptomatology, pain and haemoptysis are frequently the precipitating cause of an urgent consultation.

There is some variation in the length of history related to the histological types which are:

(1) adenocarcinoma;
(2) small-celled, anaplastic carcinoma;
(3) squamous-celled carcinoma;
(4) large-celled (giant cell) carcinoma.

Usually the most dramatic picture is produced by the small-celled (oat-celled) carcinoma which is rapidly growing and produces metastases at an early stage. Brain secondaries are common and may be responsible for the presenting symptoms. This tumour is radiosensitive but control is difficult because of its dissemination. The squamous-celled variety is very rare. Bronchogenic adenocarcinoma is relatively rare but commoner in females and is usually situated peripherally with subsequent delay in symptoms. The squamous-celled carcinoma is usually a central tumour and consequently presents at an early stage.

There are several generalized syndromes associated with lung cancer. Hypertrophic pulmonary osteoarthropathy is the best known and this can give intense pain in the small joints of the hands and feet, often with tenderness along the long bones of the lower arms and legs and swelling around the small joints of the hands and feet. This is not very common, but is a troublesome syndrome and difficult to deal with symptomatically although improvement may follow effective treatment of the primary tumour. Similar regression of symptoms may occur in the rarer neuropathies, myopathies and ectopic hormone effects which may be produced.

Whatever the mode of presentation and whichever histological category is involved, the disease is progressive except in that small group where effective curative surgery is indicated. With a short clinical course the terminal stages of the disease are reached rapidly, and as with other malignancies the manifestations of this period are variable. There is, however, normally a deterioration in general condition with increasing weight loss and lassitude and anorexia, eventually resulting in almost complete restriction of activity.

INVESTIGATION

Confirmation of the diagnosis is essential wherever possible since the exact definition of the tumour type may have some influence on the management of the patient, but it is also essential to confirm that a neoplasm is present because there are other conditions, especially in the younger age groups, which may mimic malignancy. Although the diagnosis can only be established absolutely by histological examination, in those patients where this is not possible there are investigations which provide circumstantial evidence. Once the possibility of a neoplasm has been raised, an attempt should be made to establish the diagnosis by the simplest means, bearing in mind that the patient may be quite ill. Complicated and time-consuming tests are not justified since it is desirable to spare the individual as much inconvenience as possible, and in some instances the confirmation of the diagnosis may be an unnecessary academic exercise. The diagnosis can usually be made by simple chest radiographs and additional information can be provided by sputum cytology, although this carries a high failure rate. Other investigations could include tomography, bronchography and CAT scanning if the appropriate apparatus is available. The great advantage of CAT scanning is that information is provided on the extent of the disease, as well as the actual diagnosis. Ultimately bronchoscopy or thoracotomy may be required if histological confirmation is essential. Bronchoscopy is a relatively simple procedure but it has limitations – mainly anatomical. Thoracotomy is only justified where an absolute diagnosis is essential, or where curative surgery is contemplated. In addition it may be important to have information on the presence of distant occult metastases, although this information may not have great influence on management as metastases may be presumed in many cases. This may be provided by means of skeletal radiographs, bone scans, liver scans and biochemical investigations. Such tests are justified if a radical treatment is planned, but seldom otherwise. Tests should be carried out as expeditiously as possible so that treatment may be instituted as necessary.

MANAGEMENT

Optimum management will be achieved if there is a realistic appreciation of the facts and it is essential to establish a definite policy which acknowledges the problems of this disease. Essentially management must be tailored to the individual patient's needs but the general intention should be the desire to provide the greatest good for the largest number of patients. Unfortunately those who present themselves for treatment are the problem patients, either recurrent after radical surgery, or with untreated disease requiring symptomatic and supportive treatment. The philosophy of approach is of paramount importance as most patients will be destined for a very short lifespan and treatment is unlikely to influence the length of survival. On the other hand a minority of the patients will be potentially curable and should not be deprived of this possibility. Radiotherapy is of proven value as a palliative treatment and cytotoxic drugs may also have a place in relieving symptoms, but the timing and extent of treatment requires careful thought. In these circumstances the underlying aim of treatment is to improve the quality of life and careful planning is required to ensure that symptoms are relieved and the treatment does not add to the patient's discomfort. The correct approach is therefore to provide minimal effective treatment without upset to the patient. There is no evidence that more prolonged and aggressive treatment has given enhanced symptomatic relief or longer survival. In order to provide optimum support it is important that all concerned in management accept this basic philosophy and this includes the relatives and the patient, and although the communication of these views to the relatives is often difficult, without their wholehearted cooperation it will be difficult to achieve good palliation. Although it is not possible to offer a cure it is important that hope is not abandoned, because good palliative support is an acceptable alternative. There is no need for a patient to be in discomfort no matter how advanced or progressive the disease.

PALLIATION

Palliation is essentially the relief of symptoms and can by definition be offered only if there are significant symptoms present. This is, therefore, one of those situations where no treatment may be the right treatment, and it is justifiable to await the onset of symptoms before embarking on any form of treatment.

Palliation falls into two distinct parts. Firstly there is the general support of the patient to help and relieve non-specific problems. This part of management, which is frequently badly carried out, may be the most important part of the treatment. Initially the need for general supportive treatment may be minimal because many patients with quite extensive disease are reasonably fit at the time of presentation. As the disease progresses they will need increasing support. It is important to provide adequate nutrition, antibiotics, sedatives, tranquillizers, anabolic steroids, antispasmodics, mucolytics and many other symptomatic measures, all of which provide a satisfactory base on which to graft the specific treatments which are needed to produce an acceptable quality of life.

SPECIAL SYMPTOMATIC PROBLEMS

Patients with bronchogenic carcinoma experience a great variety of symptoms so that it is impossible to be dogmatic about treatment and it is also essential to know which symptoms are likely to be relieved. An attempt has been made to deal with specific symptoms in order of importance.

Breathlessness
This is by far the commonest complaint, and may vary from slight dyspnoea on extreme exertion to marked distress, even with minimal movement, for instance, turning over in bed. The mechanism of the symptom is three-fold. Probably the commonest cause is a major airway obstructed by a large mass of tumour, which may be in the lumen or compressing it externally. In order to produce dyspnoea the tumour must impinge on one of the major bronchi or the lower trachea. Parenchymatous infiltration is not as common but produces a particularly troublesome breathlessness which progresses relentlessly and is difficult to relieve. Large effusions within the pleural cavity also give rise to breathlessness by reducing respiratory capacity but it is possible to give relief by aspiration of the fluid. Both the obstructive and parenchymatous problems may be accompanied by infection which in addition to causing a troublesome productive cough also contributes further to the breathlessness. It is usually possible to relieve the obstructive problems by irradiation, which is effective and can be localized. Treatment is of short duration and causes little upset. Cytotoxics have been used with good results but the side-effects are more pronounced. It is usually impossible to get relief from the parenchymatous infiltration but occasionally antibiotics and steroids may produce temporary improvement.

Pain
This is a particularly difficult problem. It may be associated with the primary tumour or with distant metastases and the mechanisms of pain production are so varied that it is difficult to give definite guidelines on management. The severity of pain can vary from the ill-defined tightness and discomfort associated with dyspnoea, which may be alleviated by the effective relief of breathlessness, to the severe pleuritic type pain due to pleural infiltration, or the pain associated with rib erosion or nerve damage. These different pains are difficult to control but it is sometimes

possible to achieve temporary relief by local irradiation or by cytotoxics, though often the pain persists in spite of such intervention. In these circumstances it is reasonable to use adequate analgesics, including opiates, even in the earlier stages of the disease. Pain control is frequently poorly executed and often there is delay in exhibiting analgesics of the right calibre because of the fear of addiction. Obviously such considerations are irrelevant when the natural history develops, and inadequate initial analgesia merely allows the pain problem to become firmly established with subsequent difficulty in obtaining relief. Simple analgesics should be tried, but if they fail to give relief they must be replaced by diamorphine or drugs of similar action, either alone or in combination with other agents to provide effective relief. There is no need for a patient to suffer pain; a pain-free patient is a more cooperative patient and future management will be facilitated.

It is also reasonable to use some form of nerve block or section if the appropriate facilities are easily available.

The pain due to distant metastases, usually in bone, is often an easier problem. The pain in long bones is rapidly relieved by short courses of irradiation and vertebral pain may often be controlled in the same way. Occasionally metastases in vertebral bodies have nerve compression as part of the pain component and in these circumstances the symptom is more persistent but bedrest and occasionally a supporting brace, may be helpful. Rarely – in patients in whom survival is likely to be prolonged – a laminectomy may be justified.

Distant metastases in less obvious sites do not often give rise to pain but hepatomegaly due to metastases can be painful and usually does not respond to specific measures. In these circumstances the correct management is suitable and adequate analgesia.

Haemoptysis

Whether in large or small amounts, this is a dramatic and worrying symptom, causing the patient great apprehension and consternation among the relatives, as with haemorrhage from any site. Even when the patient is extremely ill it is worthwhile attempting to control bleeding because it brings great relief and peace of mind. Control is usually permanent. Irradiation is particularly effective and control is rapid with minimal side-effects. Cytotoxics have also been used and have a place particularly in the patients where radiation tolerance has already been exceeded. Side-effects of cytotoxic treatment may be upsetting.

Cough

This is often a troublesome symptom but may not be produced primarily by the malignant process. It is usually a manifestation of infection or retained secretions resulting from obstructed airways. Relief of obstruction may help to relieve the symptom but it is usually necessary to use antibiotics as well.

The non-productive cough is more of a problem and usually results from the pressure of a tumour mass on the lower trachea or a major bronchus. It may also, unfortunately, be a sequel of irradiation therapy which produces dryness of the bronchial and tracheal mucosa. Treatment is difficult and often ineffective because it is impossible to relieve the irritation of the bronchus or trachea completely. Usually it is necessary to rely on purely symptomatic measures such as the sedative linctus or antibiotics because irradiation may not give relief and may make the problem worse. Steam inhalations are often useful and general physiotherapy with some postural drainage may help. Cytotoxics do not help.

Stridor

This is not a common symptom and can vary from a minor wheeze to the disturbing full-blown obstructive phenomenon which may require emergency or urgent treatment. It usually arises from encroachment of the growth on the lower bronchi or trachea with subsequent narrowing. Relief by removing the obstruction can usually be achieved by local irradiation or occasionally by means of cytotoxics, especially where the tumour is of the sensitive type.

Hoarseness

This gruffness or weakness of the voice is unfortunately a common symptom in patients with bronchogenic carcinoma. In a high proportion of patients it is often the presenting symptom and is one of the more distressing and frustrating aspects of the disease leading to increasing difficulty in communication. The patient is always anxious to know whether his voice will return to normal. Hoarseness is due to involvement of the recurrent laryngeal nerve as it passes round the arch of the aorta or through the upper mediastinum and it is usually impossible to reverse this troublesome nerve damage. Unfortunately, because there is an emotive problem, treatment is often given only to result in disappointment when the voice is unchanged. Obviously, in many circumstances hoarseness is only part of a group of symptoms and it is fortunate that the decision regarding treatment does not have to be made on this symptom alone. It is possible to inject teflon paste lateral to the paralysed vocal cord which moves medially as a result. This allows the mobile cord to approximate to the paralysed one and in some patients the hoarseness is relieved.

OTHER PROBLEMS

The other problems which arise in the management of the patient with lung cancer are either those due to local or distant spread, or to the many complications or associated syndromes which arise in this disease. In many instances the fundamental management is the treatment of the primary condition but there are other ways of helping and it is important to recognize the syndrome as part of this disease so that appropriate treatment can be given.

Lymphatic spread

Nodal metastases
These are an early manifestation of spread. Obviously the nodes most commonly involved are those in the mediastinum but it is also common to find enlarged nodes in the supraclavicular fossae and the lower cervical chains. Less commonly they can be found in the upper para-aortic group of nodes and in the axillae. In all sites they may, unfortunately, give rise to troublesome problems. Usually there is some pain and pressure effects may be produced. Obviously enlarged nodes in the more critical anatomical sites will be responsible for increasingly severe symptoms and the most dramatic situation is the production of the superior vena caval obstruction due to rapidly enlarging nodes in the upper part of the chest and pressure upon the major vessels. The resulting oedema of the head, neck, upper limbs and trunk, accompanied by increasing breathlessness and a feeling of constriction, is very distressing. The skin assumes a dusky, plethoric tint and there are usually grossly dilated veins in the neck with leashes of tiny vessels in the skin of the chest wall, demonstrating an attempt to establish a collateral circulation. The severity of the syndrome may vary from a situation of intermittent swelling of the head and neck to a rapidly progressive and disturbing bloatedness of the upper trunk. In all circumstances there is a troublesome cerebral anoxia. Fortunately patients who develop this syndrome are usually suffering from the more rapid form of lung cancer and therefore with such sensitive tumours there is a dramatic response to irradiation or cytotoxics. It is satisfying, therefore, to see a patient's symptoms relieved after relatively simple treatment, often

within hours. In a small proportion of patients the oedema will not subside because of thrombosis of the superior vena cava either due to prolonged pressure and venous stasis or because of invasion of the lumen of the vessel by tumour. In these circumstances it is usually impossible to relieve the symptoms, and although the use of anticoagulants has been advocated they are seldom of much value.

Nodal metastases in the mediastinum
These can be responsible for difficulties with swallowing, although this symptom may also be due to direct invasion of the oesophagus by the primary tumour. Fortunately this is not common but it is extremely distressing when it is progressive. In these circumstances where there is a sensitive tumour type, relief may be obtained by local irradiation or cytotoxics, but with the slower progressing lesions there is great difficulty in relieving the pressure effects by this means. In this event it may be justifiable to insert some form of feeding tube, such as Mousseau Barbin or Celestin tube, through the obstruction in order to re-establish a reasonably normal swallowing mechanism. Such intervention would have to be carefully considered in the context of the patient's general condition and the likely prognosis.

Cervical and supraclavicular nodes
These are usually troublesome because of their proximity to major nerve pathways. Pressure on the trunks of the cervical and brachial plexuses can give rise to intractable pain and motor changes in the upper arm – it is also likely that a troublesome Horner's syndrome may be produced because of involvement of the cervical sympathetic. Unfortunately these symptoms are difficult to relieve and pain, once established, is often not relieved although there may be regression of the tumour mass. As in other sites, response will depend upon the histological type of tumour but the more slowly growing cancer tends to be relatively resistant to cytotoxics and irradiation, and there will usually be residual disease in the treated site after treatment has been completed. Pain relief in these circumstances must be achieved by some form of nerve block or section.

Similar symptomatology is produced by the Pancoast syndrome which results from the extension of a tumour arising in the apex of the upper lobe which erodes the upper ribs and causes intense pain, partly by the bone destruction and partly due to nerve involvement. This pain is also difficult to relieve and does not respond well to treatment by cytotoxics and irradiation.

Nodal metastases in the neck
Occasionally these may produce local symptoms due to mechanical interference within the upper respiratory and alimentary passages. Treatment
by cytotoxics or irradiation in the sensitive tumours will usually provide
relief.

Secondary involvement of the brain
This is not uncommon in the natural history of the oat-cell carcinoma of
the bronchus. Symptoms from such metastases vary considerably from
minor personality changes to episodes of focal epilepsy and the progressive
features of increased cranial pressure. The high incidence of metastases in
this sanctuary area has led some authorities to suggest prophylactic
irradiation to the brain at the time of primary treatment. There is evidence
to suggest that this manoeuvre may increase survival time but so far it has
not been shown to increase survival rate. Brain metastases are protected
from the action of cytotoxic agents (with the exception of the nitrosoureas)
by the blood–brain barrier and effective treatment has to be by irradiation
which unfortunately produces complete epilation of the scalp. This must
be borne in mind when considering the advisability of irradiation in a
patient who is approaching the terminal stages of the disease.

   Where there is intracranial pressure the non-specific use of high doses of
dexamethasone is usually dramatic in relieving symptoms and this
effective simple measure may be all that is required to tide the patient over
the acute episode. Following such treatment there may be no need for
further intervention. In some patients with a localized neurological deficit
rehabilitation along the lines usually provided following a CVA may
produce great symptomatic improvement, so that suitable supportive
measures, and particularly simple physiotherapy, are often of great
psychological value. Obviously it is impossible to describe all the various
symptoms which may arise from cerebral metastases and management
must depend upon the impact of the symptoms and the general condition
of the patient.

   It is interesting that the presence of cerebral metastases does not always
predict a rapid demise – patients may sometimes survive for months in
spite of obvious metastases in this vital organ.

Skin metastases
These are common in the more anaplastic and rapidly growing lung
cancers. They are usually more troublesome because of their appearance

and number rather than the unpleasant effects which they produce. The usual clinical appearance is of multiple tiny pea-size nodules distributed widely over the skin of the body. They are usually painless unless they reach a large size, and if they do continue to grow they may ulcerate and become infected. Usually the indication is for some form of cytotoxic therapy but the response may only be minimal, even in sensitive tumours.

Bone metastases

Bone is often the site of metastases in lung cancer and the symptomatology of such lesions will be related to the anatomical site and the proximity of vital structures. Symptoms are often produced by lesions in the bodies of the vertebrae and sacroiliac joints, and also the long bones. It was noted earlier that pain must be a prominent feature of such metastatic deposits and this is usually of chronic, nagging character which may be relieved by rest, but may be persistent and difficult to control with drugs.

Spinal metastases are often associated with pain on movement and increasing stiffness of the spine, with rigidity and loss of the lumbar lordosis. Long bone metastases give rise to similar intractable pain and also may be the site of pathological fractures. Treatment will depend on the severity of the symptoms and the general condition of the patient but since there is such difficulty in controlling this type of pain with analgesics, it is usually necessary to resort to some other form of management. Non-mechanical pain in vertebrae or long bones can usually and rapidly be controlled by means of local irradiation. Treatment causes little upset and relief is often rapid. Mechanical pain due to joint involvement or pathological fracture usually requires orthopaedic intervention, but it may be possible to achieve pain relief by complete bedrest if the spinal and pelvic bones are involved. Pain relief may then be maintained by the use of a brace when the patient is mobilized. Pathological fractures should be dealt with by traction or internal fixation, depending upon the site and condition of the patient. If these measures fail and analgesics are not entirely adequate, it is possible to use a nerve block or section.

The particular character of bone pain makes it difficult to control, even with the stronger analgesics which are used for pain control in malignancy. More effective pain relief can usually be obtained by using simpler drugs particularly of the antirheumatic type, which deal effectively with this chronic pain and may be augmented with the relaxants like diazepam (Valium). If control can be achieved by such simple measures it may not be necessary to resort to the more complicated procedures.

The presence of widespread bony metastases should always raise the possibility of hypercalcaemia which is much more common than was formerly recognized. The hypercalcaemia in carcinoma of the bronchus is more often due to hormonal effects than to multiple metastases but the management is similar in both situations.

The most difficult problem associated with the presence of bone metastases is the occurrence of major neurological damage due to pressure on the spinal cord or the major nerve tracks. Such damage, usually associated with vertebral collapse, leads to at least paresis but more commonly paraplegia or quadraplegia, depending upon the site of the damage. The onset of such symptoms may be dramatic, occurring over hours or days, but occasionally may develop much more slowly. There is also a second mechanism producing nerve damage, the presence of intrathecal metastases which enlarge or constrict the spinal cord.

Management of these patients is difficult and depends on the age of the block as well as the general condition of the patient. Obviously in the patient who is approaching the terminal stages of the disease there is little to do apart from adopting symptomatic measures. In the fitter patient it may be necessary to make a decision on the advisability of laminectomy but this should only be considered if the neurological damage is less than 48 hours duration, since it is unusual to achieve recovery of nervous tissue after that length of time. In favourable circumstances, therefore, laminectomy should be seriously considered because it usually results in relief of the neurological signs and the patient can be mobilized. In the more extreme situations it eases the nursing problems in those patients who are confined to bed. Where the patient is already hemiplegic, para-plegic or quadraplegic it has to be accepted that permanent nursing has to be undertaken and in these circumstances there is no indication for local irradiation unless pain continues to be a prominent factor. Local irradiation is sometimes a useful treatment in patients with intrathecal deposits since it may cause regression of the tumour mass and relieve symptoms without laminectomy, but this is a rare situation.

Myopathies, neuropathies and encephalopathies
Various types of these may accompany the progressive symptoms of bronchogenic carcinoma. The symptoms and signs from these syndromes are bizarre and variable and it is impossible to be dogmatic about their occurrence or progress. Improvement may follow the treatment to the primary lesion or metastases, but often management has to be purely symptomatic. It is not possible to correlate the severity of the symptoms with the extent of the malignant process.

Ectopic hormones

As with some other forms of malignancy, bronchogenic carcinoma may produce ectopic hormones which lead to a variety of clinical syndromes. The two prominent problems are those associated with the production of antidiuretic hormone leading to the inappropriate syndrome (IADH) and the parathormone-like substance producing hypercalcaemia. These secretions are usually associated with the small-celled carcinomas of bronchus, and symptoms resulting from ectopic production of ACTH, melanogen-stimulating hormone, and chorionic gonadotrophin have also been recorded. They are rare, and it is common for the biochemical abnormalities to precede the clinical problems.

The treatment of the hypercalcaemia is important since the symptoms are distressing but may be reversible. The clinical signs which suggest the diagnosis are polydypsia, disorientation, drowsiness and often coma. Recognition of the syndrome at an early stage means that simple treatment may be effective before the situation becomes too advanced. Simple measures with rehydration and appropriate amounts of steroids often produce dramatic results and clinical improvement usually precedes the restoration of normal blood chemistry. If this fails, more upsetting treatment is justified using phosphates or mithramycin. Unfortunately although it is possible to achieve symptomatic relief the syndrome ultimately recurs and is uncontrollable.

Hepatic metastases

Reference has already been made to hepatic metastases and the pain which may arise from them. Fortunately such secondaries only appear in the later stages of the disease and treatment does not have to be considered in isolation from other symptoms. The appearance of overt hepatic extension is a grave prognostic sign but occult metastases are probably present in the early stages of the disease and it is relevant that a considerable proportion of the liver needs to be involved before signs of liver malfunction appear. The gross distension which accompanies the development of these metastases causes a particularly unpleasant type of pain due to stretching of the capsule and it is extremely difficult to achieve relief. Normally irradiation and cytotoxics are of little value and it is necessary to resort to symptomatic measures. An additional problem associated with liver involvement is the production of ascites due to pressure on the inferior vena cava. The earliest method of achieving relief is by simple tapping but occasionally irradiation of the porta hepatis or systemic cytotoxics may be of value.

Cardiac involvement

This is rare but can be troublesome. Depending on the anatomical site of the tumour, a variety of syndromes may be produced. Pericardial effusion is not uncommon and may lead to disturbances of cardiac function. Fortunately aspiration is a relatively easy method of relieving the situation if the problem can be recognized early. Deposits within the myocardium and particularly those within the vicinity of the conducting tissue, lead to a variety of bizarre arrhythmias and are extremely difficult to control. Usually symptomatic measures alone are the main method of treatment.

Pleural effusions

These often arise in the progressive disease, either because of pressure on a major vessel or more commonly because of an exudate from the pleural surfaces involved by nodules seeded from the original primary site. Effusions are troublesome, producing breathlessness, and often aggravate dyspnoea arising from parenchymatous infiltration or collapse. Relief is obviously achieved by aspiration, but repeated aspirations are depressing and unpleasant and eventually result in loculation with subsequent difficulty in emptying the pleural cavity. Local irradiation or cytotoxics may reduce the size of a large mass blocking a major vessel but the exudative type of effusion is best treated by intracavitary radioactive gold (^{198}Au) or yttrium (^{90}Y), or a suitable cytotoxic agent – usually nitrogen mustard (mustine hydrochloride). The latter is preferable because it does not involve radiation hazards. The treatment is simple and effective in approximately 50 per cent of patients.

This symptomatology demonstrates the many and varied clinical problems which may arise in the patient with bronchogenic carcinoma. Obviously the rarities have been included as well as the common presentations, but it is essential to understand that with such a spectrum of symptoms any new development should be regarded as part of the basic pathological process until proved otherwise. A knowledge of the various clinical presentations will also enable the clinician to make a clinical diagnosis and institute the appropriate therapy without recourse to complicated, disturbing and expensive tests. These diagnoses can and should be made by the general medical practitioner and save the patient a journey to the outpatient department or admission to hospital.

TREATMENT

Accepting that the general policy should be to provide treatment only when there are significant symptoms, it is essential to examine the type of treatment available.

Radiation therapy and cytotoxic therapy

Radiation therapy is the mainstay of palliative management but there is a definite place for the cytotoxic drugs. There is no single method of delivering radiation therapy and the particular method will depend on the specific clinical problem. These patients have a short lifespan and therefore treatment should be as short as possible and should produce very little in the way of side-effects. Most symptoms, whether related to the primary tumour or metastases, can be dealt with by means of a short course of megavoltage or orthovoltage irradiation, using a simple arrangement of fields. This is completed within 2 weeks at the most, and provided the patient is fit he may attend daily as an outpatient.

Cytotoxic therapy varies from the use of a single agent to the more popular multiple-drug regimes. Some single-agent therapy, particularly cyclophosphamide, may be given on an outpatient basis, and is well tolerated either orally or by injection. Most multiple-drug regimes require hospital admission and are given on a cyclical basis which requires repeated attendances. As with radiation therapy, it is not possible to give definite treatment regimes because there are so many varieties.

Both forms of therapy have significant and unpleasant side-effects. Both produce anorexia, nausea and vomiting and there may be dysphagia with irradiation due to oesophagitis, and epilation and oral ulceration due to the cytotoxic agents. It is not easy to make a choice between their untoward effects but it is important to remember that cytotoxic regimes mean repeated admissions and cause alopecia, and this would seem to be a distressing regime for a dying patient. In the last analysis, however, if significant symptoms are present it is essential to use the most appropriate form of therapy, but to ensure that the upset is kept to a minimum.

It is impossible to lay down dogmatic guidelines for the management of these patients. Obviously treatment will have to be tailored to the type of tumour and to the clinical course which unfolds. In view of the poor prognosis, however, and the fact that treatment does not influence survival, it is important to treat only when symptoms become difficult or troublesome. Care should be community-based wherever possible but traditionally such patients have been referred to hospital for opinion, and once the diagnosis has been established they have proceeded to treatment and remained on follow-up until the terminal stages of the disease. Obviously there are situations where this is desirable but the well-informed general medical practitioner, with the support of an under-standing and clinically alert community team, should be able to provide more care than the hospital for a variety of reasons.

In addition to the clinical problem there is also the great psychological problem of communication with the patient and relatives and this is much better done in the community than in hospital, and is an important point in improving the quality of life.

For the foreseeable future the lung cancer sufferer will continue to present a problem of management because with our present knowledge we can only expect to see a fall in incidence as cigarette smoking comes under control. Frustrating and distressing as the management of these patients would appear to be at first sight, there is no doubt that provided that there is a comprehensive understanding of the complex disease with its short natural history and relative resistance to all methods of modern treatment, the management of the patient can be extremely rewarding for all concerned. With the right sort of approach it is possible to achieve a symptom-free patient enjoying a reasonable, if not excellent, quality of life until the onset of what should be a short and controlled terminal illness.

8

Palliation of malignant disease of the gastrointestinal tract

John R. Bennett and Peter W. R. Lee

Determining the extent to which palliation should be employed in a patient when malignant disease is clearly killing him is difficult because, although the difficulty and discomfort of the palliative procedure is clinically predictable, the rate of advance of the disease, the likelihood of certain complications arising before other factors cause the patient's death, and the amount of distress likely to be caused by those complications to the patient and those caring for him, can be estimated only approximately. The problem is particularly great where the palliative procedure is surgical. Fortunately new techniques, particularly endoscopic ones, are replacing some surgical operations.

MECHANICAL OBSTRUCTION

Malignant neoplasms will eventually obstruct that part of the alimentary tube in which they grow, late in their course in capacious segments like the caecum, but early in the bile ducts or pylorus. Palliation may be by resection, surgical bypass, intubation, or reduction of the tumour by radiation or chemotherapy.

Oesophagus
The first symptoms of carcinoma of oesophagus or cardia frequently occur when the tumour is advanced, because dysphagia only occurs when about two-thirds of the circumference has been involved. This means that progress to complete dysphagia often follows soon after the first symptom.

Nutrition suffers quickly, and eventually even fluids cannot be swallowed. Palliation can be offered in several ways:

(1) palliative extirpation;
(2) repeated dilatation;
(3) operative intubation;
(4) endoscopic intubation;
(5) feeding intubation;
(6) gastrostomy;
(7) irradiation.

Palliative extirpation
Some surgeons, notably McKeown (1972), believe that the best palliation is achieved by radical surgery, and demonstrate that enthusiastic and intensive care, with particular attention to nutrition preoperatively, may reduce operative mortality to 12 per cent.

It is reasonable that, where operability or even cure is possible, a full-blooded attempt should be made, and resection may be performed even if curability is thought impossible at the time of surgery. However, if the patient clearly cannot be cured, not only is surgery expensive in medical resources, but the procedure gives the patient discomfort and anxiety (and, perhaps, hope) which are not justified.

Repeated dilatation
It is possible to restore swallowing temporarily by bougie dilatation of the malignant stricture, and this can be repeated in order to maintain adequate nutrition (Heit *et al.*, 1978). The disadvantages of this technique is that dilatation needs to be done frequently – sometimes as often as once a week – with the associated discomfort and the repeated risk of instrument perforation. If dilatation of a long, malignant stricture is carried out, the hazard of instrument perforation is best avoided by using the Eder–Puestow dilators with a wire guide to keep the bougies in the lumen (Price, Stanciu, and Bennett, 1974).

Operative intubation
Attempts have been made for 50 years to maintain patency of the oesophageal lumen by inserting tubes.

In recent years the most popular technique has been to introduce either the Mousseau–Barbin or Celestin tube by laparotomy and gastrostomy. The tube is pulled into place from below, sutured to the gastric wall to prevent proximal displacement, and the wound closed. Relief of dysphagia is good, semi-solids and minced food being swallowed easily. Unfortunately, although the operation is relatively minor, the morbidity and mortality are formidable, mainly because of infection in the malnourished patients (Amman and Collis, 1971; Johnson, Balfour, and Bourke, 1976).

Feeding intubation

Permanent placement of a wide tube by the endoscopic techniques (see below) is the best palliation (short of extirpation) for an obstructed gullet because it allows ingestion of near-normal food and drink, with an acceptably low morbidity and mortality, and with little patient discomfort. This may not be possible, perhaps because the growth extends too far distally in the stomach, or because the patient's frailty makes it unwise. It may still be possible to insert a fine feeding tube of the Stoke Mandeville type. This is a radio-opaque polyethylene tube of 1 mm internal diameter provided with a stiffening wire which can be guided through a narrow lumen under radiological screening. Liquid diet can then be given by drip or using a simple portable pump.

Gastrostomy

If a laparotomy is carried out and palliative excision is impossible it is worth attempting the operative insertion of a Mousseau–Barbin or Celestin tube via a gastrostomy. Should this prove technically impossible then the tumour is better considered inoperable and no further procedure performed. Gastrostomy as a definitive procedure is not acceptable because it does not restore swallowing or prevent the distressing respiratory problems due to spill over of mucus and food.

Endoscopic intubation

To reduce the hazards of introducing a tube through a constricting tumour, methods have been devised to accomplish this by endoscopic techniques. Atkinson and Ferguson (1977) devised an instrument with which an armoured latex tube could be placed into a previously dilated tumour. This is now sold as the Nottingham introducer (KeyMed Limited, Southend) (Atkinson, 1980).

Using either diazepam sedation or general anaesthesia (according to the general condition and nervousness of the patient) the constricting growth is dilated (to 45–50 French) using Eder–Puestow dilating bougies over a guide-wire (Price, Stanciu, and Bennett, 1974). The length of the stricture is assessed by passing the endoscope through it. A Celestin tube cut to appropriate length or an Atkinson tube (KeyMed Limited) is then held on the staff of the Nottingham introducer by an expandable plastic bobbin which slides over the guide-wire, a 'rammer' assisting by pressure from behind. The well-lubricated tube with the introducing device is slid over the guide-wire into the lesion under radiological control. When the tube is firmly in place the introducer is released and withdrawn followed by the rammer and the guide-wire.

A lateral chest radiograph next morning confirms that the tube remains in position. The patient may then eat and drink relatively freely. Large solid boluses need to be avoided, food must be chewed well, and frequent effervescent drinks taken to wash debris from the tube.

Perforation may occur at the time of intubation – in up to 8–10 per cent – but this can be managed conservatively. Later perforation, due to tube erosion, has occurred occasionally.

The technique is useful when there is tracheo-oesophageal fistula, the tube effectively sealing the fistula.

Two alternative systems for introducing Celestin tubes have been devised by Roger Celestin (personal communication). In the first of these, a latex 'rammer' slides over an endoscope introduced into the dilated malignant stricture, driving a Celestin tube into place before it. In the second a stiff plastic mandril holds the Celestin tube by an inflatable balloon, the device sliding over a guide-wire. Results of this technique are not so far published.

Radiation

For squamous carcinoma of the oesophagus irradiation offers the possibility of rapid reduction in size and restoration of swallowing; 4500–6000 r is given. There may be a 2–3 week delay in improvement because of oedema and swelling of the tumour, and the prior insertion of a feeding tube or a Celestin tube may be advisable. Adenocarcinoma responds less well because it arises in the gastric fundus which is less accessible to irradiation than the intrathoracic oesophagus.

Stomach

Carcinoma of fundus

Fundal carcinoma often causes dysphagia by infiltration of the cardia. This may best be palliated by endoscopic intubation (see above) provided the growth does not extend too far distally into the body of the stomach.

For polypoid tumours not causing dysphagia, resection probably offers the best palliation, reducing the likelihood of bleeding and anaemia, and allowing the patient to eat.

Body of stomach

The symptoms of advanced gastric carcinoma – anorexia, vomiting, pain, and cachexia – are so unpleasant that palliative resection (short of total gastrectomy) is justified if at all practicable (Lawrence, 1976). Radiation and chemotherapy have been used, but as even the most optimistic reports show only slight benefit, it does not seem justified.

Vomiting in gastric malignancy may be due to diminished capacity and loss of compliance, rather than to total obstruction. A change from standard meals to a continual 'sipping' regimen often helps, using a liquid or semi-solid diet. Palatability is important, and while homemade liquid diets (based on Casilan or Complan) are economical, proprietary 'build-ups' (such as Carnation foods) are often preferred by patients. If the patient is too weak to keep up a sipping regimen, a slow continuous flow of nutrition through a 1 mm feeding tube often helps.

Pylorus and antrum

Neoplasms of the antrum and pylorus are best treated by distal gastrectomy whenever possible. Although technically simpler the results of gastroenterostomy alone as a means of palliation are disappointing; abdominal discomfort, nausea and vomiting continue to be a problem after the operation (Griffin, Humphrey, and Sosin, 1969). If the tumour is too extensive to allow safe distal gastrectomy, then gastroenterostomy with antral exclusion should be considered. This procedure, by diverting the food flow away from the tumour, allows the inflammation to subside and the remaining stomach digests better with less regurgitation.

Carcinoma of the colon

Neoplasms of the colon should be removed whenever possible; there is little place for bypass procedures, or colostomy alone. The presence of lung or liver lesions is not a contraindication to resection. A conservative resection with end-to-end anastomosis in one stage should be carried out where there is evidence of distal spread.

Solitary metastases of the liver from large bowel tumours are amenable to resection with improved survival times (Blumgart, 1980). It must be emphasized, however, that such solitary lesions are rare, and preoperative assessment with hepatic arteriograms, liver scan and ultrasound is essential. There seems at present to be little evidence that intraoperative perfusion with chemotherapeutic agents is of benefit in advanced colorectal cancer with liver metastases (Taylor, 1978).

Carcinoma of the colon presenting with obstruction
Intestinal obstruction is commonly the presenting feature of large bowel cancer in the elderly. The conventional management of defunctioning colostomy followed by staged resection and closure of colostomy has now been challenged. Fielding, Stewart-Brown, and Blesovsky (1979) have shown that primary tumour resection has a similar mortality to the staged resection with half the duration of stay in hospital, provided the operation is performed by an experienced surgeon. The place of total colectomy and ileorectal anastomosis for obstructing left-sided neoplasms, which avoids an anastomosis involving grossly dilated ends of bowel, is at present under evaluation.

Carcinoma of the rectum

Except in the very old or grossly medically unfit, neoplasms of the rectum should be resected whenever possible. The pain, bleeding and discharge associated with a lesion left *in situ* (with either defunctioning or end colostomy) is not acceptable as palliation. With the advent of the circular stapling instrument (Goligher *et al.*, 1979; Heald, 1980), many lesions previously requiring abdominoperineal resection (with the consequent problems of colostomy management in the elderly) can now be resected and a sphincter-saving anastomosis performed. As with cancer of the colon, liver and lung metastases are not a contraindication to resection.

In the elderly and unfit, especially those patients in whom distal spread has been confirmed by ultrasound and laparoscopy, some form of local resection is more appropriate. Better palliation is achieved by electro-coagulation (Madden and Kandalaft, 1971) than cryosurgery, although some groups favour the latter (Osborne, Higgins, and Hobbs, 1978).

Severe discomfort can arise from local pelvic recurrence; it is rare for further surgery to be helpful but a course of local radiotherapy may be of benefit in alleviating pain (Williams, Shulman, and Todd, 1957). Infrequently it may be necessary to employ intrathecal alcohol or phenol injections or even chordotomy in those cases with tumour involving the sacral plexus of nerves with resulting severe sacral, perineal or sciatic pain (Robbie, 1969; O'Connell, 1969).

Squamous carcinoma of anal canal

If the patient is sufficiently fit to tolerate the operation and is capable of colostomy management, then the most satisfactory palliation for squamous carcinoma of the anal canal is abdominoperineal excision of the rectum (Beahrs and Wilson, 1976; Stearns and Quan, 1970). This procedure not only relieves the patient of his symptoms completely but also gives a better chance of long-term survival.

In the elderly or medically unfit, some palliation can be offered for even the most advanced lesion by local excision or diathermy followed by radiotherapy. Papillon (1974) has claimed excellent results (for both palliation and attempted cure) from the use of interstitial Curie therapy by the local implantation of radium needles.

Obstructive jaundice

The symptom associated with obstructive jaundice which gives most distress is pruritus. Relief of the obstruction is the best palliation, but if this cannot be done, or while waiting for the procedure, some help may be obtained from the bile-salt binding resin cholestyramine. This is most effective where obstruction is incomplete. It is unpalatable, but the preparation Questran (Bristol, Slough) is tolerated by most patients in doses up to 4 g four times daily. Steatorrhoea is made worse because of inactivation of the bile-salts, and reduction of fat intake may help if the patient has diarrhoea.

Methyltestosterone, 25 mg sublingually, relieves itching, as does norethandrolone 10 mg twice daily by mouth. Both drugs *increase* jaundice because they cause cholestasis, but they are useful when biliary obstruction is complete. Norethandrolone is preferred for women as its masculinizing effects are less marked.

If biliary obstruction is prolonged, vitamin K malabsorption may lead to spontaneous haemorrhage. This can be quickly corrected by parenteral vitamin K, followed by a maintenance dose of 10 mg i.m. each week.

A possibility not to be overlooked is that drugs, rather than malignancy, may be the cause of obstruction. Chlorpromazine is the most likely culprit, and jaundice will diminish if the drug is stopped.

Intrahepatic metastases

Obstructive jaundice sometimes results from multiple small hepatic metastases. Nothing useful can be done to relieve this mechanically.

Chemotherapy by hepatic artery perfusion is a possibility, but the likely gain rarely justifies the patient's discomfort and the expense.

Carcinoma of the bile ducts

Tumour of distal end of common bile duct

Surgery – If possible this tumour should be resected by performing a pancreaticoduodenectomy. If this is not possible, palliation can be produced by local diathermy excision of the tumour via a transduodenal approach. An alternative is division of the common bile duct proximal to the tumour with anastomosis to a loop of jejunum to form a choledochojejunostomy.

Operative dilatation and intubation of the malignant stricture – The common bile duct is opened and the stricture gradually dilated using increasing sizes of Bake's dilators. A silastic tube is then placed through the stricture by drawing it through the liver substance from outside to inside in the dilated hepatic ducts (Knight and Smith, 1977).

Niloff (1972) described a special vitallium prosthesis to be inserted after dilating the growth with Bake's dilators, and Terblanche and Louw (1973) favour a U-tube pulled into the stricture from the outside surface of the liver (Terblanche, Saunders, and Louw, 1972).

Carcinoma of the hepatic duct

Primary carcinoma of the hepatic duct, or at the junction of the two hepatic ducts is an uncommon but difficult cause of obstructive jaundice. Resection is usually impossible, but the tumour may be slow-growing so that relief of obstruction may produce useful palliation. The following techniques have all been used.

Intrahepatic cholangiocholecystostomy – This procedure is an alternative to palliative dilatation and transhepatic intubation. For the procedure to be performed the gallbladder and common bile duct must be normal and the junction of these two well below the porta hepatis. The gallbladder is anastomosed side to side to a dilated intrahepatic duct.

If the gallbladder is unsuitable for this procedure, or the tumour is encroaching on the common bile duct, then an alternative is to create a Roux loop of jejunum and anastomose this to the dilated intrahepatic duct (Knight and Smith, 1977).

Percutaneous transhepatic procedures – The dilated bile ducts proximal to an obstruction may readily be cannulated by a needle, or trocar and a cannula passed percutaneously into the liver under local anaesthesia. For diagnostic purposes the favoured technique currently uses the slender Chiba needle (Okuda *et al.*, 1974). This will drain bile only slowly, and for most manipulations larger cannulae are used, though the initial diagnostic radiology may be done with a Chiba needle first.

Simple drainage. A thin polyethylene catheter may be introduced over a 13 cm No 18 needle, the needle withdrawn and a guide-wire placed into the catheter which is then withdrawn. The wire then serves as a guide for a drainage catheter (such as Kifa green 1.22 mm ID) with several side holes to be placed in the dilated duct (Mori *et al.*, 1977; Tylen, Hoevels, and Varg, 1977). This is only suitable for short periods of drainage; bile tends to leak around the catheter and there may be pain at the catheter site.

Cannulation of the stricture – Pereiras *et al.* (1978) described a technique in which a 0.635 mm guide-wire is passed *through* the stricture enabling the standard percutaneous cholangiogram Teflon sheath to pass through the stricture. A thicker guide-wire (0.965 mm) replaces the thinner one, and then an 8 French Teflon catheter is passed through the stricture. Over this whole assembly a larger Teflon catheter (12 French) is advanced to dilate the stricture. After withdrawing this a prosthesis is created from the Teflon 12 French tubing with a flared proximal end, and placed in position, pushed by a catheter. Such prostheses have lasted with good drainage up to 20 weeks.

A similar technique in which a polyethylene catheter was inserted over a wire without prior dilatation (Burcharth, 1978) had a higher failure rate.

Carcinoma of the head of the pancreas
The most effective form of palliation is removal of the tumour; provided the patient can tolerate the operation then resection, either by a pancreatic-duodenectomy (Whipple's operation) or total pancreatectomy, should be considered in every patient in whom the carcinoma has not invaded the wall of the portal vein (Smith, 1978). If resection is not possible then some form of palliation is usually indicated for the following reasons.

Relief of obstructive jaundice – Biliary bypass is best achieved by cholangiojejunostomy either in the form of a Roux loop or as a simple jejunal loop with enteroanastomosis below it. Spread of tumour may make this operation technically impossible. A variety of ingenious manoeuvres have been used to create a bypass using substitutes for the bile duct such as ureter, vein, artery, nylon mesh, teflon or dacron.

Relief of duodenal obstruction – Occasionally the tumour is found to be obstructing the duodenum at the time of operation and certainly the possibility of such obstruction developing later must be considered. Gastroenterostomy should, therefore, be performed, in addition to any other procedure.

Pancreatic pain – Proximal obstruction of the pancreatic duct by the tumour is responsible for some cases of pancreatic pain. The body of the pancreas can be incised distal to the tumour and decompression provided by T-tube drainage of the main pancreatic duct into either the stomach or the jejunum.

Cancer of the body and tail of pancreas
The resectability and long-term survival rate of such tumours is so poor as to lead some surgeons to recommend avoiding laparotomy if the diagnosis is certain. Palliation can be provided by chemotherapy via the coeliac artery and is indicated for persistent pancreatic pain. The place of combined chemotherapy and radiotherapy is currently under study.

Steatorrhoea in pancreatic carcinoma
Fat malabsorption due to lack of pancreatic enzymes leads to steatorrhoea, which may cause distress because of frequent, loose stools or because of their offensiveness. Although the addition of pancreatic enzymes supplements (such as Pancrex, Nutrizym) seems the logical treatment – and may help – they may further inhibit an already jaded appetite. Reduction of the fat content of the diet to 40–50 g daily is often as effective and more acceptable to the patient.

Multiple intestinal obstruction
Metastatic malignancy affecting the peritoneum, or primary mesothelioma, may eventually result in multiple sites of intestinal obstruction. These are not amenable to surgical relief because of their multiplicity, but obstruction is often incomplete, allowing benefit to be obtained from the

use of low-fibre diets (Clinifeed, Vivonex, Trisorbon), sometimes given by the 1 mm enteral tube technique so that the rate of infusion may be slow enough, spread over 24 hours, to allow assimilation without the volume causing obstructive symptoms.

NON-OBSTRUCTIVE PROBLEMS

Primary hepatoma

Attempts at palliation of primary hepatocellular carcinoma are worthwhile, provided that coexisting cirrhosis is not so severe that any direct therapy to the liver will result in hepatocellular failure.

Hepatic artery ligation (Almersjö *et al.*, 1972; Balasegeram, 1977) (because hepatomas are supplied direct by the artery) does not produce good results. Infusion of 5-fluorouracil into the hepatic artery has met with more success, and ligation can be combined with chemotherapeutic infusion (Fortner *et al.*, 1973). These procedures necessitate laparotomy, and the treatment may be complicated by hepatocellular failure, haemorrhage from the catheter, or alimentary bleeding.

The advent of doxorubicin (Adriamycin) may make direct attack on the liver unnecessary. There have been good reports of remission obtained by intravenous infusions of 60 mg/m^2 at 3-weekly intervals to a total of 550 mg/m^2. White cell counts and electrocardiograms must be carried out before each infusion because of the high risk of cardiotoxicity. Response may be followed by falling fetoprotein levels (Johnson *et al.*, 1978; Olweny *et al.*, 1976; Tormey *et al.*, 1973).

Secondary carcinoma of liver

Evidence that any therapy usefully prolongs survival or improves the quality of life in the presence of multiple metastases in the liver is small, and the use of chemotherapy cannot often be justified. If there is some special reason for wanting to prolong life for a short while, 5-fluorouracil, 15 mg i.v. on alternate days for 10 days and then weekly, may be used – there are relatively few side-effects.

There are often no local symptoms from metastatic liver carcinoma, but there may be back pain or pleuritic pain, which respond to analgesics, or dyspnoea, best coped with by opiates if severe enough to cause distress.

Carcinoid tumours

Carcinoid tumours spread relatively slowly, but apart from mechanical problems they may cause unpleasant symptoms as part of the 'carcinoid syndrome', the main features of which are flushing and diarrhoea. This occurs only when there are hepatic metastases, and is usually confirmed by the presence of abnormal quantities of 5-hydroxy-indole-acetic acid in the urine (though this biochemical marker may be absent in up to 30 per cent of patients).

Flushing may be controlled by phenoxybenzamine (10–30 mg daily), antihistamines or phenothiazines. Diarrhoea may respond to standard antidiarrhoeals such as codeine phosphate, or loperamide; if these are insufficient methysergide is helpful, in doses up to 4 mg four times daily (Mengel, 1965). Cyproheptadine (16–32 mg/day) may also be helpful (Berry, Maunder, and Wilson, 1974), blocking the cellular site of action of 5-HT. Methyldopa has been reported to help in a few patients.

In some cases the unpleasant carcinoid symptoms are uncontrolled by any combination of these drugs. An attempt may then be made to reduce the amount of secreting tissue in the liver by chemotherapy; 5-fluorouracil by hepatic artery infusion is usually employed. Apart from the complications of the procedure, the infusion sometimes produces a severe exacerbation of the syndrome, which can be fatal.

Ascites

Peritoneal malignancy causing exudation and ascites may cause considerable distress, with painful abdominal distension and dyspnoea.

Paracentesis

Simple drainage of the ascites may be achieved using a peritoneal dialysis cannula. The cannula is inserted, using local anaesthesia, in either iliac fossa, or in the lower midline provided the area is free of obvious masses. Fluid does not need to be drained slowly, and binders are unnecessary. The procedure may be done as a day-case.

If drainage is incomplete, due to loculation of fluid, puncture at a second or third site may be used, though frequently the compartments are small, drainage is inadequate, and the patient is little relieved.

After simple drainage the rate of reaccumulation may be observed, and further paracentesis performed as necessary. The patient's general condition usually declines during the procedure because of loss of nutrition in the ascites. Chemotherapy may slow the rate of reaccumulation if it is rapid (see below).

Ascites dialysis

The Rhodiascit apparatus (Rhône–Poulenc Corporation, Paris) dialyses ascitic fluid, so that the concentrated protein may be reinfused into the patient, thus slowing nutritional deterioration. It is intended for the treatment of ascites with cirrhosis, but has been used in malignant ascites (Parbhoo, Ajdukiewicz, and Sherlock, 1974). Blockage of the catheter and clogging of the dialysis membrane is liable to occur.

Dialysis of drained ascites may also be carried out with a dialysis technique using a standard haemodialysis coil; this is cheaper than the Rhône–Poulenc method (Manuel *et al.*, 1978).

LeVeen shunt

A peritoneovenous shunt was devised by LeVeen, primarily for treatment of ascites in portal hypertension (LeVeen *et al.*, 1976); however, it has been applied to the management of malignant ascites. Pollock (1975) used a Holter valve in the same way. There is a tendency for growth to clog the outlet of the tube, but if ascites is accumulating rapidly it is worth considering, as the procedure is relatively simple technically.

Chemotherapy and radiotherapy

Chemotherapy reduces the rate of ascites accumulation in about 50 per cent of patients. Nitrogen mustard (0.4 mg/kg), 5-fluorouracil (2–3 g) and thiotepa (60 mg in 60 ml water), infused direct into the peritoneal cavity after first draining the ascites, have all been used with some success.

Alternatively, [198]Au may be instilled. This has also been reported to control ascites, and may cause less nausea and marrow depression than chemotherapy (O'Bryan *et al.*, 1968).

Pruritus

Pruritus may occur in any malignancy, but it usually implies liver metastases. The itching is due to the accumulation of bile-salts because of intrahepatic cholestasis. Jaundice will not always be present, though the alkaline phosphatase is usually high.

Antihistamines and phenothiazines give little relief, and local applications are of little value except as placebos. Cholestyramine is the agent most likely to help, though relief is often only partial. There is a fairly palatable preparation – Questran – taken as a powder, four times daily; however, it may cause nausea, and tends to produce steatorrhoea.

Methyltestosterone and norethandrolone may also relieve pruritus, but will *cause* jaundice by cholestasis. They should only be used in non-jaundiced patients if the pruritus is extreme and uncomfortable.

Constipation

Many patients with terminal malignancy become constipated, adding the possible discomfort of abdominal distension, lower abdominal pain, anal fissures or prolapsing haemorrhoids to their other problems. The causes are:

(1) small fibre intake because of anorexia;
(2) lack of physical exercise;
(3) weakness;
(4) side-effects of drugs, especially opiates and dihydrocodeine (DF118)

Management

Initial relief may be given by glycerine suppositories, a simple soap enema, or a small 'disposable' enema (Fletcher's phosphate enemas); this can be repeated from time to time. However, patients dislike having these attentions and they take up nursing time. If a regular bowel habit can be reinstituted the patient will feel more comfortable. The chief measures, in order, should be:

(1) Keep opiates etc to a minimum – use non-constipating analgesics when possible.
(2) Encourage dietary fibre – fruit (stewed or tinned may be more palatable than fresh), vegetables, crispbreads, digestive biscuits, etc. A traditional 'light' or sloppy diet contains almost no fibre. Unprocessed bran can be stirred into Complan or scrambled egg, a teaspoonful at a time.
(3) Hydrophilic colloids may be taken by mouth. Celevac tablets 0.5 g, up to eight a day, are most convenient, but Isogel or Normacol Special granules may be preferred; Fybogel and Cologel are liquid forms. All must be taken with plenty of water to be fully effective. They tend to make the patient feel distended and may diminish appetite.
(4) Osmotic cathartics may be added. Magnesium sulphate (Epsom salts) in strong fruit juice can be titrated in dose, beginning with a teaspoonful (5 ml) at night, increasing or decreasing according to response. Some patients prefer Milpar (magnesium sulphate plus liquid paraffin) 5–30 ml at night, or night and morning. Duphalac (lactulose) is more palatable, but is expensive and has to be taken in large volumes (such as 20 ml four times daily).
(5) A stimulant cathartic may be needed in addition. Senokot (tablets or

granules) at night gives fewest side-effects. Bisacodyl (Dulcolax) tends to cause griping pains and is best avoided.

References

Almersjö, O., Bergmark, S., Rudenstam, C. M., Hajstrom, L. and Nillson, L. A. V. (1972). Evaluation of hepatic dearterialization in primary and secondary cancer of the liver. *Am. J. Surg.*, **124**, 5

Ammann, J. F. and Collis, J. L. (1971). Palliative intubation of the oesophagus. Analysis of 59 cases. *J. Thorac. Cardiovasc. Surg.*, **61**, 863

Atkinson, M. (1981). Intubation of oesophageal malignancies. In J. R. Bennett (ed.) *Therapeutic Endoscopy and Radiology of the Gut* (London: Chapman and Hall)

Atkinson, M. and Ferguson, R. (1977). Fibreoptic endoscopic palliative intubation of inoperable oesophagogastric neoplasms. *Br. Med. J.*, **1**, 266

Balasegeram, M. (1977). Complete hepatic dearterialization for primary carcinoma of the liver. *Am. J. Surg.*, **124**, 340

Beahrs, O. H. and Wilson, S. M. (1976). Carcinoma of the anus. *Ann. Surg.*, **184**, 422

Berry, M., Maunder, C. and Wilson, M. (1974). Carcinoid myopathy and treatment with cyproheptadine (Periactin). *Gut*, **15**, 34

Blumgart, L. H. (1980). Hepatic resection. In: S. Taylor (ed.) *Recent Advances in Surgery* (Edinburgh: Churchill-Livingstone)

Burcharth, F. (1978). A new endoprosthesis for non-operative intubation of the biliary tract in malignant obstructive jaundice. *Surg. Gynecol. Obstet.*, **146**, 76

Fielding, L. P., Stewart-Brown, S. and Blesovsky, L. (1979). Large bowel obstruction caused by cancer: a prospective study. *Br. Med. J.*, **2**, 515

Fortner, J. G., Mulcare, R. J., Solis, A., Watson, R. C. and Golbey, R. B. (1973). Treatment of primary and secondary liver cancer by hepatic artery ligation and infusion chemotherapy. *Ann. Surg.*, **178**, 162

Goligher, J. C., Lee, P. W. R., McFie, J., Simpkins, K. C. and Lintott, D. J. (1979). Experience with the Russian gun for rectal anastomosis. *Surg. Gynecol. Obstet.*, **148**, 517

Griffin, W. O., Humphrey, L. and Sosin, H. (1969). The prognosis and management of recurrent abdominal malignancies. *Curr. Prob. Surg.*, **April,** 12

Heald, R. J. (1980). Towards further colostomies – the impact of circular stapling devices on the surgery of rectal cancer in a district hospital. *Br. J. Surg.*, **67**, 198

Heit, H. A., Johnson, L. F., Siegel, S. R. and Boyce, H. W. (1978). Palliative dilatation for dysphagia in esophageal carcinoma. *Ann. Intern. Med.*, **89**, 629

Johnson, I. R., Balfour, T. W. and Bourke, J. B. (1976). Intubation of malignant gastro-oesophageal strictures. *J. R. Coll. Surg. Edin.*, **21**, 225

Johnson, P. J., Thomas, H., Williams, R., Sherlock, S. and Murray-Lyon, I. M. (1978). Induction of remission in hepatocellular carcinoma with doxorubicin. *Lancet*, **1**, 1006

Knight, M. and Smith, R. (1977). Operation for carcinoma of the common hepatic duct. In: C. Rob, R. Smith and H. Dudley (eds.) *Operative Surgery, Abdomen*, pp. 379–89. (London: Butterworths)

Lawrence, W. (1976). Surgical management of gastrointestinal cancer. *Clin. Gastroenterol.*, **5**, 703

LeVeen, H. H., Wapnick, S., Grosberg, S. and Kinney, M. J. (1976). Further experience with peritoneo-venous shunt for ascites. *Ann. Surg.*, **184**, 574

Madden, J. L. and Kandalaft, S. (1971). Electrocoagulation in the treatment of cancer of the rectum: a continuing study. *Ann. Surg.*, **174**, 530

Manuel, M. A., Saiphoo, C. S., Keith, R. and Evans, J. (1978). Treatment of ascites by ascitic fluid ultra filtration and re-infusion. *Dialysis Transplant.*, **7**, 710

McKeown, K. C. (1972). Trends in oesophageal resection for carcinoma. *Ann. R. Coll. Surg. Engl. Wales*, **51**, 213

Mengel, C. E. (1965). Therapy of the malignant carcinoid syndrome. *Ann. Intern. Med.*, **62**, 587

Mori, K., Misumi, A., Sugiyama, M., Okabe, M., Matsuoka, T., Ishii, J. and Akagi, M. (1977). Percutaneous transhepatic biliary drainage. *Ann. Surg.*, **185**, 111

Niloff, P. H. (1972). A prosthesis for palliative treatment of obstructive jaundice due to cholangiocarcinoma. *Surg. Gynecol. Obstet.*, **135**, 610

O'Bryan, R. M., Talley, R. W., Brennan, M. J. and San Diego, E. (1968). Critical analysis of the control of malignant effusions with radioisotopes. *Henry Ford Hosp. Med. J.*, **16**, 3

O'Connell, J. E. A. (1969). Anterolateral chordotomy for intractable pain in carcinoma of the rectum. *Proc. R. Soc. Med.*, **62**, 1223

Okuda, K., Tanikawa, K., Emura, T., Kuratomi, S., Jennouchi, S., Urabe, K., Sumikoshi, T., Kanda, V., Fukuyama, Y., Mush, H., Mor, A., Shimokawo, Y., Yakushi, I. F. and Mastawara, Y. (1974). Non-surgical percutaneous transhepatic cholangiography – diagnostic significance in medical problems of the liver. *Am. J. Dig. Dis.*, **19**, 21

Olweny, C. L. M., Toya, T., Katongole-Mdibbe, E., Mugerwa, J., Kyalwazi, S. K. and Cohen, H. (1976). Treatment of hepatocellular carcinoma with Adriamycin. Preliminary communication. *Cancer NY*, **36**, 1250

Osborne, D. R., Higgins, A. F. and Hobbs, K. E. F. (1978). Cryosurgery in the management of rectal tumours. *Br. J. Surg.*, **65**, 859

Papillon, J. (1974). Radiation therapy in the management of epidermoid carcinoma of the anal region. *Dis. Colon Rectum*, **17**, 181

Parbhoo, S. P., Ajdukiewicz, A. and Sherlock, S. (1974). Treatment of ascites by continuous ultrafiltration and reinfusion of protein concentrate. *Lancet*, **1**, 949

Pereiras, R. V., Rheingold, O. J., Hutson, D., Mejia, J., Viamonte, M., Chiprut, R. O. and Schiff, E. R. (1978). Relief of malignant obstructive jaundice by percutaneous insertion of a permanent prosthesis in the biliary tree. *Ann. Intern. Med.*, **89**, 589

Pollock, A. V. (1975). The treatment of resistant malignant ascites by insertion of a peritoneo-atrial valve. *Br. J. Surg.*, **62**, 104

Price, J. D., Stanciu, C. and Bennett, J. R. (1974). A safer method of dilating oesophageal strictures. *Lancet*, **1**, 1141

Robbie, D. S. (1969). General management of intractable pain in advanced carcinoma of the rectum. *Proc. R. Soc. Med.*, **62**, 1225

Smith, R. J. (1978). Cancer of the pancreas. *J. R. Coll. Surg. Edin.*, **23**, 2, 133

Stearns, M. W. and Quan, S. H. Q. (1970). Epidermoid carcinoma of the anorectum. *Surg. Gynecol. Obstet.*, **131**, 953

Taylor, I. (1978). Cytotoxic perfusion of colorectal liver metastases. *Br. J. Surg.*, **65**, 109

Terblanche, J. and Louw, J. H. (1973). U-tube drainage in the palliative therapy of carcinoma of the main hepatic duct junction. *Surg. Clin. N. Am.*, **53**, 1245

Terblanche, J., Saunders, S. J. and Louw, J. H. (1972). Prolonged palliation in carcinoma of the main hepatic duct junction. *Surgery*, **71**, 720

Tormey, D. C., Bergevin, P., Blom, J. and Petty, W. (1973). Preliminary trials with a combination of Adriamycin (NSC-123127) and bleomycin (NSC-125066) in adult malignancies. *Cancer Chemotherap. Rep.*, **57**, 413

Tylen, U., Hoevels, J. and Varg, J. (1977). Percutaneous transhepatic cholangiography with external drainage of obstructive biliary lesions. *Surg. Gynecol. Obstet.*, **144**, 13

Williams, I. G., Shulman, I. M. and Todd, I. P. (1957). The treatment of recurrent carcinoma of the rectum by supervoltage x-ray therapy. *Br. J. Surg.*, **44**, 506

9

The management of refractory disease (myeloma, the lymphomas and gonadal tumours)

J. M. A. Whitehouse

INTRODUCTION

Advances in medical care rarely occur suddenly. Exceptions, such as the introduction of antibiotic therapy which radically transformed the management of infectious disease, happily do arise and give encouragement to those faced with patients for whose problems only palliation is at the moment available. Cancer was for a long time regarded as essentially untreatable and since it represented for the clinician the prime example of his fallibility, tended to be feared by patient and doctor alike. Over the past few years there has been a profound change in cancer management, not as immediately obvious as that following the introduction of antibiotics, but nonetheless significant. The long dependence on surgery has illustrated its limitations, despite greater technical expertise or a move to more and more radical techniques in an attempt to achieve cure.

Radiotherapy has the added advantage over surgery that local sterilization of the tumour may be effected yet function retained and disfigurement largely avoided. Unfortunately a simple understanding of the biology of cancer highlights the weakness of depending solely on local treatment, however effective this may be. By the time a simple primary nodule is apparent, it contains some 1×10^9 cells. These neoplastic cells have proliferative potential and are motile – the ideal cells to infiltrate through tissue planes and blood or lymphatic vessel walls. It is, therefore, not surprising that there is a tendency for many tumours to relapse at distant sites at some time after apparently effective therapy for the primary. It is this characteristic – the proliferation of previously dormant

169

cells remote from the primary which constitutes the real threat of a cancer. One or more 'micrometastases', as these have been called, is almost certainly present very early in the natural history of the disease and this led to the aura of hopelessness, which has frequently surrounded the patient once malignancy was confirmed.

The discovery of drugs effective against certain cancer cells – predicted by Paul Ehrlich – raised hopes that tumours might be eradicated. Unfortunately tumours vary considerably in behaviour depending on the tissue of origin. Both the site of the primary tumour and the individual patient's clinical state appear to influence its natural history. Other variables such as drug metabolism, drug access and toxicity have meant that of many hundreds of thousands of drugs screened, less than 30 are in common use (Figure 1). None have total specificity for the cancer cell. Virtually all have significant toxicities, and in order to achieve maximum benefit, their use has become more and more specialized, so removing much therapy from the domain of the general clinician.

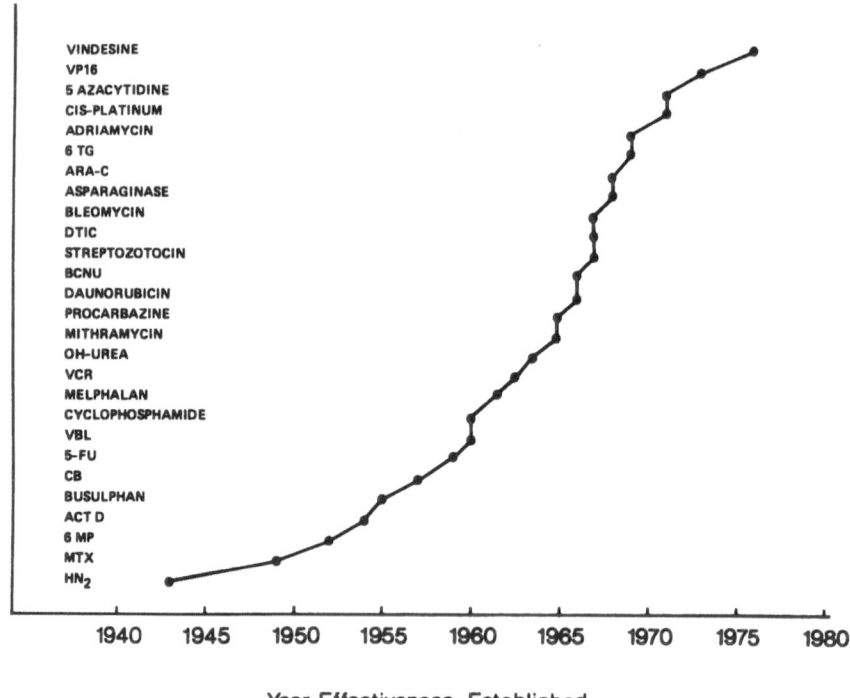

Figure 1 Introduction of anticancer drugs (after Frei)

Despite its failings, however, the advent of chemotherapy has been responsible for the major change seen in attitudes to the cancer patient. It has restored hope of real therapeutic benefit to the doctor and patient and while there is no doubt that such optimism must be tempered by caution, where once only palliation was possible, now sometimes cure results. More valuable than the occasional cure is the generally increased interest in the overall care of the cancer patient at every level. No longer need the patient be abandoned at any stage of his disease. Support should be available from the community, the social worker, nurse and doctor, even when specific anticancer therapy promises little. In specialist units, surgeons, radiotherapists and physicians, work side by side to provide optimum management and to avoid the morbidity of an irrelevant and unnecessary treatment. Since there is no ideal therapy for any cancer, not only must those treatments that are useless and harmful be eliminated, but the best available treatment must be improved.

New drugs, new drug combinations, new techniques of surgery or radiotherapy, used alone or in combination, must all be evaluated. This is a slow and painstaking process which many centres in the United Kingdom and the United States have willingly undertaken. Multicentre or single-centre studies (predominantly the latter) have been responsible for those areas of greatest progress in conditions such as acute lymphoblastic leukaemia of childhood and Hodgkin's disease. No doubt further progress will come from some of the studies already in progress.

It is now possible to define a clear policy of management when the patient's assessment is complete. There are three major options. Firstly, where cure is a possibility, secondly, where prolongation of life is possible but cure unlikely and, thirdly, where neither of the first two options can be contemplated and when palliation becomes of primary importance. Although it is tempting to think of cure as the most important management option, the patient who is unresponsive to therapy needs the commitment, judgement and skill of the clinician just as much, if not more, than the patient whose ultimate cure reduces his dependence on medical care.

As will be appreciated in those circumstances where a tumour is truly localized, surgery alone will effect a cure. So too may radiotherapy. However, Table 1 summarizes those conditions where, as is more often the case, local therapy alone is frequently insufficient to cure, but where chemotherapy has now made this a possibility. Also listed are those conditions where chemotherapy may assist in the prolongation of life. Of course such distinctions are somewhat artificial for there may be patients who are in theory potentially curable, but in whom relapse ultimately

Table 1 Conditions where chemotherapy may contribute to cure or prolongation of life

Normal lifespan	Improved survival
Choriocarcinoma	Acute leukaemia
Testicular tumours	Other lymphomas
Hodgkin's disease	Multiple myeloma
Histiocytic lymphoma	Neuroblastoma
Skin cancer	Cancers of:
Childhood tumours	Ovary
Leukaemia	Breast
Rhabdomyosarcoma	Endometrium
Ewing's tumour	Prostate
Wilm's tumour	
Retinoblastoma	

Table 2 Toxicities of commonly used anticancer drugs

Drugs		Side-effects
Antimetabolites	B	
6-Mercaptopurine	O	Nausea
6-Thioguanine	N	Nausea
Cytosine arabinoside	E	Nausea, abdominal discomfort
Methotrexate		Nausea
	M	
Alkylating agents	A	
Mustine	R	Nausea, thrombophlebitis
Cyclophosphamide	R	Nausea, alopecia, haemorrhagic cystitis
Busulphan	O	Pulmonary fibrosis, Addisonian-like syndrome
Melphalan	W	
Antibiotics	S	
Daunorubicin	U	Nausea, alopecia, thrombophlebitis, cardiotoxicity
Adriamycin	P	
	P	
Plant alkaloids	R	
Vinca alkaloids	E	Peripheral neuropathy, autonomic neuropathy
Epipodophyllotoxins	S	Nausea, alopecia
	S	
Miscellaneous	I	
L-Asparaginase	O	Nausea, hypofibrinogenaemia, diabetes mellitus,
	N	hypoalbuminaemia
Prednisolone		As for corticosteroids

occurs, and others who fail to respond to therapy.

Most patients who attend a cancer centre, do so with an 'expectation of life'. This is in complete contrast to those patients admitted to terminal care or to continuing care institutions, who are gradually accustomed to an 'expectation of death'. This chapter will concern itself primarily with those patients whose expectations are in a state of flux because they have failed primary treatment, either because their disease is unresponsive to therapy, or because of eventual relapse and disease progression through secondary treatment. Specific diseases will be considered. Failure of therapy becomes apparent in two ways: as disease progression through treatment or a gradual failure of therapy despite dose escalation or drug substitution. The indications for therapy in such circumstances are confined to palliation, and consequently an appreciation of potential drug toxicities is vital, for if misused cancer chemotherapy may produce significant morbidity and in consequence the terminal phase of the illness may be even worse for the patient (Figure 2). The major toxicities of commonly used drugs are summarized in Table 2.

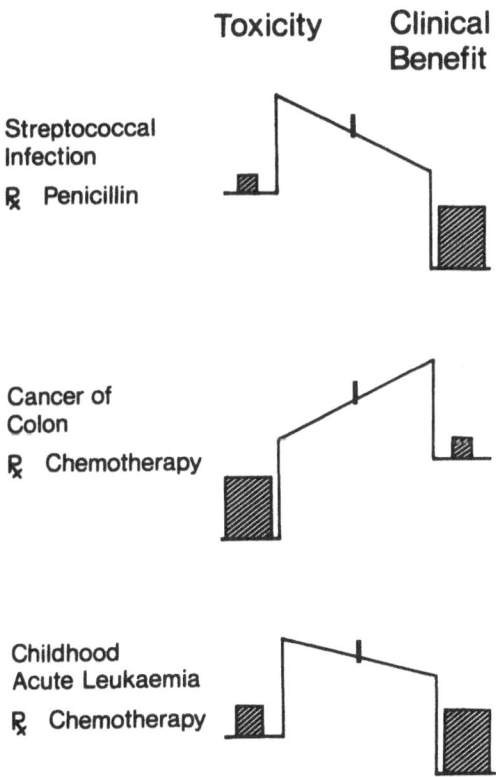

Figure 2 Morbidity versus benefit in the application of treatments

MULTIPLE MYELOMA

Multiple myeloma is the commonest neoplasm of plasma cell origin. Rarely, apparently solitary plasma cell tumours – plasmacytomas – may present as an isolated skeletal tumour, either of soft tissue or intraosseous origin. Although careful examination may substantiate the tumour's isolated development, frank multiple myeloma eventually follows in most cases.

Marrow infiltration by myeloma cells is responsible for the clinical features of multiple myeloma. Infiltration of the marrow tends to be patchy but may nonetheless result in anaemia or thrombocytopenia. Growth of the myeloma cells in short-term culture has shown that these cells cause resorption of bone. The factor responsible for this appears similar to the osteoclast activating factor which is secreted by normal leukocytes. The practical complications of myeloma cell proliferation are in the production of lytic lesions of bone, particularly in the skull, vertebrae and ribs, or of widespread osteoporosis, producing the hypercalcaemia found in about 30 per cent of patients at presentation. Metabolite production by the abnormal cell population may be detected in the urine as Bence–Jones proteinuria. Tubular deposition of protein or amyloidosis may produce renal damage and ultimately renal failure. The course of the disease is very variable. Patients may present with any combination of features including bone pain, which may or may not be related to an overt underlying lesion, anaemia, thrombocytopenia, tumour mass, symptoms of hypercalcaemia, or infection.

Radiological change and serum immunoglobulin electrophoresis may both suggest myeloma, and indeed, where the 'M' band is IgG >3.4 g/% or IgA >2 g/% with a reduction in background gammaglobulins, and where the urinary kappa (x) or lambda (λ) excretion exceeds 1 g/day, this is diagnostic. Bone marrow examination is essential, but infiltration with myeloma cells tends to be patchy, so that a doubtful bone marrow examination should be followed by a further aspiration from a different site. The degree of infiltration required for the diagnosis is somewhat arbitrary but plasma cells in excess of 5–10 per cent with large, immature and multinucleated forms is highly suggestive of the diagnosis, and when 15–20 per cent are present as clusters or sheets, with a large proportion of immature and abnormal forms, the diagnosis is virtually certain. Radiological evidence alone may be suggestive, but without other features of myeloma is not diagnostic. Where a plasmacytoma is diagnosed as a result of tissue biopsy, a careful search for bony lesions and immunoglobulin abnormalities should be initiated. Once the diagnosis of myeloma is established, renal function should be assessed, hypercalcaemia excluded, and anaemia and thrombocytopenia documented. A skeletal survey provides a useful baseline from which to monitor the course of the disease.

A three-tier system of staging has been proposed by Durie and Salmon (1977) which is related to measurements of cell mass in a group of patients. This appears to correlate well with prognosis, and may form the basis of additional comparative studies.

There is an increased risk to the patient with multiple myeloma of developing acute myelogenous leukaemia. Whenever this condition arises in association with another malignancy, it tends to be more refractory to treatment, but nonetheless may be controlled for a period of time. Plasma cell leukaemia has been identified as a distinct entity and may present as a frank leukaemia with white cell counts in excess of 15 000 of which 15 per cent are plasma cells. Hepatosplenomegaly is usually present. The cells in the peripheral blood range from mature plasma cells to immature and atypical forms. Abnormalities of immunoglobulins may be similar to those of myeloma.

Treatment
Although a variety of drug combinations have been tried, the treatment of choice remains a combination of melphelan and prednisolone given intermittently. A useful regimen is melphelan 10 mg daily plus prednisolone 40 mg daily given in combination for 5 days. This can be repeated at 6-weekly intervals, and the course prolonged to 7 days provided this is well tolerated. Melphalan and cyclophosphamide appear comparable as single agents, and intermittent therapy is simpler to manage than when the drugs are given continuously. A 70 per cent response can be anticipated in patients receiving melphalan and prednisolone together, and the effect is to increase the median survival from 12 months in untreated patients to between 24 and 30 months in those receiving treatment. Continuous steroid administration may help to control the hypercalcaemia which also responds to the intermittent alkylating agent therapy, thus removing the need for prolonged steroid administration. Renal functional impairment is rarely reversed, but progressive damage may be halted. Maximum reduction in disease bulk is paralleled by a gradual reduction in the 'M' band achieved over a 6–9 month period. Substituting alternative drugs at this point has little effect in further decreasing the size of the 'M' band. In patients who respond initially to treatment the 'M' band plateaus for a period of time which varies between individuals. Although many

clinicians continue to administer melphalan and prednisolone for long periods, the 'M' band eventually begins to rise again despite therapy. Substitution of high-dose cyclophosphamide therapy at this point may produce a transient response in a minority of patients, but is unlikely to produce lasting benefit. This resistance to chemotherapy has prompted some clinicians to discontinue melphalan and prednisolone once the plateau phase has been established for a period of 2 months or more in the hope that the plasma cells will remain sensitive to chemotherapy when renewed disease activity occurs. The justification for this procedure awaits a clinical trial.

Attempts to inhibit the osteoclastic activity, which is significant in some patients with myeloma, with mithramycin have only been partially successful, but combining sodium fluoride and calcium carbonate did appear to increase bone density which was assessed by microradiography and videodensitometry. Both procedures remain to be evaluated satisfactorily, however, and are not yet current practice.

Solitary plasmacytoma is best treated by local radiotherapy, but as these lesions are very rarely truly localized, treatment should be followed by prolonged and careful follow-up. Minor regression of amyloid infiltrates may follow alkylating agent therapy, but no effective treatment is yet known which will eradicate the deposition of amyloid material (comprising portions of immunoglobulin molecules and a non-immunoglobulin protein and glycoprotein).

In assessing the patient with a presumptive diagnosis of multiple myeloma, it is essential to exclude a benign monoclonal gammopathy. The latter occurs principally in the elderly, and is usually a chance finding on immunoglobulin electrophoresis which reveals the presence of an 'M' band without significant reduction in the background immunoglobulins. The 'M' band is usually fairly stationary for a period of years, and while recent studies suggest that the cells responsible are dispersed throughout the bone marrow, this does not compromise the patients nor usually progress to overt myeloma. Treatment of this condition is not indicated.

Primary treatment failure

Escape from melphalan and prednisolone control of disease may not be apparent for many months or even years after the 'M' band has stabilized at a lower level. The first indication of disease progression may be the rising 'M' band, but frequently this is only confirmed after the patient has presented with falling blood counts. Melphalan depresses both the white blood counts and the platelet count, but the nadir of this depression is at 2–3 weeks. At 6 weeks when the next treatment with melphalan and prednisolone is due, the full blood count is a fairly accurate representation of the degree of bone marrow compromisation by disease rather than therapy. A gradual trend downwards of blood counts at this time, indicates both a refractoriness to therapy and advancing disease. Alternative treatment at this stage either with single agents or with combinations, rarely alters the course of the disease. The rate of progression varies significantly from patient to patient and while it is tempting in some patients, because of their general state, to conclude that there is little to offer, some may derive considerable benefit from minimal intervention. It is important that reversible complications of the disease are dealt with early. Hypercalcaemia is distressing and may well contribute to bizarre mental changes making management more stressful for those closely involved in the home. Adequate hydration and steroids may produce satisfactory control, but if not admission to hospital may be required.

The extent of bone changes on X-ray (osteoporosis, lytic lesions) are not always a helpful indicator of prognosis, and a fracture in such a patient may imply a situation of hopelessness. Local stabilization, local therapy (such as radiotherapy), and subsequent mobilization may transform the clinical situation even though the radiological evidence discourages optimism. The author had just such a patient, presenting with a collapsed vertebra, who was bedridden, in considerable pain and was assumed by his relatives and his family doctor to have little chance of leaving his bed again. Certainly, even short-term immobilization puts such a patient at considerable risk. Satisfactory pain control was obtained with diamorphine, and gentle but regular mobilization was achieved, so that he was able to attend for radiotherapy in a chair. More than a year later he is mobile and has recently written to say that he does all that he wishes to do with the exception of playing golf.

Not all patients are so fortunate, for while stabilization of fractures, local treatment and mobilization may bring rewarding results, generalized disease progression may rapidly overwhelm all attempts at supportive therapy. Once there is evidence of advancing renal failure or the consequences of severe bone marrow suppression, survival is short and the full emphasis of management should go towards symptomatic relief. Continued mobilization should be encouraged where possible. Relief of pain, particularly when focal, can be achieved even at this stage by local radiotherapy. An analgesic should be prescribed at the level necessary to reduce pain to a minor symptom.

THE LYMPHOMAS

This classification includes a broad spectrum of disease types, ranging from Hodgkin's disease to a heterogeneous group of conditions which are collectively labelled the non-Hodgkin lymphomas.

Hodgkin's disease

This condition is often quoted as the prime example of progress in the management of malignant disease. Indeed, some 40 years ago only 10 per cent of those presenting with the disease survived for 2 years. In those now treated at major centres some 60 per cent are still alive after 10 years, and most of these are probably cured. Nonetheless, even with such expert management 40 per cent are still dead at this time, emphasizing the importance of this condition being managed by clinicians who are totally familiar with all aspects of the disease and the improvements in management.

Four histological types of Hodgkin's disease are recognized: lymphocyte predominant; nodular sclerosing; mixed cellularity and lymphocyte depleted. Although these subcategories were originally thought to have prognostic significance, only the patients with lymphocyte-depleted histology are now recognized to have a poorer prognosis even with present treatment. It would appear that Hodgkin's disease arises in one group of lymph nodes spreading to involve contiguous lymph node groups. This behaviour has made it possible to define therapy in a much more logical

Table 3 The currently used staging procedure for Hodgkin's disease

Stage I	Involvement of a single lymph node region (I) or of a single extralymphatic organ or site.
Stage II	Involvement of two or more lymph node regions on the same side of the diaphragm (II) or localized involvement of extralymphatic organ or site and one or more lymph node regions on the same side of the diaphragm (II_E).
Stage III	Involvement of lymph node regions on both sides of the diaphragm (III) ± involvement of the spleen (III_S) or localized extralymphatic organ or site (III_E).
Stage IV	Diffuse or disseminated involvement of one or more extralymphatic organs or tissues, for example, liver, marrow, pleura, lung, bone and skin.

Systemic symptoms – weight loss >10 per cent in 6 months, fever, sweating. If absent = 'A'. If present = 'B'.

way than is feasible in many other malignancies. Local radiotherapy is highly effective in the treatment of localized Hodgkin's disease. Treatment is designed to encompass associated nodes which might include disease. A staging system has been devised based on disease spread and this is summarized in Table 3. This staging plays a critical role in defining treatment policy and depends on the careful identification of disease spread. Progressively more invasive evaluation, commencing with clinical examination and then lymphangiogram and bone marrow aspirate and trephine, determine the need to progress to laparotomy and splenectomy. The latter is a highly specialized investigation and is only applicable to those patients whose disease appears confined to lymph nodes despite the earlier investigations. It can be appreciated that the patient with widespread disease undetected by an inadequate staging laparotomy who then receives local treatment will certainly relapse and the disease may then prove difficult to manage. Where disease is confined to sites above the diaphragm, radiotherapy is given to all lymph nodes including the mediastinum, axilla, cervical, submandibular and occipital nodes in what is termed the 'mantle' area. Below the diaphragm radiotherapy is given to the para-aortic, splenic hilum and parailiac nodes in an 'inverted Y' distribution. In patients who have stage III disease, but are asymptomatic, it is necessary to treat both the 'mantle' and the 'inverted Y' areas. Symptoms of greater than 10 per cent weight loss over 6 months and frequent night sweats are recognized to indicate more extensive disease and, indeed, patients with these symptoms and stage III disease treated by local radiotherapy alone have an unacceptable relapse rate. Fortunately, combination chemotherapy is highly effective at producing complete remission, and indeed long-term cure, in those with extensive disease. Originally combinations including MOPP (mustine, vincristine, pro-carbazine and prednisolone) were used, but this has an appreciable morbidity, if only temporary, and is likely to be superseded by newer alternative chemotherapy combinations once these are proven to be equally effective.

Failure of primary treatment
Sadly, there are still some patients who relapse despite appearing to have eminently curable disease. A proportion of patients whose primary treatment is radiotherapy can, in the event of relapse, still be rescued by chemotherapy, but the remaining patients in whom relapse becomes apparent are rarely cured. Disease truly refractory to primary treatment is rare, and in these patients remorseless progression of disease, leading to the classical terminal state, seen less and less commonly, of generalized wasting and cachexia is inevitable. Many patients who relapse after initially successful treatment exhibit varying degrees of disease chronicity

so that in some, survival may be prolonged for many years and even decades. Almost all such patients eventually die of the consequences of their disease. The skilful combination of second-line chemotherapy, either in combination or given cyclically as single agents with appropriate radiotherapy, may minimize the consequences of the illness and allow the patient to lead a virtually normal life. In the later stages of the disease, there may be recurrent regional lymphadenopathy but extranodal involvement is also much more common. This may become apparent as widespread infiltration of the lungs, as hepatomegaly or pancytopenia from bone marrow infiltration. Although the cycling of single agents may contain this situation for a while, eventual progression is inevitable, and while troublesome symptoms such as pruritus and fevers may have been contained by single-agent therapy, eventually they become apparent once more. At this point prednisolone in doses of 40 mg/day or more may help to contain these symptoms and also to improve wellbeing. Where deposits are troublesome either as bulky lymphadenopathy, as painful lesion of bone or in causing mediastinal obstruction, local radiotherapy may be the only means of relief. The chronic phase of this illness may last for several months during which time the patient will require considerable support. Unfortunately the level of nursing required terminally often means hospital admission. Death usually occurs from an overwhelming infection or renal or hepatic failure either separately or in combination.

Table 4   Classification of the non-Hodgkin lymphomas (after Rappaport)

Nodular	*Diffuse*
*Lymphocytic, poorly differentiated *Mixed, lymphocytic and histiocytic *Histiocytic	*Lymphocytic, well differentiated Lymphocytic, poorly differentiated Mixed, lymphocytic and histiocytic Histiocytic Pleomorphic (undifferentiated or stem cell)

*'Good' prognosis

The non-Hodgkin lymphomas

Unfortunately the proliferation of subclassifications for the non-Hodgkin lymphomas far from clarifying the situation has instead resulted in an unhealthy confusion. Although the Rappaport classification of this group of conditions is set out in Table 4, it is perhaps helpful to remember that a follicular or 'nodular' pattern to the node and the presence of 'well-differentiated' cells is associated with a better prognosis than when the lymph node architecture is destroyed and the disease is labelled 'diffuse'. This means that although the architecture of the lymph node may be diffuse the presence of well-differentiated lymphocytes in the 'well-differentiated diffuse' lymphoma is a favourable feature. Indeed if the lymph nodes from a patient with chronic lymphocytic leukaemia are examined histologically, many would be reported as 'well-differentiated diffuse lymphomas'. Furthermore, despite the fact that the cells are only poorly differentiated in a 'poorly differentiated nodular lymphoma', the presence of a nodular pattern in the lymph node indicates a good prognosis and this is borne out clinically. In crude terms, the median survival of many lymphomas in the good-prognosis groups exceeds 6 years, whereas that of 'diffuse', bad-prognosis groups is less than 2 years.

Staging procedures are less important in this group of conditions, for most patients have widespread disease at the outset and local radiotherapy as primary treatment is therefore almost never indicated. Unlike Hodgkin's disease, there is, as yet, no known curative treatment for the good-prognosis lymphomas. Paradoxically, approximately one-quarter of the patients with histiocytic diffuse lymphomas can be cured when given appropriate treatment. As for Hodgkin's disease, because of the complexity of management, treatment should not be planned outside special centres, although once defined, some patients can be managed close to their home. In certain patients with good-prognosis lymphomas, no treatment may be required at the time of presentation provided that the patient is asymptomatic and has minimal evidence of disease. Therapy can be reserved until there is evidence of disease progression or deterioration. At the present time there is no obvious advantage of combination chemotherapy over single-agent therapy in this group of lymphomas, but the whole approach to management is being critically evaluated by those centres actively involved in treatment.

The bad-prognosis lymphomas require much more intensive management along the lines of that given to patients with acute leukaemia. Careful clinical and haematological assessment of the disease extent is made, followed by intensive chemotherapy until complete eradication of disease is apparent – complete remission. This latter term is somewhat meaningless since most patients later relapse anyway. However, there is now clear evidence of an improved survival among those patients achieving complete remission compared with those who do not.

In particular, as has been mentioned, cure may be achieved in a proportion of patients with histiocytic diffuse lymphomas.

Primary treatment failure

In the good-prognosis lymphomas, disease progression may become apparent either as increasing lymphadenopathy or be indicated by a gradual and progressive fall in the peripheral blood count. Fluctuating lymphadenopathy is a frequent feature of the follicular lymphomas and usually responds over a period of years to treatment with single-agent chemotherapy. A progressive fall in the blood count is a more ominous feature and when combined with lymphadenopathy refractory to treatment is usually an indication of the terminal phase of the illness. Occasionally a frankly leukaemic transformation occurs. Combination chemotherapy may temporarily arrest the process, but usually offers little respite. Death generally results from the consequences of bone marrow suppression often as an infective episode or occasionally a fatal haemorrhage.

Disease progression of the diffuse lymphomas mimics that of acute leukaemia either as an obvious leukaemic phase with abnormal primitive cells in the peripheral blood, anaemia, neutropenia and thrombocytopenia, or by profound bone marrow suppression. Generalized lymphadenopathy is also common. Retreatment with the original intensive chemotherapy may result in second and third remissions, but eventually overwhelming disease refractory to treatment becomes apparent, with rapid decline and death from infection or haemorrhage. The terminal features of these conditions are often sufficiently severe to warrant hospital admission. Judicious use of blood transfusions, antibiotics and anticancer drugs may make home management possible for a large part of the terminal phase.

CARCINOMA OF THE OVARY AND TESTICULAR TERATOMA

These two conditions justify discussion together since carcinoma of the ovary is the second commonest cancer in women and testicular tumours are the commonest malignancy in young men. Furthermore, the outlook in both conditions is gradually changing with the advent of effective chemotherapy. While it is fairly rare for a family doctor to be faced with a patient with a malignant teratoma, he epitomizes the problems of managing a young adult with a potentially fatal disease. Most doctors in the community are, at one time or another, involved in the management of a middle-aged women with carcinoma of the ovary.

Testicular teratoma

This condition frequently presents as a swelling of the testis which may or may not be painful. It has been clearly shown that inguinal orchidectomy reduces the incidence of scrotal relapse. Many teratomas produce βHCG and alphafetoprotein and these are helpful indicators of disease activity. Immediate preoperative levels may be compared with those taken 14 days postoperatively. A fall to normal limits may indicate a possibility of total resection. However, a lymphangiogram, whole lung tomograms and a whole-body CAT scan are important techniques for defining disease extent since components of the tumour may be non-secreting, and the markers are thus of little value in assessment of disease extent. Management policies are being continually reviewed, but since chemotherapy is capable of producing cures in patients with small-volume disease this has tended to become the first line of treatment when residual disease is known to be present following surgery, although radiotherapy is still given by some clinicians. Many patients who have localized tumour are cured by surgery alone.

Bulk disease indicates a poorer prognosis and the role of surgical debulking, local radiotherapy to areas of bulk disease, and the use of both

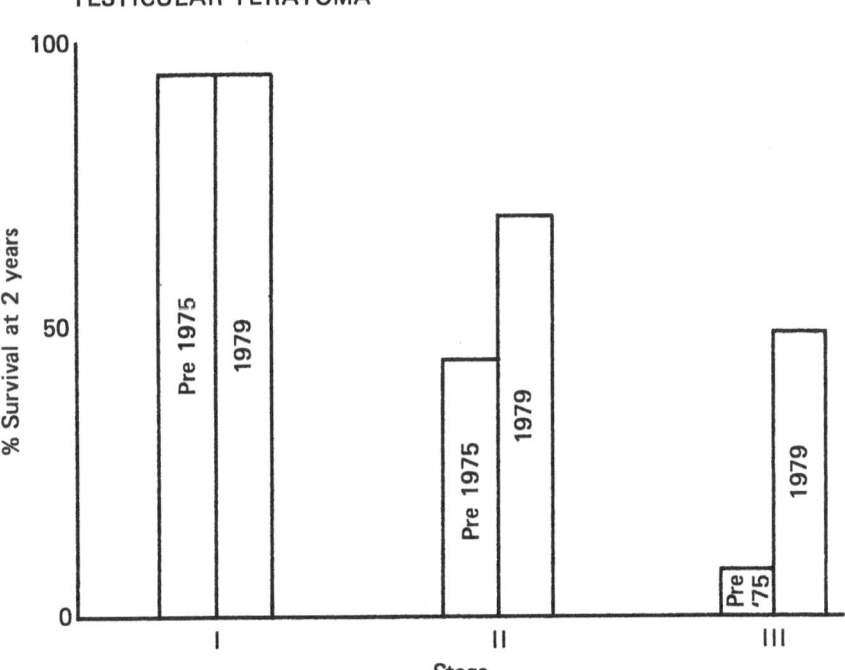

Figure 3 Change in prognosis for patients with testicular teratoma

in combination with chemotherapy, all have to be evaluated.

Although chemotherapy can now produce a high percentage of remissions and definitive cures (Figure 3) it is at the expense of short-term but serious morbidity. Treatment requires admission to hospital and throughout the period of hospital care the patient will be considerably dependent on the supportive care of medical and nursing staff. To the patient it may later have no more significance than a bad memory, but there is no doubt that for many this time represents a period of very considerable stress. In the individual whose disease responds only partially to therapy or in whom relapse occurs, this stress is amplified.

The continuing morbidity resulting from treatment, the constant dependance on hospital care and the need for frequent admissions, take their toll. Pulmonary metastases or recurrent abdominal tumours are common, and death may actually occur from respiratory failure. Once the disease is so far advanced very little respite can be obtained and symptomatic relief may only be achieved by progressively larger doses of analgesics and the judicious use of diamorphine. Occasionally abdominal masses may enlarge very slowly, but where this has happened in the face of previous chemotherapy and radiotherapy symptoms should be treated as they arise. Surgery in the management of local relapse has not yet been adequately assessed.

Carcinoma of the ovary

Many women present with this condition as a result of noting abdominal swelling, discomfort or even pain. Unfortunately, because of the situation of the primary cancer, 60 per cent have advanced disease at the time of presentation. The apparent hopelessness of the situation led to an acceptance of palliative treatment with single-agent chemotherapy – usually cholorambucil or cyclophosphamide. Newer combinations of drugs indicate that even large tumour masses may regress leaving microscopically normal tissue. Unfortunately the toxicity of some of the most effective drugs makes the treatment unsuitable for widespread use. As in the testicular tumours, the initial treatment is associated with an appreciable, if temporary, morbidity but there is now a clear association between the achievement of complete remission and survival. It is too early to identify whether cure can become a reality in this condition but the impact of combination chemotherapy on disease-free survival is encouraging. In those patients whose disease appears localized at operation, local radiotherapy or chemotherapy may have a place, while some patients are cured by surgery alone.

Relapse or progressive disease are characterized by enlargement of the abdominal masses, hepatic enlargement and often recurrent ascites. Where previous chemotherapy has been given, it is unusual to achieve any benefit with a combination of drugs. However, some control, if only temporary, may be effected in patients who have received radiotherapy only.

Ascites is particularly troublesome. In some patients the introduction of bleomycin following paracentesis may help to delay reaccumulation. However, fever and abdominal discomfort may accompany the instillation and only a proportion of patients benefit. Newer chemotherapies may help to control this distressing symptom. It is certainly helpful to relieve the abdominal symptoms where possible, for many patients are then able to lead fairly normal lives for periods which may range from weeks to months.

CONCLUSIONS

The management of the patient with malignant disease which is advancing despite therapy places considerable stress on the patient, close relatives and involved medical and nursing staff. Unfortunately medical training prepares doctors poorly for what is a fairly common problem in clinical practice, and most doctors learn to deal with this situation only when faced with the reality of the many problems that exist. The development of newer and more complex management techniques has unfortunately meant that frequently the significance of treatment is not immediately apparent to the patient's family doctor. Where treatment is successful a failure of communication is less important, but where disease is obviously progressing, the justification for continuing therapy must be clearly stated. Communication between clinicians responsible for different aspects of patient care is vital and the specialist clinician has, because of the rapid development in cancer management, a particular responsibility for ensuring that the patient's doctor has a complete understanding of management policy. It is important too that conflicting views on therapy are discussed, and some responsibility falls on the patient's doctor to discuss his anxieties about therapy directly with the cancer physician (to do so with the patient obviously undermines confidence) so that the fullest commitment to the patient's care can be obtained.

While medical services concentrate resources on patient care, the closest relative is largely ignored, but almost certainly suffers stresses and strains as great, if not greater, than the patient. Anxiety about the future, the patient's suffering, pain, the symptoms of disease, prognosis and many other factors mean that time must be given to them to explain situations and both to support and to reassure. No substitute exists for this, but all too often such discussions are avoided or handled rather remotely. Where one exists the early involvement of the continuing-care physician can help greatly.

All symptoms merit attention – the skilful use of analgesics is crucial to the comfort of the patient, but the judicious use of radiotherapy or chemotherapy in the management of pain from infiltrating or bulky disease may considerably reduce the need for analgesics. Pleural effusions and ascites should be tapped to increase comfort. Steroids too may be useful in patients with terminal lymphomas for their euphoriant and anti-tumour activity. Therapy which may help to maintain the patient's mobility and his enjoyment of life around him should be given serious consideration and not discarded lightly. The last few weeks or months of life demand much from those surrounding the patient and this is after all the greatest challenge to the physician's art.

References

Calman, K. C. and Paul, J. (1978). *An Introduction to Cancer Medicine.* (London: Macmillan Press)

Durie, B. G. M. and Salmon, S. E. (1977). Multiple myeloma, macroglobulinaemia and monoclonal gammopathies. In: *Recent Advances in Haematology (2).* (Edinburgh: Churchill Livingstone)

Kaplan, H. S. (1972). *Hodgkin's Disease.* (Cambridge, Mass.: Harvard University Press)

The non-Hodgkin lymphomas (1979). *Clin. Haematol.,* **8(3)**

Germ cell tumours. In: *Seminars in Oncology VI(1)* (1979)

Proceedings of the National Cancer Institute Miami Symposium on Ovarian Cancer. (1979). *Cancer Treat. Rep.,* **63(2)**, 225

10

The control of pain
I: by drugs; II: by non-drug methods

Susan M. Tempest and Ian M. C. Clarke

The control of pain in the patient with a limited life-expectancy is, in many ways, simpler than the management of pain due to non-terminal disease. Many of the most effective methods of pain relief are either uncomfortable or carry a risk of unpleasant or even dangerous side-effects which would be unacceptable in a patient who may survive 20 or 30 years. The risk of addiction from narcotics or long-term side-effects from other drugs are not seen when these are given for a few weeks or months, and adjuvant drugs to potentiate analgesia or minimize other symptoms are the rule rather than the exception.

Physical methods may produce better relief than drugs but require sophisticated equipment and considerable technical expertise which is not generally available.

Since drugs are available to all, and it is in drug therapy that the 'therapeutic revolution' in terminal pain control has been most apparent, these will be discussed first.

DRUG THERAPY

In the minds of many people a 'label' of terminal cancer is synonymous with a severe unrelenting pain which is relieved only by death. However, up to 50 per cent of patients with disseminated malignant disease experience only a mild degree of pain. The remaining 50 per cent have significant pain and about 10 per cent will probably require management by experts. It is this group of patients that present the physician who is not familiar with the treatment of the terminally ill with many perplexing problems, the chief of which is usually the control of pain.

The pain experience

Pain is not purely a physical phenomenon, but a delicate interaction between the perception of pain and the patient's emotional response to it. It follows that there are many modulating factors which will affect a patient's pain experience. This is especially true of terminal patients who are usually under great psychological stress for a prolonged period. Some of the more obvious 'pain modulators' are insomnia, fear, frustration, anger, depression, and mental and physical isolation. Thus it follows that pain cannot be relieved solely by the administration of analgesics. By paying attention to the relief of these other factors it is possible to raise the pain threshold and therefore reduce the dose of the 'conventional analgesic' and, with it the accompanying side-effects. The use of adjuvant medication and co-analgesics is discussed elsewhere (page 193).

Acute and chronic pain

It is appropriate to emphasize the differing nature of acute and chronic pain.

Acute pain is transient, diminishing, has a limited time-span, with a usually attributable cause. Chronic pain, on the other hand, especially that of terminal illness, is a semi-permanent state, thus occupying much of the patient's attention, lacks meaning and frequently increases progressively. As a consequence the treatment rationale for these two conditions must be different.

Acute pain is relieved 'on demand' usually by injection of a standard drug within a restricted dosage regime. Sedation is an acceptable side-effect. In total contrast, analgesics given for the relief of chronic pain should *never* be given 'on demand'. The dose of analgesic must be carefully titrated against the patient's pain so that the next dose of analgesic is given before the pain has been allowed to return. Thus the pain is always anticipated. In practical terms the pharmacokinetic behaviour of most potent analgesics means that they are given every 4 hours 'by the clock'. There is no place for p.r.n. prescribing in the relief of chronic malignant pain.

The dose is increased rapidly until pain is completely relieved and relief is maintained until the next dose. This is usually somewhat more than is actually required. The dose is then reduced in small increments without increasing the dosage interval until the pain just breaks through. Then returning to the previous slightly higher dose establishes the base level of analgesia. As the patient realizes that the pain is not going to break through before the next dose is given, his tension and depression will start to lift and it is then often possible to reduce the dose, which then helps to cut down side-effects.

Unfortunately, analgesic clinical trials in human volunteers deal with the relief of pain in the acute situation and it is often difficult, if not impossible, to extrapolate this data to the chronic situation. It follows from this that analgesic doses used in the acute, usually postoperative situation, only provide the barest guideline for analgesic dosage in the control of chronic pain. The only guideline for effective dosage in this situation is the patient himself. The optimum dose of an appropriate drug for a patient is that dose which gives that particular patient pain relief in that particular situation. The only dosage ceiling is that set by practical problems such as unacceptable side-effects or large dosage volumes.

The Brompton cocktail

The continued inclusion in the *BPC* and *BNF* of both morphine, diamorphine and cocaine elixirs with and without chlorpromazine is a lamentable state of affairs. Inclusion of these mixtures in such standard works would seem not only to vouch for their efficacy but also encourage their use. This is almost always borne out when one asks a house officer why he has prescribed that particular mixture. He inevitably replies that he got it from some old formulary, but on close questioning cannot think of any pharmacological rationale for the inclusion of the cocaine, alcohol or syrup. This is not surprising, since there is none.

The Brompton cocktail has a variety of titles all equally morbid and mis-leading – Haustus E, Mist Euphoriens, Mist pro moribundo, Mist pro euthanasia, Mist Brompton. Under its various guises this mixture is, regrettably, still used in many hospitals and in general practice throughout the country, and is partly responsible for many patients dying in a semiconscious state with a degree of unrelieved pain.

Snow (1896) first reported the use of a morphine and cocaine elixir for the relief of pain in terminal malignant disease. Cocaine was included ostensibly for its mood-elevating effects. Financial pressures subsequently led to its removal.

The next record in the literature of the use of this mixture is about 30 years later at the Brompton Hospital where it was used primarily as a post-thoracotomy analgesic; the local anaesthetic properties of cocaine were obviously an added advantage in those patients with buccal or pharyngeal carcinoma. However, the inclusion of gin as a preservative and honey to help mask the bitter taste of the morphine would largely have counteracted the beneficial local effects of cocaine in these patients. When the morphine and cocaine elixir used at the Brompton Hospital first appeared in print in 1952 as a supplement to the *National Formulary*, the gin and honey had been replaced by alcohol and syrup. The mixture had the following formula and was known as Haustus E:

> Morphine hydrocholoride ¼ grain (15 mg)
> Cocaine hydrocholoride ⅙ grain (10 mg)
> Syrup 60 minims (4 ml)
> Alcohol 90% 30 minims (2 ml)
> Chloroform water to ½ fl. oz. (15 ml)

This formula was subsequently included in the 24th edition of *Martindale's Extra Pharmacopoeia*.

As if a mixture containing five ingredients, some of doubtful value, was not enough, later variants of the Bromptom cocktail contained a phenothiazine as an antiemetic, usually chlorpromazine. Now, having briefly summarized the possible contents of a Brompton cocktail, it is prudent to consider the pharmacological rationale for their use.

Morphine or diamorphine?

There is much debate as to whether it is preferable to give morphine or diamorphine to patients with disseminated malignant disease. In a randomized controlled trial (Twycross, 1977) involving nearly 700 patients at St Christopher's Hospice, London, it was shown that patients who received individually determined doses of a solution containing either morphine or diamorphine fared equally well with regard to pain and other symptoms. Patients who were well enough were given the alternate opiate in appropriate dosage after 2 weeks. It is interesting to note that female patients generally required a smaller dose of opiate to control their pain, but significantly more females received an anxiolytic.

Diamorphine is rapidly deacetylated *in vivo* to 6-O-monoacetylmorphine and morphine, and thus only has a transient pharmacological action of its own.

A study of the urinary excretion of morphine (Twycross, Fry, and Wills, 1974) in patients receiving morphine or diamorphine by mouth showed that diamorphine is completely absorbed from the gastrointestinal tract, whereas morphine is only about two-thirds absorbed. One can, therefore, conclude that the oral potency ratio of diamorphine and morphine 1:1.5

may simply reflect differing properties of absorption from the gastrointestinal tract and, that provided equianalgesic doses are given, the two may be regarded as interchangeable when being given by the oral route. The relative merits of morphine and diamorphine injections are discussed below.

Cocaine

Two trials (Twycross, 1977; Melzack, Mount, and Gordon, 1979) have shown that the 10 mg of cocaine normally used in 'Brompton mixtures' rapidly produces tolerance.

In a controlled trial either equianalgesic morphine or diamorphine-containing elixirs with or without cocaine 10 mg per dose were given to terminally ill patients. It was found that the introduction of cocaine caused a statistically significant increase in alertness. There was no detectable effect when the cocaine was withdrawn.

Twycross (1977) postulated that at this dosage cocaine was of borderline efficacy and tolerance occurred within a few days. However, some elderly patients can become restless, agitated and confused when given cocaine, whereas others exhibit characteristic withdrawal symptoms when deprived of a routine cocaine-containing elixir.

It is therefore concluded that there is no benefit in adding cocaine to mixtures for terminally ill patients. It does not, as previously believed, elevate mood, potentiate analgesia or obviously reduce drowsiness.

Antiemetic

Patients normally only need an antiemetic for the first week of treatment with a narcotic. Phenothiazines are usually used as antiemetics, but although they potentiate the analgesic activity of narcotics by blocking the reuptake of dopamine, they are extremely sedative, have a long half-life and many active metabolites. (Chlorpromazine, for example, has some 168 metabolites, many of which are pharmacologically active.) In addition to sedation, phenothiazines have anticholinergic properties and may therefore cause difficulty in micturition, dry mouth and impaired accommodation. The dose of chlorpromazine (12.5 mg in 10 ml) in the *BNF* formulation is probably not large enough to control emesis. The need for an antiemetic should be continually reviewed. Haloperidol 0.5 mg by mouth or 2.5 mg by injection is the antiemetic of choice. Prochlorperazine is a suitable alternative and is less sedative than chlorpromazine. Antiemetics should always be given separately from the narcotic; if they are included in the mixture, an increase in dose of narcotic means an automatic increase in the dose of antiemetic, inevitably accompanied by enhanced sedation.

Alchohol and syrup

The Montreal study (Melzack, Mount, and Gordon, 1979) showed that 0.75 ml of 98 per cent alcohol per 10 ml in a syrup-containing mixture was sufficient to inhibit bacterial growth. However, some patients find the alcoholic bite of such mixtures unpleasant. For patients with buccal or pharyngeal carcinoma it may cause more pain by a direct action on the ulcerated area. Probably an equal number of patients find that the honey or syrup produces a feeling of nausea.

Stability of solutions

At 25 °C an aqueous solution of diamorphine 500 mg in 10 ml was estimated to show 10 per cent hydrolysis within 10 days (Davey and Murray, 1969) but precipitation of 6-O-monoacetyl morphine occurred at about 7 per cent hydrolysis. The rate of degradation is not constant and increases rapidly below pH 4, acetic acid being one of the breakdown products. Other workers (Twycross and Gilhodey, 1973) looked at a more standard mixture – diamorphine 10 mg, cocaine 5 mg, ethanol 95 per cent 1.25 ml, syrup 2.5 ml, chloroform water to 10 ml and variations on this. The standard formulation showed 10 per cent hydrolysis of diamorphine after 8 weeks storage at 22 °C.

Higher temperatures increased hydrolysis and refrigeration reduced it by half. Increasing or decreasing the ethanol concentration respectively increased or decreased stability. Substitution of honey or dextrose for sucrose syrup decreased stability. Addition of chlorpromazine reduces the time for 10 per cent hydrolysis from 8 to 2 weeks.

Because of the variation in rates of degradation, precipitation problems and presence of other ingredients, extrapolation of these results to normal concentrations used and cocktail formulations is difficult.

Conclusion

An increasing number of hospitals and hospices are using simple solutions of morphine hydrochloride/sulphate or diamorphine hydrochloride in chloroform water. Diamorphine appears to be most stable to hydrolysis at pH 4 which is the pH of chloroform water. Although data is not yet fully evaluated, such mixtures would appear to be stable for at least 2 weeks. Chloroform water also helps to inhibit microbial growth.

Co-analgesics
Many drugs potentiate the analgesic effects of narcotics.

Chlorpromazine has been used for many years but is really too sedative and cumulative for regular use. Haloperidol is a much more potent antiemetic and also has narcotic sparing effects like chlorpromazine (probably related to the dopamine receptor blockade produced by both these drugs and the narcotics).

The use of tricyclic drugs to relieve certain types of non-malignant pain has prompted their use in terminal patients. Methylated tricyclics such as amitriptyline and clomipramine appear to be the most potent as analgesics and are best given as a single dose at night to minimize side-effects (mainly anticholinergic in type).

Amitriptyline combined with perphenazine is a particularly potent combination and produces analgesia, sleep, and lifting of mood; the perphenazine has a mild antiemetic effect.

Suitable doses are shown below:

Amitriptyline 25–75 mg nocte
Haloperidol 0.5 mg. b.d. – t.d.s. (antiemetic dose)
Amitriptyline 25 mg + perphenazine 2 mg (Triptafen DA) 2–3 nocte

Analgesic preparations of proven efficacy are now considered in the following order:

(1) Non-narcotic analgesics
(2) Non-steroidal anti-inflammatory drugs (NSAID)
(3) Weak narcotic analgesics
(4) Strong narcotic analgesics
         oral
         rectal
         injectable

Some commonly used preparations have been omitted as it is impossible in a single chapter to attempt an exhaustive study of all drugs ever used to treat malignant pain. Rather we propose to concentrate on drugs which have stood the test of time and to deal with these in detail. It is more important for the clinician to become familiar with a few drugs in each group rather than to dabble with many.

Non-narcotic analgesics
The usefulness of mild analgesics should not be underestimated, for they are highly effective in some patients. Moreover, the patient receiving

potent analgesics for severe pain will still require a mild analgesic for headaches, etc.

Aspirin is a peripherally acting analgesic and a potent inhibitor of prostaglandin synthetase and thus has anti-inflammatory activity. Its use is solely restricted by side-effects, the most prominent of which is gastrointestinal irritation. Both codeine and paracetamol are centrally acting analgesics but the mode of action of paracetamol has yet to be fully elucidated. Basic data of common preparations is given in Table 1.

Table 1 Common non-narcotic analgesics

Approved name/ trade name	Presentation	Typical dose	Comment
Aspirin (Nuseal aspirin)	tablet, soluble, 300 mg tablet, enteric-coated, 300 mg, 600 mg	300–600 mg 300 mg every 4 hours	no value in visceral pain; take after food to minimize gastric irritation; increases methotrexate blood levels; enhances effect of oral anticoagulants
Aspirin with codeine (Codis)	tablet, soluble, aspirin 500 mg, and codeine phosphate 8 mg	2 tablets every 4 hours	as for aspirin; codeine may cause constipation
Paracetamol (Panadol)	tablet, 500 mg tablet, soluble, 500 mg	1 g every 4 hours	caution in liver impairment
Paracetamol with codeine (Paracodol)	tablet, soluble, paracetamol 500 mg and codeine phosphate 8 mg	2 tablets every 4 hours	as for paracetamol

Non-steroidal anti-inflammatory drugs (NSAID)

These are specifically indicated for the relief of bone pain (Table 2). Osseous metastases are a common cause of pain in many patients with carcinoma of the breast, bronchus and thyroid and in multiple myeloma. The growth of secondary deposits appears to be linked with induced bone resorption. Prostaglandins may play a part in tumour spread and growth in bone. It follows from this that the non-steroidal anti-inflammatory drugs which are potent inhibitors of prostaglandin synthetase should be effective in relieving bone pain, although it does not appear that clinical efficacy is proportional to a drug's relative potency at inhibiting prostaglandin synthesis. Thus flurbiprofen is no more efficacious in relieving bone pain than is aspirin. Corticosteroids prevent the release of prostaglandins by their stabilizing effect on cell membranes. However, they do not inhibit prostaglandin synthesis and are not an effective treatment for bone pain, although they do modulate other facets of the inflammatory process and are effective in relieving pain due to nerve compression.

Table 2 Common non-steriodal anti-inflammatory drugs (NSAID)

Approved name/ trade name	Presentation	Typical dose	Comment
Diflunisal (Dolobid)	tablet, 250 mg 500 mg	500–750 mg every 12 hours	excellent for bone pain; twice daily dosage only; less gastric irritation than aspirin; may enhance effects of oral anticoagulants
Salsalate (Disalcid)	capsule, 500 mg	1 g every 8 hours	good for bone pain; take after food to minimize gastric irritation; may enhance effects of oral anticoagulants and hypoglycaemic agents
Indomethacin (Indocid)	capsule, 25 mg; sustained release capsule, 75 mg; syrup, 25 mg/5 ml	25 mg every 6 hours; 75 mg once or twice daily	good for bone pain; potent gastric irritant; causes frontal headache in 50 per cent of chronic users

Weak narcotic analgesics

When non-narcotic analgesics fail to give pain relief a weak narcotic should be tried (Table 3). Even weak narcotics cause constipation due to occupation of endorphin receptors in the gut, so laxatives should always be given to patients taking regular doses of narcotics. Distalgesic (dextropropoxyphene 32.5 mg, paracetamol 325 mg) has been deliberately omitted from the discussion as there is no evidence that it gives any better analgesia than does paracetamol alone. It is unlikely that enough dextropropoxyphene is absorbed from a single dose to significantly potentiate analgesia produced by paracetamol. It enjoys considerable popularity, perhaps partly due to the fact that it is easy to swallow and only available on prescription. According to the logic of many patients analgesics available only on prescription must be more potent pain relievers than those available over the counter. As a starting point, codeine (Houde, Wallenstein, and Beaver, 1958) is about one-twelfth as potent, and dihydrocodeine (Seed *et al.*, 1958) is one-sixth as potent as morphine.

Soluble aspirin and papaveretum is a much-neglected preparation. As the tablets tend to froth excessively and require at least half a tumbler of water in which to dissolve, this occasionally limits their use. It is not a controlled drug which is some advantage, but its use should nevertheless be monitored if long-term therapy is envisaged. Generally speaking, fixed combinations of drugs in a single-dose unit are to be avoided. Increasing the dose to obtain more benefit from one constituent may produce unwanted effects from the other(s).

Table 3 Common weak narcotic analgesics

Approved name/ trade name	Presentation	Typical dose	Comment
Codeine phosphate	tablet, 15 mg, 30 mg, 60 mg; syrup, 15 mg in 5 ml (codeine linctus BPC)	30 mg–60 mg every 4 hours	if a single dose of 60 mg fails to relieve pain larger doses rarely succeed but may cause restlessness; causes less respiratory depression than morphine
Dextro-propoxyphene (Doloxene)	capsules, dextro-propoxyphene napsylate 100 mg (equivalent to 65 mg hydrochloride salt)	2 capsules every 4 hours	large doses may cause drowsiness; similar onset and duration of action to codeine; little antitussive activity
Paracetamol with dihydro-codeine (Paramol 118)	tablet, paracetamol 500 mg with dihydro-codeine 10 mg	2 tablets every 4 hours	see under paracetamol and dihydrocodeine
Dihydro-codeine (DF118)	tablets, 30 mg dihydro-codeine acid tartrate; syrup, 10 mg in 5 ml	2 tablets every 4 hours	caution in asthmatic patients and those with impaired liver function; effective cough suppressant
Aspirin and papaveretum	tablet, soluble; aspirin 500 mg; papaveretum 10 mg	2 tablets every 4 hours	excellent combination for pain of central and peripheral origin; doses in excess of 2 tablets not practicable

Strong narcotic analgesics

There is no maximum dose of a strong narcotic, only that determined by practical parameters such as number of tablets or volume of solution. Doses should be determined on an individual basis, the right dose being that which gives relief for at least 3 or preferably 4 or more hours. Tolerance and addiction to opiates does not occur in patients taking these drugs for the relief of cancer pain. If the dose of an opiate has to be increased to maintain pain control it indicates a change in the underlying pathological process and *not* the development of tolerance. Some patients whose disease is stable have been kept pain-free on the same dose of opiate for up to 2½ years. Patients receiving large doses of opiates, who then have a cordotomy or pituitary ablation which totally relieves their pain, are usually able to stop narcotics immediately.

Contraindications for pentazocine and pethidine

Pentazocine (Fortral) and pethidine have *no* place in the treatment of chronic cancer pain. By mouth 50 mg of either are less potent than two tablets of Codis. Pethidine is a potent emetic and pentazocine causes an unacceptable level of psychomimetic side-effects which appear to be dose-related. The one study comparing oral and parenteral pentazocine (Beaver, 1968) showed that 90 mg orally was equivalent to 30 mg parenterally. The recommended adult parenteral dose is 40–60 mg. With an oral bioavailability of 18 per cent this suggests a dose increase of five times when switching from the parenteral to the oral route. Therefore, a patient receiving the recommended oral dose of 50 mg every 3–4 hours is considerably underdosed. However since there is considerable intersubject variation in bioavailability, standard oral doses of pentazocine even if increased five times would still be unsuitable for some patients.

Dextromoramide

This is a potent analgesic; 5 mg is approximately equivalent to diamorphine 10 mg/morphine 15 mg in terms of peak effect, but it only gives pain relief for 1–2 hours, and is therefore not suitable for the maintenance of analgesia. However, it is useful as an additional 'as required' analgesic for intermittent severe breakthrough pain.

Methadone

The disposition of methadone has not been fully characterized. On repeat dosing the drug accumulates in the body reaching a steady-state level after 4–6 days indicating a half-life of about 20 hours and possibly up to 56 hours. Studies have shown that plasma concentration is linearly related to dose on multiple dosing. The drug is extensively metabolized, only 12 per cent of the dose being recovered unchanged in the urine and faeces. Although the plasma concentration of the drug increases with increasing dose, on repeat dosing pharmacological response as judged by changes in miosis does not. Pupillary tolerance to the drug develops after 8–10 days and the response decreases for a given plasma concentration. However this smaller response correlates well with changes in plasma concentration.

Whether a similar effect exists in connection with pain relief is not known.

Chronic use of methadone thus causes excessive sedation and variable analgesia. It is not suitable for elderly debilitated patients.

Dipipanone

This is a potent analgesic with a rapid onset of action whose effects last 4–6 hours. Unfortunately it is only available in the United Kingdom in combination with cyclizine as Diconal. There is no evidence that dipipanone causes any more nausea than other narcotics and the inclusion of a fixed dose of cyclizine means that as the dose is increased to maintain pain control patients become more and more sedated until finally they become semiconscious. Diconal, therefore, is of limited use except at the lower end of the dose range.

Nepenthe and aspirin

This combination is much favoured by some clinicians. However, despite a good pharmacological rationale it has practical drawbacks. Nepenthe is an alcoholic extract of opium containing a standard amount of morphine. Each 1 ml of undiluted nepenthe contains 10 mg morphine. It is generally

Table 4 Strong oral narcotic analgesics

Approved name/ trade name	Presentation	Typical dose	Comment
Diamorphine	powder (hydrochloride)	2.5 mg upwards every 3–4 hours	1.5 times as potent as morphine when taken orally
Morphine	powder (sulphate)	5 mg upwards every 3–4 hours	both diamorphine and morphine should be given in a simple solution of chloroform water
MST-1	tablet, slow-release morphine 10 mg	10 mg, twice daily as starting dose	slow-release tablet only needs to be given twice daily; use limited by small dose unit; larger dose unit will probably be available soon
Phenazocine	tablet; sublingual 5 mg	5–20 mg every 4–6 hours	must be given sublingually for full effect; least sedative of all the narcotics; three times more potent than diamorphine on a weight-for-weight basis

prescribed as a 10 per cent or 20 per cent solution. Precipitation occurs at higher concentrations. Aspirin is unstable in solution and is supplied separately, being added to the nepenthe mixture just before administration. Such a complicated manipulation is highly undesirable for patients at home. An equally efficacious and far simpler alternative is diamorphine and diflunisal, as the latter only needs to be given *twice* daily.

There are three strong oral narcotic analgesics which are eminently suitable for control of severe pain: diamorphine, morphine and phenazocine (Table 4).

Rectal preparations
Most patients are able to take analgesics by mouth for the greater part of their life. When dysphagia, intestinal obstruction and persistent vomiting make this impossible, suppositories provide a useful alternative, especially for patients at home. Injections should only be used as a last resort. Three narcotic analgesics are available as suppositories: dextromoramide, oxycodone and morphine (Table 5).

Table 5 Narcotic analgesics used as suppositories

Approved name/ trade name	Presentation	Typical dose	Comment
Dextro- moramide (Palfium)	suppository, 10 mg	10–20 mg every 3–4 hours	too short a duration of action to be useful
Oxycodone pectinate (Proladone)	suppository, 30 mg slow release	30–60 mg every 6–8 hours	limited availability (see note)* 30 mg oxycodone pectinate approximately equivalent to 20 mg morphine PR
Morphine hydro- chloride	suppositories, 10, 15, 20, 30, 60 mg	10 mg upwards every 3–4 hours	10 mg and 20 mg available as a 'special' from Macarthys

*Oxycodone pectinate suppositories, although previously freely available from Boots are now made only as a 'special' through hospital pharmacies or branches of Boots. Practitioners should therefore check on current availability before prescribing.

Injectable preparations
Towards the end of their lives, some patients have to receive analgesic medication by injection. Most of them are cachectic with very little muscle mass left, so a small volume injection is both desirable and humane (Table 6). The greater solubility of diamorphine hydrochloride (1 g in 1.6 ml) gives diamorphine an important practical advantage over morphine

sulphate or hydrochloride (1 g in > 20 ml). In practice this means that patients need never be given an injection of greater volume than 0.5 ml. As it is unstable in solution diamorphine is manufactured as freeze-dried pellets whereas morphine is supplied in solution with a minimum volume of 1 ml. In the patient who is receiving antiemetics concurrently by injection the diamorphine can be dissolved in this solution, further reducing the volume to be given. This is at least half, usually far less than the volume which would need to be given by injection if morphine were used. Thus, diamorphine is always the agent of choice for parenteral use.

Table 6 Injectable analgesic preparations

Approved name/ trade name	Presentation	Typical dose	Comment
Diamorphine	ampoules, freeze-dried, 5, 10, 30 mg	10–60 mg every 3–4 hours	very soluble, 300 mg may be dissolved in 0.5 ml
Dextro-moramide (Palfium)	ampoules, 5, 10 mg per ml	10 mg every 2–3 hours	short duration of action, large volume of injection, and high inciaence of side-effects, make it unsuitable
(Cyclimorph)	ampoules, morphine tartrate 10 mg, cyclizine 50 mg per ml; morphine tartrate 15 mg, cyclizine tartrate 50 mg per ml		fixed dose for cyclizine gives unacceptable degree of sedation at higher dosages necessary for pain relief
Levorphanol (Dromoran)	ampoules, levorphanol tartrate 2 mg in 1 ml	2–4 mg every 4–3 hours	2 mg equivalent to 7.5 mg diamorphine by injection; no advantage over diamorphine
Methadone (Physeptone)	ampoules, 10 mg per 1 ml	10 mg every 6–8 hours	cumulation, and profound sedative effects make this unsuitable

NON-DRUG THERAPY

Radiotherapy or chemotherapy

Pain due to solitary secondary deposits or to growth of primary tumour may respond rapidly to 'single-shot' doses of radiation or to short courses of chemotherapy. Many patients may be maintained pain-free for long periods in this way without analgesics.

Surgery

Reduction in total tumour mass either by palliative surgery or radio-therapy or chemotherapy may delay the onset of pain due to nerve compression. Where secondary deposits have produced spinal cord compression a laminectomy may reverse neurological signs temporarily and relieve pain.

Pathological fractures are a common source of pain and are best treated by fixation. Healing of such fractures is uncommon and internal fixation is preferable to other methods even when life-expectancy may be only a few weeks.

If the patient is too ill for surgery, fixation may be achieved by plaster of paris, firm strapping, slings, or by careful use of pillows or plastic foam cut to shape. Care when changing position to support the broken bones can minimize discomfort.

The use of bypass procedures for tumours of the gut may greatly reduce obstructive symptoms which contribute to distress and lower pain tolerance. Similarly a colostomy or indwelling urethral catheter may enhance mobility and social acceptability and thus reduce distress.

Psychological measures

The importance of psychological support and reassurance cannot be over-stated. An anxious, frightened, lonely patient experiences much greater pain from his or her symptoms than one who is cared for in an atmosphere of trust and compassion. This implies the presence of people who will listen and discuss the patient's problems, both physical and emotional, in an honest and sympathetic manner whenever asked. The caring community contributes greatly to the management of pain.

Special techniques

While drugs may interfere with the central perception of pain, modify the emotional response to it, or mimic naturally occurring peptides like morphine, it is difficult to achieve total relief of pain by drugs alone.

Physical interruption of nerves along classical pain pathways may produce complete analgesia but at the expense of anaesthesia and even some motor weakness. Such may be the intensity of terminal pain that this is often acceptable to the patient. Nerves may be interrupted by surgical section, by cryogenic neurolysis or by chemical neurolytic agents. Surgical section is probably the most certain and long-lasting but may involve extensive exploration to gain access to the nerves involved. An alternative technique is to freeze the nerve with liquid nitrous oxide using the cryoprobe. This disrupts the nerve fibres as they defrost and the resultant analgesia may last 8 weeks or more.

Injection of nerves with aqueous phenol or absolute alcohol can also produce either nerve destruction with analgesia lasting 8–12 weeks, or a chemical neuritis resulting in an increase in pain.

These techniques are suitable for individual peripheral nerves and have the merit of being simple. However cancer pain occurs more often in the distribution of several nerves, and multiple injections, even at root level, may be unacceptable. It may be better to attempt neurolysis either in the epidural or subarachnoid spaces. The use of a neurolytic agent in the epidural space has considerable disadvantages. Not only does it require skill to confidently identify the space, but localization of the solution to the desired segmental levels can be very difficult and unpredictable. Aqueous phenol injected into the sacral hiatus can be helpful for sacral pain but the success rate is not high. A variable amount of the solution can escape from intervertebral foramina, so larger volumes of solution must be used, increasing the risk of systemic toxic effects if there is absorption into epidural vessels.

In contrast, subarachnoid injection of neurolytic agents has been used for many years following the pioneering work of Maher. Several substances are used. Neurolytic agents may be hypobaric (less dense than the CSF) or hyperbaric (heavier than the CSF) and the technique of use varies depending on the solution.

Hypobaric solutions rise in the CSF and the patient must be positioned with the painful part uppermost. Injection is made at the level where nerves leave the spinal cord rather than at the level of exit through intervertebral foramina. The level of injection is critical since the usual hypobaric agent, ethyl alcohol, is rapidly fixed and the position cannot be changed once the agent has been injected. Alcohol is said to last longer than hyperbaric solutions. The maximum dose at any session is 2 ml in 0.5 ml increments.

Most practitioners now use hyperbaric solutions since their use is technically easier than hypobaric solutions; 5 per cent phenol in glycerine is the most commonly used agent, and this is injected above the level of the painful segments with the patient lying on the painful side and tilted 45° backwards so that the solution bathes the sensory roots and enters the intervertebral foramina. The use of glycerine, in addition to increasing density, also delays the release of the neurolytic agent so that relief occurs more slowly than with alcohol but also allows some alteration in position to be made after injection. Alternatives to phenol have been 2 per cent chlorocresol or silver nitrate (0.5 mg in 1 ml of 4 per cent phenol in glycerine). These solutions are considerably more toxic than 5 per cent phenol but in experienced hands may give longer-lasting results. Occasionally 10 per cent phenol may be employed for the relief of spasticity or where nerve roots are protected by malignant infiltration.

Complications of intrathecal neurolytic agents are generally related to destruction of sensory nerves producing anaesthesia and paraesthesia, motor nerves producing weakness (usually transient), or sphincter disturbance. The latter is especially common with lumbar or sacral blocks, although less than 5 per cent overall where the block is unilateral and there were no problems before injection. Neurolytic block is less effective the longer pain has been present and the greater the general disability.

A special situation exists in the cervical region where intrathecal injection is especially hazardous, even with X-ray monitoring. For pain in the cervical and upper thoracic dermatomes a subdural injection may be performed. For this technique a short-bevel spinal needle is introduced (with X-ray monitoring), usually at the C6/7 level, until the point lies beneath the dura but just outside the arachnoid. Phenol 7.5 per cent in myodil injected here ascends against gravity in a thin straight line. The X-ray appearances are characteristic. Increments of 0.2 ml may be injected to a total of 1 ml. This is usually sufficient to relieve the pain of an apical lung tumour within 30 minutes.

In cancer patients most neurolytic blocks give pain relief for 8–10 weeks and can always be repeated. It should be noted that since the disease is often progressive the duration of pain relief may be shorter than expected. Where patients already have a colostomy and bladder disturbance due to disease (for example, pelvic recurrence after abdominoperineal resection of the rectum), a sacral block may give relief of pain without serious effects. The concurrent introduction of a permanent urinary catheter can restore social mobility and comfort.

Pain in the head and neck may respond to block of the trigeminal nerve, although extensive growth may demand additional block of the appropriate cervical nerves. Tumours involving the floor of the mouth may also require alcohol or phenol block of the glossopharyngeal or vagus nerves.

Visceral pain due to cancer of intra-abdominal organs such as pancreas or stomach may be effectively relieved by destruction of the coeliac plexus with alcohol or phenol. This requires the patient to lie prone while two 16 cm needles are introduced just below the 12th rib about 4 cm lateral to the spine of L1 on each side. The needles are advanced until the tips lie anterior to the body of D12 and anterior to the aorta. The position is checked by X-ray (ideally using TV image intensification) and loss of resistance to the injection of a little air and contrast medium (water-soluble). The neurolytic solution usually employed is 50 per cent ethyl alcohol. The injection can be very painful, so is sometimes performed under general anaesthesia. The discomfort can be reduced and general anaesthesia avoided if the neurolytic solution is made up of absolute alcohol and local anaesthetic (usually bupivicaine 0.5 per cent) in equal parts. A total of 50 ml is injected. Splanchnic vasodilatation produces postural hypotension for about 24 hours until the vascular space is filled by redistribution. Bedrest is thus essential and the patient stays in hospital at least overnight. Relief lasts up to 6 months and the injection can be repeated.

Pain at any level below about C6, which is unilateral with no midline or bilateral component, and which does not respond to simple analgesic measures, may be best controlled by section of the anterolateral spino-thalamic tract on the contralateral side. Classical pain theory states that the anterolateral spinothalamic tract is the primary nociceptive pathway for somatic pain. Although there is now considerable experimental and clinical evidence to suggest that this is too naive a view, alternative pathways (such as the dorsal columns) appear to require up to 2 years to become dominant. Thus interruption of the spinothalamic tract can provide total relief of pain in the region supplied by the nerves sectioned for up to 2 years.

Nerve fibres in the spinothalamic tract are classically laminated, with fibres being more anterior the higher they originate. This is also too simple since, although there is some grouping of fibres from adjacent dermatomes, there is great variation between individuals. The original technique of open cervical cordotomy relied on classical anatomical descriptions and a surgical section was made according to that description. The lesion made was usually greater than that absolutely necessary and, of necessity, required a laminectomy. The introduction of percutaneous radiofrequency coagulation of the spinal cord in 1965 (Rosomoff, 1974) not only allowed cordotomy without exposure of the cord, but also permitted precise control of the site of the lesion. Under local anaesthesia a needle is introduced into the subarachnoid space between C1 and C2 and through it a fine wire, insulated except at the tip, is stereotactically placed in the anterolateral part of the cord. A stimulating current is passed through the wire and the patient experiences a tingling or hot/cold sensation in part of the body. Correct placement is indicated when the stimulated sensation corresponds to the painful part. A coagulating current is briefly applied and a small thermal lesion made. This can be progressively enlarged until pain relief is complete.

At this high level of the cord neurones are involved in the automatic control of respiration. These are frequently damaged by the cordotomy and if bilateral lesions are made at the same level about 4% of patients lose the power of automatic respiration (sleep apnoea or Ondine's curse); this is permanent in half of those affected. Bilateral cordotomy may be employed so long as there are several segments between the lesions but there are considerable technical difficulties in making lesions below C1/2. Some workers use an anterior approach to the cord especially for the second side but this is much more difficult than the lateral technique.

The principal complication is that of postcordotomy dysaesthesia which occurs in about 1 per cent of patients 6 months or more after the cordotomy. This is experienced as a severe burning sensation in the previously hypaesthetic area. It can be virtually impossible to relieve and is comparable to the anaesthesia dolorosa which may follow coagulation or section of trigeminal rootlets.

Patients who have widespread, bilateral or midline pain may obtain relief from alcohol injection of the pituitary gland. This was developed following the observation that patients undergoing open hypophysectomy as part of hormone ablation therapy for cancer of the breast or prostate often obtained analgesia, whether or not there was regression of metastases. Experience with the technique suggests that hormone suppression is not essential for the analgesic effect and some non-hormone-dependent metastases may become pain-free.

The method involves the introduction of a specially strengthened trocar and cannula through the nose and sphenoid sinus into the pituitary fossa. It is important that the cannula is kept in the midline since the cavernous sinus and internal carotid artery lie laterally. A small hammer is used to drive the cannula through the floor of the pituitary fossa and into the gland. After injecting a little radio-opaque contrast medium to confirm the position, a maximum of 1.0 ml absolute alcohol is injected in 0.1 ml increments. After each incremental dose the pupil size and reaction to light are checked since spillage of alcohol outside the fossa is usually first manifest by its effects on the III cranial nerve. After the cannula is removed the nose is packed with gauze for a few hours although bleeding is rarely a problem.

Pain relief often occurs immediately although it may take up to 24 hours to develop. About 40 per cent of patients are rendered pain-free, and a further 30 per cent obtain significant reduction in analgesic requirement. Complications increase if the dose of alcohol exceeds 1 ml at each session. Most complications are simple, such as nasal bleeding or transient CSF rhinorrhoea, or are related to involvement of cranial nerves with alcohol. Transient visual disturbances may also occur but are rarely permanent.

Diabetes insipidus occurs in 10–15 per cent of patients but is easily managed with carbamazepine or vasopressin (DDAVP). Hormone replacement with corticosteroid is always required although other hormones are not replaced unless survival exceeds 6 months. Beyond that time it may be necessary to supply thyroxine.

The whole procedure can be easily completed in 25–30 minutes. An overnight stay in hospital is required in case diabetes insipidus occurs and urine output must be carefully observed for the first 24–48 hours.

Traditional methods of pain relief in cancer, other than drugs, have involved the destruction of nerve pathways. The use of stimulation to relieve pain has a long history in the East, for example, acupuncture, but has only recently been used in the West. Although acupuncture is highly effective for some types of non-malignant pain, and some European acupuncturists have found it to be useful for pain in terminal patients, this has not been confirmed by all British workers.

Transcutaneous nerve stimulation, using machines which produce a low frequency (20–100 Hz) electrical pulse applied through skin electrodes may be useful for pain due to nerve irritation and can give considerable relief with no side-effects. An electrode jelly is usually used and this must not be allowed to dry out or deep burns can occur. A tingling sensation replaces the pain and, theoretically, interferes with onward transmission of pain impulses in the spinal cord through the 'gate' mechanism. Electrical stimulation of the central nervous system by directly applied electrodes is a recent concept. It has been known from animal experiments that stimulation of the dorsal columns of the spinal cord or parts of the hypothalamus or periaqueductal grey matter can produce analgesia. Recent work suggests that this is due to release of endorphin by the brain and the analgesia produced can be reversed by naloxone, a specific narcotic antagonist.

Dorsal column stimulation may be achieved by direct introduction of electrodes at laminectomy or percutaneously through epidural needles. Cerebral stimulation requires the making of at least one burr-hole and a stereotactic procedure to place the electrode in the correct position.

Although the cost of a fully implantable system, including a subcutaneous aerial and external radio transmitter, is £1000–3000 at current prices, for relief of pain in terminal patients it is usually unnecessary to have an implanted system and the electrodes may be led out through the skin to an external stimulator. For short-term use infection is not a great problem and the disturbance to the patient is minimal.

References

Bates, T. (1978). Radiotherapy in terminal care. In C. Saunders (ed.) *The Management of Terminal Disease.* (London: Arnold)

Bates, T. and Vanier, T. (1978). Palliation by cytotoxic chemotherapy and hormone therapy. In C. Saunders (ed.) *The Management of Terminal Disease* (London: Arnold)

Beaver, W. T. (1968). A clinical comparison of the effects of oral and intramuscular administration of the analgesics pentazocine and phenazocine. *Clin. Pharmacol. Ther.,* **9,** 582

Bond, M. R. (1976). Pain and personality in cancer patients. In Bonica, J. J. and Albe-Fessard, D. (eds.) *Advances in Pain Research and Therapy.* Vol. 1, p. 311 (New York: Raven Press)

Davey, E. A. and Murray, J. B. (1969). Hydrolysis of diamorphine in aqueous solutions. *Pharmaceut. J.,* **203,** 5538, 739

Fairman, D. 1976. Neurophysiological basis for the hypothalamic lesion and stimulation by chronic implanted electrodes for the relief of intractable pain in cancer. In Bonica, J. J. and Albe-Fessard, D. (eds.) *Advances in Pain Research and Therapy.* Vol. 1, p. 843 (New York: Raven Press)

Ganz, E. and Mullan, S. (1977). Percutaneous cordotomy. In S. Lipton (ed.) *Persistent Pain.* (London: Academic Press)

Houde, R. W., Wallenstein, S. L. and Beaver, W. T. (1965). Clinical measurement of pain. In de Stevens, G. (ed.) *Analgesics.* (London: Academic Press)

Katz, J. (1974). Current role of neurolytic agents. *Adv. Neurol.,* **4,** 471

Lipton, S. (1979). The treatment of cancer pain. In *Relief of Pain in Clinical Practice.* (Oxford: Blackwell Scientific Publications)

Lipton, S., Dervin, E. and Heywood, O. B. (1974). A stereotactic approach to the anterior percutaneous cervical cordotomy. *Adv. Neurol.,* **4,** 689

Lipton, S., Miles, J. B. and Williams, N. E. (1979). Pituitary injection of alcohol for inoperable and intractable cancer pain. In Bonica, J. J. *et al.* (eds.) *Advances in Pain Research and Therapy.* Vol. 3, p. 905 (New York: Raven Press)

Maher, R. and Mehta, M. (1977). Spinal and epidural anaesthesia. In S. Lipton (ed.) *Persistent Pain.* (London: Academic Press)

Meyerson, P., Boethius, J. and Carlsson. A. M. (1979). Alleviation of malignant pain by electrical stimulation in the periventricular-periaquadctal region. In Bonica, J. J. *et al.* (eds.) *Advances in Pain Research and Therapy.* Vol. 3, p. 525 (New York: Raven Press)

Melzack, R. Mount, B. M. and Gordon, J. M. (1979). The Brompton Mixture vs. morphine orally: effects on pain. *Can. Med. Assoc. J.,* **120,** 435

Merskey, H. (1976). Psychiatric aspects of the control of pain. In Bonica J. J. and Albe-Fessard, D. (eds.) *Advances in Pain Research and Therapy.* Vol. 1, p. 711 (New York: Raven Press)

Moricca, G. (1974). Chemical hypophysectomy for cancer pain. *Adv. Neurol.,* **4,** 707

Moricca, G. (1977). Pituitary neuroadenolysis in the treatment of intractable pain from cancer. In Lipton, S. (ed.). *Persistent Pain.* (London: Academic Press)

Parker, R. G. (1974). Selective use of radiation therapy for the cancer patient with pain. *Adv. Neurol.,* **4,** 491

Rosomoff, H. L. (1974). Percutaneous radiofrequency cervical cordotomy for intractable pain. *Adv. Neurol.*, **4**, 683

Seed, J. C., Wallenstein, S. L., Houde, R. W. and Belville, J. W. (1958). A comparison of the analgesic and respiratory effects of dihydrocodeine and morphine in man. *Arch. Int. Pharmacodyn. Ther.*, **116**, 293

Snow, H. (1896). Opium and cocaine in the treatment of cancerous disease. *Br. Med. J.*, **2**, 718

Twycross, R. G. (1977). Value of cocaine in opiate-containing elixirs. *Br. Med. J.*, **2**, 6098, 1348

Twycross, R. G. (1977). Choice of strong analgesic in terminal cancer: diamorphine or morphine. *Pain*, **3**, 93

Twycross, R. G. and Gilhodey, R. A. (1973). Euphoriant elixirs. *Br. Med. J.*, **4**, 5891, 553

Twycross, R. G., Fry, D. E. and Wills, P. D. (1974). The alimentary absorption of diamorphine and morphine as indicated in urinary excretion studies. *Br. J. Clin. Pharmacol.*, **1**, 491

Ventafridda, V. and Martino, G. (1979). Clinical evaluation of subarachnoid neurolytic blocks in intractable cancer pain. In Bonica, J. J. and Albe-Fessard, D. (eds.) *Advances in Pain Research and Therapy.* Vol. 1, p. 699 (New York: Raven Press)

White, J. C. and Sweet, W. H. (1979). Anterolateral cordotomy vs. closed comparison of end results. In Bonica, J. J. *et al.* (eds.) *Advances in Pain Research and Therapy.* Vol. 3, p. 911 (New York: Raven Press)

Williams, M. R. (1978). The place of surgery in terminal care. In Saunders, C. (ed.). *The Management of Terminal Disease.* (London: Arnold)

Note: *Advances in Pain Research and Therapy,* Vol. 2 (1979) (New York: Raven Press) reports the proceedings of an international symposium on pain of advanced cancer and provides a comprehensive view of the subject.

11

Management of other common symptoms of the terminally ill

A. G. O. Crowther

An awareness of the problems of our patients, for whom a cure cannot be achieved, is an important attribute to any physician. We have concentrated for far too long on making a diagnosis so as to produce a cure, to the near exclusion of the symptom control of those patients who cannot be cured; for too long these patients have been considered a 'thorn in our side', to be passed by with an embarrassed acknowledgement of the day, rather than a kindly understanding of their problems and proper attempts to control their symptoms.

In this field we have a shift from quantity of life to one of comfort and quality of life; with this slightly different concept of treatment there should be no need for our patients to ask for voluntary euthanasia. This shift in attitudes does not, however, rule out the need for acute procedures, which if used appropriately will enhance the patient's quality of life; we must always be prepared to consider these. The decisions needed are sometimes easy and obvious, but they can be far from straightforward and may well require discussion with the other professions involved with the patient's care, the relatives and the patient himself.

Many terminally ill patients can and will be cared for at home with lesser or greater involvement and support from other disciplines. For the patient this is perhaps the most natural and relaxed way of spending the remaining days, weeks or months of life, with relatives, friends and familiar surroundings. However, the problems, which may be medical, social or most commonly a combination of both, may be such that admission to hospital, nursing home or hospice is desirable, where and when such a bed is available. Many of these patients will be suffering from malignant disease but we must also consider those with terminal respiratory, cardio-vascular or neurological disease. It can be difficult to prognosticate with malignant disease, but it can be even more difficult with non-malignant terminal diseases and this uncertainty may well add to the problems facing these patients and their relatives.

Many symptoms can be helped or completely alleviated by an awareness of simple nursing principles and procedures long before the doctor's armoury of drugs and skills is required. A gentle caring approach to the patient by relatives and staff, and by staff to relatives will go a very long way to help with symptom control in our terminally ill patients.

ANXIETY AND FEAR

The problem here is that many of us assume that our patients are anxious about their impending death. However, this expected anxiety is less common and easier to treat than a much more deepseated one which frequently manifests itself by making other symptoms worse and consider-ably resistant to treatment.

Much of the anxiety or fear that our patients have is not that of dying, but rather of what is going to happen to them up to death, at death and very occasionally after death. Many patients have said to me, 'I am not afraid of dying, it is what happens if . . .'. The sentence trails off and is not finished; it is the unknown that produces so much fear. If we ask the patients to finish the sentence, it is often, 'what happens if I die alone, choke when there is no one there to help, start vomiting or get severe pain'. It is this aspect of anxiety and fear which sometimes makes symptom control at home more difficult than in hospital and may even make the situation at home quite impossible for both patient and relatives. Many patients are anxious and fearful because they only suspect what is wrong or what is happening to them. They may have asked and had any semblance of truth denied to them. Patients who ask what is wrong with them are often seen as a threat to our position, and yet with few exceptions a denial of the truth simply increases patients' fears and anxieties by isolating them from us. We have lied to them and all too often they know this. The most powerful weapon against anxiety and fear is to give the patient confidence; not that cure is round the corner, but that we are aware of the problems, that we are going to help these problems and that we are prepared to talk to the patient on equal terms truthfully.

Cicely Saunders compares truth in this context to a crystal with many facets on it, and which facet of truth we use, from the more distant ones at the back to the bald truth at the front, depends on many factors, mostly controlled by the patient. We may move forward on the crystal as the patient indicates a desire or need to know more. Patients are very skilful at changing the subject of conversation when they have the information with which they wish to cope; they may ask for further details at a later stage, or they may not feel the need for more direct information. With few exceptions, a denial of truth to our terminally ill patients makes their burden very much more heavy, and certainly makes for more difficult symptom control. Generally, I feel that we underestimate our patients' ability to cope with knowledge regarding their situation.

Along with an honest approach to our patients, an attitude of helping them with their problems to the best of our ability will in itself give the patient hope, not of survival, but of comfort and dignity. This approach does more than anything else to establish good rapport with patients under our care, and this must surely form a substantial basis for every brand of medicine, but none more relevant than in the field of symptom control for the terminally ill patient.

Seldom are drugs needed for anxiety alone, rather the morphine or diamorphine used for pain control are also useful for their strong anxiolytic effects. Because of respiratory suppression, these will be contra-indicated in patients with respiratory failure and yet there seems little or no problem with malignant respiratory problems. Alternatively a phenothiazine may be used for the anxiety, for this also potentiates any opiate analgesic being administered along with, in some cases, an antiemetic effect. The benzodiazepines are probably of more limited use, but may help particularly if the patient is tense as well as anxious during nursing procedures.

Phenothiazines
Prochlorperazine (Stemetil) mild anxiolytic, more powerful antiemetic
Chlorpromazine (Largactil) strong anxiolytic, good antiemetic
Promazine (Sparine) good anxiolytic, poor antiemetic

These drugs can be administered orally, in tablet or syrup form, by intra-muscular injection or by suppository (not promazine).

The dose will vary from patient to patient and with the particular problem. They have the disadvantage of causing some degree of Parkinsonian effects (stiffness, tremor, flat facial expression, etc.) particularly in the elderly. Generally these effects are more common with chlorpromazine than prochlorperazine, and promazine is least likely to cause problems.

Of the benzodiazepines perhaps diazepam (Valium) is the most commonly used at the present time. It can be given orally by tablet or syrup or by intramuscular injection – with this latter route it is useful to remember that with the patient requiring injections of diamorphine, this latter dissolves directly into the injectable diazepam, thus reducing injection volume. It also has a place when used intramuscularly in larger doses, or more particularly by the intravenous route, for patient management for acute severe anxiety state or difficult painful short procedures (such as manual removal of faeces in a particularly frightened patient, or where local pain precludes bowel clearance any other way).

Haloperidol (Serenace) is a butyrophenone derivative useful for nausea and vomiting (0.5 mg orally b.d. or t.d.s.); it has an anxiolytic effect which is more pronounced in supraemetic doses, for example, 5–10 mg 8 hourly by mouth or even by injection. In these doses, however, it has a fairly strong sedative effect.

NAUSEA AND VOMITING

A reasonable fluid intake is probably more important here than our drugs. Good and adequate nursing care will frequently allow a patient to avoid the need for intravenous hydration with very frequent small sips of fluid (which may be any flavour the patient likes), avoiding milk which tends to coat the mouth so much; it is easy to forget that icy drinks or even sucking of ice may help to maintain some fluid intake. Patients often feel that they must eat at all costs ('otherwise I've lost, haven't I?'), and yet we all know that at this stage fluids are much more important to life and comfort than food. An explanation of this can transform a nausea and vomiting problem.

Before trying to solve a vomiting problem, we must consider the cause.

Is it due to intestinal obstruction or subacute obstruction?
This may be extrinsic (tumour deposits) or intrinsic (severe constipation). If the latter is the problem, intensive attention to getting the bowels moving must be instituted ('resuscitation by enema' – Lamerton). If it is extrinsic, then one must consider whether the patient is well enough to withstand surgery and indeed whether surgery can help or is even morally justified. It is amazing how canny nature is in very ill patients; how with attention to fluids (small amounts and often) and the passage of time, the obstruction, even in the presence of massive intra-abdominal tumour deposits, will settle without surgical intervention. The colic of this

obstructive process is probably best dealt with by giving pethidine intramuscularly, rather than morphine or diamorphine, as pethidine relaxes smooth muscle more than the latter. If the patient is already on an opiate for additional pain problems, then pethidine may need to be given in between the opiate analgesia. Of course we must be alert to other surgical conditions arising anew and not directly connected to the known disease process.

Is it due to hypercalcaemia?
This is always a possibility in any patient with bony metastases who for some reason suddenly gets severe and intractable nausea and vomiting. A serum calcium will clinch the clinical diagnosis but the laboratory result need not be awaited before instituting treatment. This should be with prednisolone 10–15 mg t.d.s., but if this does not improve the symptoms (within a week) and the laboratory results confirm the diagnosis, then there are several courses open:

(1) increase the fluid intake along with a loop diuretic (frusemide or bumetamide) in high dosage;
(2) give Sandoz-phosphate tablets 1 b.d. or t.d.s.;
(3) give aspirin, phenylbutazone or indomethacin;
(4) give mithramycin in a subcytotoxic dose of 1.5–2.0 mg by slow intravenous injection;
(5) start a course of calcitonin.

Is it due to ionizing radiation or cytotoxic therapy?
This is not nearly as common as is supposed unless radiotherapy has been given over a wide tissue area or to the abdomen. Treatment by increased fluid intake and antiemetic drugs, as outlined below, will usually alleviate the problem.

Is it due to other drugs?
Morphine and diamorphine can and do cause nausea particularly in the ambulant patient. It is not as a rule so severe as to require other than routine medication with antiemetic drugs, but if severe, a change to other analgesics (dextromoramide – Palfium, or dipipanone – Diconal) may have to be considered.

The drug management of nausea and vomiting lies with the butyrophenone derivative haloperidol (Seranace) in a dose 0.5 mg b.d. or t.d.s. orally, or selected phenothiazines. These are prochlorperazine (Stemetil) 5 mg or chlorpromazine (Largactil) 10, 25 or 50 mg given 8 or even 4 hourly by mouth in a tablet or syrup. By intramuscular injection the dose of chlorpromazine is similar but prochlorperazine is given at a dose of 12.5 mg i.m. 8 hourly. Suppositories are also available (prochlorperazine 25 mg; chlorpromazine 100 mg) for nocturnal and morning control or when oral administration is not feasible and where regular injections are difficult (if the patient is at home, or very cachectic).

The vomiting from carcinoma of the stomach, particularly at the pyloric end, may be eased by the use of metoclopramide (Maxolon) 10 mg before meals, but apart from that use, it has disappointing results in nausea.

Having tried this group of drugs there will be patients who still have a vomiting problem. These need support in a general sense and many accept that they will continue to vomit periodically. A few patients are happier eating their chosen food and accepting that they will lose it later, rather than be compelled to stay on a fluid diet and still be nauseated.

The vomiting of raised intracranial pressure can often be helped by a course of dexamethasone. This is discussed further under coma (page 229).

BREATHLESSNESS

Progressive dyspnoea is perhaps the most frightening symptom that a terminally ill patient may have to face. The feeling of total inability to get one's breath is quite terrifying; it has been likened to a fit person closing off fully one nostril and half the other nostril, closing their mouth firmly and trying to exist on the inspiration and expiration possible through the half-patent nostril.

The causes range from a simple lack of tolerably normal lung tissue, as in multiple lung deposits, chronic lung disease or longstanding cardiac disease with associated pulmonary congestion, to mechanical obstruction anywhere in the respiratory system.

The latter group can quite well be helped by the normal medical methods for congestive causes, bronchospasm, pleural effusion, and anaemia.

Congestive causes and bronchospasm
For the former, diuretics are advised, and for the latter either broncho-dilators (orally or parenterally or by inhaler), or corticosteroids (orally or by i.m. injection).

Pleural effusion

This should be drained if the patient's condition is such that the procedure will be of benefit and if the lungs are normal. No more than 1 l at a time should be taken off; this reduces the chances of mediastinal shift, which may be lethal or at best frightening to the patient, and of overexpansion of the lung with consequential severe coughing bouts. If an attempt is to be made to stop the effusion returning or reduce the speed at which it reaccumulates, then a pleural irritant (nitrogen mustard or bleomycin 60–120 mg in 100 ml normal saline) can be used. Unfortunately, in the later stages of terminal malignant disease with effusion pleural aspiration is often disappointing, either because the fluid has loculated (often after previous aspiration) or because the real cause of the symptoms is grossly thickened pleura with malignant infiltration and the effusion is almost irrelevant.

Anaemia

Occasionally blood transfusion may be justified, but generally the results are poor. In the patients where dyspnoea is caused by sheer lack of normal lung tissue, then the problem is far from easy.

Oxygen has limited use, but may help whatever the cause, particularly in the patient who is used to having the oxygen near at hand. In these distressed patients, it is not good medicine (art) to withhold what they are used to or have faith in. Attention to the temperature and humidity of the air being breathed is the simplest and most important area of help for these patients.

Without a doubt the treatment of choice for the patient who has severe pulmonary malignant disease (wherever the primary site) which is causing sudden distressing and severe attacks of dyspnoea, is an immediate i.m. or s.c. dose of diamorphine or morphine (5–10 mg) so as to relieve the terror. This will allow the patient to die in a relaxed manner, or survive comfortably until the next attack.

CONSTIPATION

Apart from the fact that many of these patients are not eating well and are less mobile than normal, many are on diuretics and opiates, therefore much of the constipation problem is iatrogenic. This does not mean it has to be accepted with a complacent or defeatist attitude, but rather that it should be tackled with care, consideration and vigour.

The treatment of constipation as with many other symptoms starts with the nursing of the patient. An adequate fluid intake, suitable diet with fruit and roughage along with regular aparients: Normax (dioctyl sodium), Duphalac (lactulose) syrup, and Dorbanex (danthron) readily come to mind. Enemata, suppositories (glycerine or bisacodyl) or even manual evacuations may have to be used either initially when the problem presents or later, particularly if the patient is on large doses of opiates. It should be remembered that the commonly used disposable phosphate enema is only of use for a loaded rectum. If the rectum is empty than an enema with 1–2 l of normal saline with 30 ml glycerine is called for to clear a loaded descending and pelvic colon. It must not be forgotten that constipation may tip the older patient – and especially the male – into retention of urine, and perhaps even more commonly the elderly can become very confused as a result of chronic constipation or incontinence.

The paraplegic patient is often nursed with twice-weekly manual evacuation. To achieve this with ease and remove the distressing faecal leak in these patients, constipation is deliberately produced, usually with a suitable dose of tablets, codeine phosphate 30–60 mg b.d.

DIARRHOEA

It is important to discount spurious diarrhoea where the patient with faecal impaction is uncontrollably leaking liquid faeces. A rectal examination will give the diagnosis, with an enema or manual evacuation as cure. This must be followed up by suitable aperients.

Genuine diarrhoea must be looked at overall; any causes from drugs or other aspects of patient care (too many aperients!) must be tackled.

If the cause is due to malignancy interfering with normal bowel function (such as intergut fistulae, ileostomy or proximal colostomy), then Lomotil 2.5–5 mg t.d.s., codeine phosphate 30 mg 1–2 q.d.s. or loperamide (Imodium) 2–4 mg t.d.s. or q.d.s. will usually help.

Pancreatic dysfunctions (from carcinomatous involvement) will cause offensive diarrhoea which seems greasy and floats on water. If the patient can manage to swallow, then pancreatic extract in its various forms will help. Highly offensive stools associated with fistulae and pancreatic disease can be alleviated, or partially so, by the use of one of the non-absorbable sulphas, such as phthalyl sulphathiazole by tablet or suspension.

INCONTINENCE

The difficulties that this problem causes, whether urinary, faecal or both, will add considerably to other burdens in the home and may well dictate the need for hospital admission. Apart from this, if the patient is aware of the incontinence, it is a tremendous loss to his dignity and to his general poise in relation to his illness.

Urinary frequency
Confirmation and appropriate treatment of any urinary infection is of obvious importance. However urinary frequency may be as a result of bladder irritation, from previous infections or nearby tumour extensions, and this can be helped by the use of emepronium bromide (Cetiprin) 100–200 mg q.d.s. Nocturnal frequency in the elderly female can be helped by the administration of a short-acting diuretic (frusemide or bumetanide with potassium supplements) in the afternoon, so as to achieve a diuresis before bedtime.

Urinary incontinence
A urinary infection should be sought and treated vigorously but there will still be occasions when incontinence continues. This in men will probably be associated with a degree of prostatic obstruction with retention of urine, alongside a general weakness associated with the progress of the malignant disease. An indwelling catheter (14 FG with 5 ml bulb) will help the situation in that wet beds with associated disturbance to the patient when changing the bed linen are a thing of the past, and also the skin is less at risk. In addition, the weak patient no longer needs to struggle to pass urine into a urinal, bedpan or commode.

Urinary incontinence may be due to malignant infiltration of the sphincter mechanisms, of the nerve supply to these mechanisms, or it may be due to vesical fistula formation. The first two will be most easily dealt with by indwelling catheter, but the problems of urinary incontinence from vesical fistula are not so easily solved. From the anatomy of the region, these fistulae are much more common in women, from cervical carcinoma in particular, but also from bladder carcinoma, with fistulous connection to the vagina. We then must consider surgery for urinary tract deviation if the patient's condition and prognosis is such as to justify what is a fairly major procedure. More often surgery is not suitable and it may well be worthwhile putting a normal 5 ml bulb indwelling catheter into the bladder, and a 30 ml bulb one in the vagina, in the hope of plugging the fistula and so causing more urine to flow down the catheter in the bladder. The large bulb is deflated for an hour twice a day. This approach does not seem to cause the expected tissue necrosis and will sometimes help the patient considerably. One patient had a proven vesicovaginal fistula which was helped considerably by a vaginal 30 ml bulb catheter; however, this fell out one day, and before it could be replaced it was noted that she was quite dry, and remained so until her death some 4–5 weeks later. The fistula had presumably been plugged with tumour and/or necrotic tissue.

Faecal incontinence
It is worth repeating that it is of fundamental importance to establish this as genuine incontinence rather than faecal overflow from an impacted rectum. Many a faecally incontinent patient's life has been transformed by suppository, enema or manual evacuation (if the anal area is very painful this may have to be done under light sedation with oral or intramuscular diazepam, or more profound but short sedation with intravenous diazepam).

Tumour involving the anal sphincters or causing rectovaginal fistula will give faecal incontinence. If the condition of the patient permits the procedure, a palliative colostomy should be suggested to the patient, and if accepted will greatly improve their quality of life.

Faecal incontinence due to severe diarrhoea, interbowel fistulae not suitable for surgery, or gross bowel involvement in tumour, are probably best dealt with by the use of Lomotil tablets 2.5–5 mg t.d.s., or codeine phosphate 30–60 mg q.d.s. or loperamide hydrochloride (Imodium) 2 mg, 1 t.d.s. or q.d.s. If the patient is near death, then rectal evacuation may not be required, but if not, then twice-weekly manual evacuation is far preferable to total faecal incontinence.

FISTULAE

If these are internal, and if surgery has nothing to offer the patient, then symptomatic treatment of the resultant problems, if any, should be attempted.

Fistulae from the inside onto the body surface are distressing to the patient and sometimes difficult to manage from a nursing point of view. If further surgery is inappropriate then it is a question of frequent cleaning of the skin and suitable protection of the skin from any injurious fluids.

Orabase is probably the best protection but Complan applied locally will help when enzymes are thought to be in the leakage. An appropriate-sized stoma bag should be considered for the management of chest wall or abdominal wall fistulae with more discharge than a gauze pad will reasonably absorb.

Oral fistulae to the submental or submandibular areas need frequent dressing and mopping with absorbent material (Netelast can be used to hold dressing pads in awkward sites). Occasionally a patient will still have a small appetite, even though food swallowed comes straight through a large malignant fistula onto the supraclavical fossa. Here a tightly rolled gauze pad prepared by a nurse, but held to the fistulous opening during swallowing by the patient, will direct food along the correct track. This may well be preferable to a nasogastric tube, although this alternative method of feeding may be appropriate with some patients.

PARAPLEGIA

The patient who has become paraplegic through malignant disease and has not responded to appropriate acute medical treatment (radiotherapy with or without laminectomy decompression) needs careful intensive nursing and considerate medical attention.

We must not sacrifice patients to their paraplegic state. Many patients cope better psychologically with their situation when it is explained that concentration is to be on the top half of the body; in other words, 'forget about yourself below the waist and let us get you sitting up, into chairs for meals and wheelchairs to get you more mobile'. In these patients an imposed paraplegic regime would be wrong.

However, other patients will respond to a further period of strict paraplegic regime in the hope of improved movement and sensation in the lower limbs. This is certainly worth considering in patients with some movement or sensation in their limbs, particularly in those with spinal secondaries from carcinoma of the breast. The natural history of this disease is often long and variable, and we can alter the hormonal treatment of the patient so that tolerably often the condition does improve, even to being able to walk again and become independent. This may need a protracted period of paraplegic care, but if the patient is psychologically able to manage this, it can be most rewarding.

Alternatively the totally paraplegic patient who has a pressure sore cannot be sat out lest the pressure area deteriorates. Even this may have to be ignored if the deterioration generally indicates that life for the patient is short.

Sometimes the difficulty in achieving pain control with patients with pelvic or upper femoral secondaries can be helped by instituting a fuller paraplegic regime, while medication or other treatment becomes more effective. How strictly this regime is applied depends on the degree of pain relief that is achieved and the patient's adjustment to the regime.

DEPRESSION

This is often difficult to assess in this group of patients, whatever the cause of the terminal illness. So often the depression seems appropriate (that is, reactive), and here doctors differ in their views as to the usefulness of anti-depressants. It may be that the division into reactive or endogenous depression is false although useful, and this is no more true than when looking after terminally ill patients.

The restrictions with diet and other drugs that are mandatory to the administration of monoamine oxidase inhibitors (MAOI) really precludes their use in the terminally ill.

Most of us are familiar with the tricyclic antidepressants imipramine and amitriptyline and they remain the most generally useful antidepressants. The side-effects of these drugs are well known and may even be of additional use; amytriptyline is mildly sedative, whereas imipramine is less so. They both tend to have anticholinergic side-effects (dry mouth, hesitancy, blurring of vision, constipation etc.) but these are not usually a problem as the dosages used are lower than in psychiatric patients. Imipramine can occasionally cause fits so perhaps should be avoided in patients with cerebral lesions.

The problem of the 10–14 day delay before antidepressants start to work applies to all groups of antidepressant drugs including the newer tetra-cyclics, although this group does seem to have fewer side-effects. In this group mianserin (Bolvidon, Norval) is probably the most useful for the terminally ill in a dose of 20–60 mg at night.

However, it is perhaps more true with antidepressants than any other group of drugs that the doctor's familiarity with a particular antidepressant is more important than any theoretical pharmacological advantage of another product. When in any doubt, we should use the drug with which we are familiar, otherwise we will get lost trying to assess and use the large number of antidepressants that are on the market today.

CONFUSION, HALLUCINATION, AGITATION, PARANOIA

It is strictly wrong to group these states together, but perhaps this can be justified in that one may complicate the other and therefore all three may have to be considered in any one patient.

If the cause of the confusion can be recognized (such as pneumonia, hypercalcaemia, toxaemia from gross sepsis, constipation etc.) then the appropriate treatment must be instituted with vigour. So often a treatable cause cannot be found so that treatment with psychotropic drugs or simple sedation must be started if only for the sake of relatives and other patients in a ward unit. If the confusion is mild and non-distressing, particularly if it is of longstanding, then no treatment is preferable. Night sedation with a chloral preparation or chlormethiazole (Heminevrin) may be required; both products can be given as a tablet or elixir.

If the confusion is more severe and distressing, then a regular dosage with chlorpromazine (Largactil), promazine (Sparine), or haloperidol (Serenace) should be given.

Before hallucination can be accepted as a symptom, we must exclude misinterpretation of normal sounds, particularly where hyperacusis is suspected; this can occur with severe weight loss, or wax in the ears. If true hallucination is the diagnosis then regular dosage of chlorpromazine, promazine, or haloperidol may be needed, often in a somewhat higher dosage than for confusion.

Agitation and paranoia can in the terminally ill patient be considered together. If the agitation is a part of the terminal phase of the illness, where support and counselling are ineffective, then an increase in the dose of opiate along with a sedative drug is called for. If the patient is not so ill, and if the regular administration of chlorpromazine, promazine or haloperidol fail to control the problem, a difficult decision must be made. The patient may need to be rapidly transferred from his or her present physical environment, either from home to hospital, or hospital to home, with maximal medical and ancillary support. If for any reason this is impossible, then heavier sedation with the above drugs given by injection or by paraldehyde (10–20 ml i.m. by glass syringe) must be used. Whichever course is taken, relatives should be warned that this mental state often heralds the final few days of life.

OEDEMA

In terminally ill patients this is often positional or associated with a low serum albumen in the debilitated patient or impaired lymphatic and venous drainage of a limb by tumour.

Position of the limb or limbs is important. Sitting with legs up on a stool or settee or an arm on one or two cushions, the foot of the bed raised 75 to 100 mm, can all produce some improvement to dependent oedema. Elastic web bandages properly applied are of more use in maintaining improvement than in reducing oedema by themselves.

The Jobst pump (American) or Flowtron pump (British) both produce an intermittent positive pressure through a cuff or sleeve to arm or leg; this helps to reduce oedema or at least soften brawny oedema, which tends to splint the limb as well as add to the patient's pain, so that it is well worth trying to soften the area.

In addition, diuretics should be used in appropriate dosage. Loop diuretics (such as frusemide or bumetanide) have the advantage of efficiency as well as speed of action. Additionally an aldosterone antagonist should be used alongside the other diuretics, but spironalactone or triamterene take longer to show effect.

Treatment with antibiotics may be needed where there is any cellulitis associated with oedema.

Occasionally cytotoxic therapy or radiotherapy may be appropriate to effect the palliative diminution in a tumour mass that is causing venous or lymphatic obstruction.

Oedema of scrotum and penis, which is secondary to tumour of bladder or prostate, adds to the discomfort of patients and to the problems of their nursing care. Particular cleanliness must be observed. An indwelling catheter inserted for incontinence of urine and occasionally a bridge of adhesive tape between the anterior aspects of the thighs, which supports the oedematous male genital organs, will help.

Pulmonary oedema should be assessed and treated vigorously with diuretics, and also with other therapy appropriate for the overall condition of the patient. A good diuresis may transform the bubbling that comes at the end of life for a patient with carcinoma of the bronchus.

ANOREXIA

It is stupid to try to increase the appetite of a patient who has intractable nausea and vomiting or one with severe dysphagia. Often by pressing patients to eat more, by giving large or even normal-sized portions of food to eat, a profound anorexia is produced. It is far better to give small, well-prepared and well-presented meals; it is surprising how soon this will produce a request for a second helping or at least the achievement of clearing a plate.

The anorexia so often associated with malignancy in the gastrointestinal tract may respond to prednisolone 5 mg once or twice a day. This drug also gives a feeling of wellbeing and so can be useful for many terminally ill patients.

Anorexia may be the result of oral monilia or just a 'dirty' mouth. Nursing care, plus nystatin 1 ml q.d.s., or amphotericin (Fungilin) oral tablets sucked 1 q.d.s., or miconazole (Daktarin) tablets or gel sucked q.d.s., should improve this. Of course, attention to adequate hydration is also important.

In malignant disease, particularly of the bronchus and colon, perhaps associated with liver metastases, patients occasionally complain of a nasty taste in the mouth – 'like chewing copper coins'. There is no reliable remedy for this interesting symptom.

DRY MOUTH

Attention to general hydration and to cleanliness of the mouth and teeth are really all we have to offer here. If mouth breathing can be avoided, this will help a lot.

If the patient's condition is such that general rehydration is not reasonable, then regular small sips of liquids (fizzy drinks for preference) or even the sucking of crushed ice will help remove the unpleasantness of a dry mouth. This symptom may be iatrogenic and attention to the drug regime is indicated. Diuretics, propantheline and tricyclic antidepressants are all possible causes of a dry mouth. Parotitis is also a possibility, and if this occurs it should be treated with an appropriate antibiotic.

EXCESSIVE SALIVATION (OR INABILITY TO SWALLOW THE NORMAL PRODUCTION OF SALIVA)

This is seen in bulbar palsy, motor neurone disease and oropharyngeal tumours (particularly if DXR has not been given). It is not easy to treat and the first line is one of providing an adequate supply of tissues for mopping up saliva.

Propantheline tablets 15 mg–30 mg b.d. can be useful, as can atropine tablets 0.6 mg ½−1 t.d.s. (but side-effects of the central nervous system must be monitored). Some people use belladonna mouthwashes or Eumydrin drops.

Antidepressants sometimes cause reduced salivation as a useful side-effect.

ASCITES

If the accumulation of ascitic fluid is such as to distress the patient, giving a feeling of abdominal tightness, discomfort or heaviness, or difficulty with breathing, then an abdominal tap can be done. If the fluid has not loculated then there can be good relief of the symptoms. Reaccumulation can be reduced or prevented by the instillation of thiotepa, but this does tend to produce loculation and hence difficulty with draining if the ascitic fluid returns. There seems some uncertainty as to how fast the fluid can be run out; if anything we tend to be too slow and conservative, and a tap of 10 l in a few hours generally has no untoward effects on the patient.

Diuretics, particularly the aldosterone antagonists, spironalactone (Aldactone) or triamterene (Dytac), seem to reduce the speed of fluid reaccumulation. However, if the patient has few or no symptoms, then there probably is no reason to drain or attempt to drain the accumulation of fluid. This attitude can similarly be applied to pleural effusions.

COUGH

If this is productive of sputum and troublesome, then help with the sputum is needed. There is doubt as to whether there is really an effective expectorant available.

However for tenacious sputum, several things can be attempted. If possible, avoidance of a dry atmosphere which is too warm (central heating) by giving adequate humidity is important. Nose breathing should be encouraged, the old-fashioned steam inhalants are helpful.

Of the drugs available for making sputum less viscid, perhaps bromhexine (Bisolvon) 9−16 mg q.d.s. is the most effective. A course of oxytetracycline at the same time may help.

The dry cough, which is so much the feature of carcinoma of the bronchus, should be suppressed with drugs, if radiotherapy to the offending tumour or gland has not helped or is thought to be inappropriate.

Codeine linctus 5–10 ml 4 hourly or the controlled drug methadone linctus 5–10 ml t.d.s. or 4 hourly are very effective. Care is needed with methadone, particularly in the elderly, since it is only slowly excreted and quickly accumulates in the body. Opiates, which may be being used for pain control, are also good cough suppressants. In a non-specific way prednisolone 5 mg t.d.s. may also help the troublesome dry cough.

INSOMNIA

This may be due to pain, fear, other symptoms or as a result of sleeping and resting more in the day than the patient used to. A warm night-time drink along with adequate sedation, usually avoiding barbiturates (unless the patient is accustomed to them and has had them for years), is required. If the patient is already on phenothiazines (such as chlorpromazine or promazine) than an increased dose at night-time or in the evening is useful. Otherwise diazepam (Valium), dichloralphenazone (Welldorm), or chlormethiazole (Heminevrin), all of which can be given in tablet or elixir form, are probably the drugs of choice.

Troublesome frequency of micturition at night causing loss of sleep in the terminally ill patient, where treatment of a urinary infection has been attended to, or emepronium bromide (Cetiprin) has been found ineffective, will best be treated by an indwelling catheter.

SMELL

It is wrong to assume that the patient's own smells are not noticed by them. Often it is not mentioned, perhaps more in shame than anything else, but with good relationships it often becomes clear that the patient is only too well aware of the problem.

It has already been suggested that offensive faecal smells can be helped considerably by giving phthalyl sulphathiazole by tablet or suspension. Malignant tumours of the female genital tract can produce a highly offensive-smelling discharge. Penotrane vaginal pessaries night and morning if the patient is not ambulant, at night only if they are, will often help. Another useful preparation is povidone-iodine (Betadine) as pessary or vaginal gel. Dental sepsis should be dealt with by a dentist if the patient's condition merits it; if not, then prolonged antibiotic cover along with nystatin suspension 1 ml q.d.s. will diminish the discomfort and odour.

Antibiotics are sometimes useful for reducing the smell from oral, nasal and pharyngeal tumours that by their anatomical position must inevitably have an element of infection associated with them. However, there is no substitute for good nursing care in oral hygiene.

If the smell is from a fungating lesion, then regular local application of plain yoghurt with the dressing will transform a stinking area into one with little or no smell. If very bad, then the dressings may need changing four times a day for the first few days before reducing to twice daily.

In addition and more basic to all these suggestions, is the provision of adequate nursing staff so the patient can have at least one bath a day, assuming he or she is well enough. It is often surprising how delighted even very ill patients are at being able to have a bath (less so the men perhaps!). Simple domestic fans or air extraction apparatus may also be useful.

DISFIGUREMENT

It goes without saying that the management of this problem lies in a total acceptance of the patient by all staff, with no sign of disgust or reticence. The patient is usually only too aware of the lesion and as professionals we must be above showing any unhelpful feelings.

HICCOUGH

The problem here is that the aetiology is almost always unknown. It may be pleuritic, local (gastric dilation) or central, due to uraemia. It is probably best to start with lay-methods of treatment which seem to consist of stimulating the posterior wall of the pharynx – that is, by swallowing dry granulated sugar, by use of a feather, cold water swallowed from the back of a quarter-full glass, or pharyngeal 'tickle' using a nasogastric tube to the level of second cervical vertebra, having decompressed the stomach.

If these methods have failed and treatable uraemia has been excluded, then the following drugs or procedures can be used:

(1) Chlorpromazine (Largactil) 25–50 mg orally or by injection.
(2) Metoclopropamide (Maxolon) 10 mg by injection first and then orally.

(3) Quinidine 200 mg q.d.s.
(4) Methylphenidate (Ritalin) 10 mg b.d. or t.d.s., or dexamphetamine sulphate 5 mg b.d.
(5) Phrenic nerve crush under local anaesthetic.

DYSPHAGIA

If this is thought to be due to oesophagitis this should be treated with antacids, cimetidine or alginic acid (Gaviscon). If there is a possibility of monilia being the cause, then nystatin, Fungilin or Daktarin should be given regularly.

If obstruction is mechanical and the patient is fit enough, we must consider having an oesophageal tube (such as Celestin's endo-oesophageal tube) put down under direct vision. If the patient already has one *in situ*, there may be food or tumour blocking it off; the treatment will then depend on how fit the patient is, whether oesophagoscopy is reasonable or whether any active treatment other than fizzy drinks is possible.

The essential part of management is an adequate fluid intake with sloppy or minced foods (the meat and vegetables minced but left separate and not mixed together). If the dysphagia is high up or pharyngeal, then apart from the fluids and minced foods radiotherapy or some surgical technique (cautery with or without regional perfusion or cryosurgery) may have to be used. The advent of the Clinifeed tube, so much more comfortable than the older nasogastric tube, makes tube feeding far more acceptable than previously, although it is surprising, with good nursing care, how rarely it is needed. Gastrostomy is very rarely justified. Local anaesthetic agents can be helpful if taken just before drinking or eating is being attempted.

PRESSURE SORES

These are traditionally nursing problems, but the doctor must know what is going on and how to manage the patient. The best treatment is by prevention with good nursing and attention to incontinence, discharges, and the skin condition. All of these still apply even after a sore has developed.

If the sore is shallow, and therefore painful, then the treatment is basically to keep the patient off the area with regular turns (including the prone position), keeping the area dry (a hairdryer is useful) and the use of infrared light to stimulate healing.

If the lesion is deep, then slough needs to be removed by cutting it away, or by the use of Aserbine, Eusol or Debrisan. Systemic antibiotics may be needed to localize an area of cellulitis. Having achieved cleanliness, Eusol and paraffin dressings will keep the lesion clean and stimulate granulation and healing.

However, we must not sacrifice the patient to the pressure sore. This may mean that when life is obviously short, and rapidly getting shorter, we may have to accept that the pressure sore may need turns every 2 hours, but we must not interfere with the use of a wheelchair or even a short car journey.

WEAKNESS, DIZZINESS, ATAXIA

Several of the drugs that are used for vomiting, anxiety or as co-analgesics may cause Parkinsonian symptoms. These are usually reversible if the drug can be stopped, but if not, benzhexol (Artane) 2 mg t.d.s., orphenadrine (Disipal) 50 mg t.d.s., or levodopa (Madopar) 100 mg b.d. or t.d.s. should be given.

Dizziness, having excluded hypertension, hypotension and vestibular causes, can be helped by prochlorperazine (Stemetil) 5 mg q.d.s., promethazine (Avomine) 25 mg t.d.s., or dimenhydrinate (Dramamine) 50 mg t.d.s. These must be used along with an explanation of changing position carefully and slowly ('growing old gracefully means changing position slowly and gracefully') and using aids (walking stick, walking frame, or strategically placed furniture).

The weakness of malignant disease is very real and often the main trouble in the preterminal phase of the illness, when other symptoms are controlled. Prednisolone 5 mg once or twice a day may help, but generally honest explanation is the best treatment. A gentle reminder that although the symptoms are better, the patient is still ill, will help in the acceptance of the weakness. Most patients have kept a dog or cat at some time and I often ask what their pet did when it was ill; the reply is usually 'They slept most of the time', which is easily turned to the present situation. On two occasions a patient has replied, 'They lick themselves', which after explaining the answer I was expecting, both conveyed the message and produced a laugh as well.

FEVER

A history and examination will often reveal the cause which, if appropriate, will require the necessary treatment. It may be due to urinary infection (often associated with rigors), cellulitis, pneumonia or impending pneumonia, or the usual viral infections contracted from other persons on the ward or at home.

If no cause is found, then we have to decide whether to treat blindly or wait 24 or 48 hours for further clues to a diagnosis.

However, it must not be forgotten that malignant disease, particularly if widespread, does sometimes cause pyrexia. This is best treated with aspirin or one of the non-steroidal anti-inflammatory drugs (NSAID), along with the supportive measures of good fluid intake, tepid sponging, and perhaps, if the central heating is fierce, a bedside fan.

COMA

This state will usually mean that the patient is very near the end of life. Nevertheless, this period may be one of several days, so care and attention is still needed, with regular turns, attention to mouth and eye care, and above all vigilant skin care. If the patient does not have an indwelling catheter *in situ*, then if the deterioration is not very rapid inserting one will help all concerned.

If bronchial secretions cause noisy breathing, which can be so distressing to other patients or the relatives, hyoscine 0.4 mg i.m. should be given every 8 hours or depending on need. If this is not sufficient, then a suction apparatus may be needed; also an increase in any opiate drugs already being given will help in reducing respiratory excursion and thereby reduce the noise.

If the coma is sudden in onset or not expected, then other causes must be considered.

The patient who remains in semi-coma can present a difficult nursing problem, particularly in maintenance of some fluid intake to prevent dehydration and discomfort. This can be overcome with an overnight rectal drip of tap water, and this is so much more acceptable than nasogastric or intravenous administration.

Where the cause is cerebral malignancy, a course of dexamethasone 8 mg i.m. b.d. may lift the coma level enough to permit some return of the patient's consciousness for a time.

Fits can be controlled in the patient in coma or semi-coma with twice-daily intramuscular injections of phenobarbitone 100–200 mg.

SKIN IRRITATION

If this is due to irritative secondary carcinoma deposits in the skin, then the radiotherapist can help with X-rays or cytotoxic drugs; occasionally non-steroidal anti-inflammatory drugs will help.

However some patients get a distressing irritation of the skin secondary to their malignancy. A trial of an antihistamine may help but is often disappointing. The skin irritation of icterus can be helped by pheno-barbitone 30 mg t.d.s., methyltestosterone 25 mg sublingually b.d., or norethandrolone (Nilevar) 10 mg t.d.s Cholestyramine is also valuable. It has recently been found that cimetidine (Tagamet) helps the trouble-some skin irritation sometimes seen with Hodgkin's disease.

TENESMUS AND RECTAL DISCHARGE

The former can be one of the most distressing of symptoms to a patient with inoperable carcinoma of rectum, or the rare secondary deposit in the distal part of the rectum. The constant desire to defaecate which produces little or no result is demoralizing, undignified and extremely tiring to the patient, his relatives and staff. In view of this, surgery to remove the lesion should be done if at all possible, even if known only to be palliative. If surgery cannot be done or is refused, then we must still try and help. Local applications are very disappointing as are spinal block procedures, and the treatment of choice appears to be chlorpromazine (Largactil) 25 mg 6–4 hourly along with an appropriate dose of an opiate.

Rectal discharge can be helped by the use of morphia and adrenaline suppositories, betamethasone suppositories, or rectal washouts with 4 per cent tannic acid phosphate.

If the patient's condition is relatively good and the discharge constant with faecal incontinence, then a colostomy should be considered so as to at least remove the faecal stream and therefore reduce the offensive nature of the discharge.

FUNGATING LESIONS

These are not common, but when they do occur, they are distressing to the patient and relatives and, on occasions, even to experienced nursing staff.

The key to the problem is regular dressings at a frequency according to the particular problem. Nursing staff have their own ideas for dressings but Sofra-Tulle must be high on the list of preferences. Netelast is invaluable for holding dressings in place, even on difficult areas like the ear or mandible.

CONCLUSION

Attention to detail is vital when it comes to controlling symptoms in the terminally ill patient. Attention to simple points, such as mouth care or fluid intake, may be at least as important as the use of drugs to control particular problems. There will be symptoms that are not relieved by drug therapy, but the patient will frequently be content to know that everyone concerned is doing their best.

One trap that is so easy to fall into is to prescribe too many pills and medicines in an attempt to help all the symptoms. We must keep a balance between reasonable symptom control and overtreatment. By using one drug that will help several symptoms (for example, many antiemetics are also anxiolytics, methadone is a good cough suppressant as well as being analgesic) the total number of medicaments can be kept down.

The ethics of giving antibiotics to dying patients is one best settled by discussion between medical and nursing staff as well as appropriate relatives. Similarly the decision to give dexamethasone to a patient with cerebral symptoms should usually be a joint one. It is most important that having made such a decision the situation be kept under constant review, and if the clinical state which led to those decisions changes, there may well be indications for taking a different view.

It is difficult or impossible to project or forecast how we should react to our own terminal illness. However, when looking after terminally ill patients, it can be a useful exercise if there are problems with no obvious solution to ponder over what we would expect if we were in that particular situation. Also in the care of these patients, perhaps above all others, a mutual sharing of expertise and suggestions between medical and nursing staff can only benefit our patients and the relatives who are soon to be bereaved.

12

The personal impact of dying

Peter Maguire

INTRODUCTION

A firm link has been established between the experiencing of stressful events and the later onset of psychiatric illness (Brown and Harris, 1978). Life events which involve or threaten an important or personal loss are especially likely to lead to a depressive illness or anxiety state. Consequently, patients who are aware that they may be dying are at considerable risk of experiencing significant mood disturbance. Studies of patients dying at home, in hospitals or other institutions have confirmed that nearly two in every five experience distressing symptoms of anxiety and depression (Hinton, 1963; Cartwright, Hockey, and Anderson, 1973). In one in six the mood disturbance is moderately severe or severe.

The patient's close relatives, who have to contend with the imminent loss of a loved one, are also at risk of psychiatric illness. While the incidence of psychiatric morbidity in relatives before death has still to be established, they are more likely than the non-bereaved to develop depressive illness, phobic-anxiety states or alcoholism after bereavement (Parkes, 1964).

As many as 80% of patients who are dying appear to be aware of this even though they may not have admitted this to medical or nursing staff (Hinton, 1980). Most relatives certainly know since comparatively few deaths are wholly unexpected. Yet, it is clear that only some patients and relatives get to the point of needing help for their depression and anxiety.

The presence of such mood disturbance in dying patients intensifies their mental suffering. It also lowers the threshold at which they experience physical distress, and can make it impossible to achieve adequate pain control. Seeing a loved one suffer in this way can also make it more difficult later for the relatives to resolve their grief. So, it is important to consider why some dying patients and their relatives cope much less well than others, as well as to discuss how to identify and help them.

THE DYING PATIENT

Age at death

Younger patients (those under 50 years of age) experience more mental and physical distress than older patients in the period before death (Hinton, 1963). They are more likely to feel very sad, angry and cheated that they will not now be able to realize their hopes and ambitions. Parents of growing children often feel especially distressed because they will not be able to complete the task of helping them become adults, leave home and make stable relationships. They fear that the family will not be able to cope when they are gone and feel desperately sad at having to part from them. They can also feel that they are letting the family down by dying.

What a time to pick! She's only 16 and taking her 'O' levels this summer. Her dad's so busy – he won't be able to give much help even if he wanted to – it's awful, just when she needs me most I have to let her down . . . sometimes I think I did not fight [the melanoma] hard enough.

The parent who is dying tends to worry most about how his or her spouse will manage the family and about any children of the same sex. Children who have yet to pass through puberty often provoke much worry. 'She hasn't started her periods yet – who'll be able to help her with that?' These worries will be much greater when the patient has not discussed them with the surviving parent and made appropriate plans.

Single parents or those who have lost their spouse are in a particularly difficult situation. They not only worry about who will be the best guardian and how the children will fare without any parent but also how to break the news. If the children are already experiencing problems the parent will feel very distressed.

They've just never got on. They're always bickering. I can't stand it. If I thought they'll be all right I'd die easy. I can't stop worrying about them. What on earth is going to happen? It's so unfair. Their father only died 4 years ago. I've told the boy but I can't tell the girl. She'd be so upset.

Relatively few people die before the age of 50. Consequently, the patients commonly wonder why they have been singled out. This may lead to their feeling extremely bitter especially if they consider they have led blameless lives. 'Why pick on me? What have I done?' They may contrast the fate that is about to befall them with the ability of others much less deserving to escape personal disaster.

Young adults who have coped with adolescence successfully may also feel especially cheated that their lives are to be cut short and can find it impossible to find any sense in what has happened to them. It can be terribly painful if they have just got engaged or have only recently married. Sometimes, they may have unfinished business with their parents. There may have been feuds or misunderstandings which caused great distress and led them to wonder if their parents really understood and loved them. They can become very preoccupied and feel very hurt and bewildered, especially if their parents and others around them fail to realize this. Young adults have often had little opportunity to form stable relationships with the opposite sex. They may not have had any sexual experience. Consequently, they may brood a lot about opportunities they declined to take up at the time.

I did have a boyfriend when I was at college. I liked him very much but I did not want to be tied down. I wanted my independence. He kept pressing me to get engaged but I refused. He was ever so upset. I have often wondered if I did the right thing. The sickening thing ... what really gets me ... is that I'll never get engaged to anyone now, will I?

Younger patients who are going through adolescence often find the prospect of death extremely difficult to accept (Adams, 1979). They were full of ideas about what they might achieve when they became independent beings. Now they are to be denied this and they may not have enough good emotional experiences to sustain them. They may become rebellious and difficult or retreat into their own world. They are often very conscious of their body image and concerned about its integrity. This can cause them to resist physical treatments which affect them adversely. They would rather die intact than risk undergoing unpleasant changes through treatment.

They said I might get better again if I had one more course of treatment – I told them what they could do with it. Last time it made me sick and all my hair fell out. I know I'm not going to make it. I want to meet my maker with my hair on. Mind you, *he's* got a lot to answer for, hasn't he?

They may also try to develop some sense of purpose in the time they have left by doing something useful if they are physically able to do so. For example, they may try to write a poem or make a model car. They commonly insist on remaining as independent as possible of any help with self-care.

Children between 6 and 9 years tend to view death as man-made and may worry that they are being punished for actual or proposed wrongdoing. Their main concern is to be with their parents and family and avoid separation. They can become very demanding of the parents and insist on them being present all the time. Anxiety about being separated from their parents also tends to dominate children aged 5 and under, although they may not view death as finite. Indeed, they may consider that death will only mean a temporary separation like a long sleep.

As with adults facing death, children and adolescents are often concerned with unfinished business. They wish to say their goodbyes to key people in their lives, give instructions about the dispersal of their personal belongings including pets, and ask previously unvoiced questions. They can become especially upset if people close to them, and medical and nursing staff fail to realize that.

I can't get over the calm way he just sat there telling me what to do with his things. He asked me to give his gun to his GP. That broke my heart 'cos it meant so much to him.

While it is generally true that younger patients find it harder to accept death it does not follow that all older people adapt more easily. When a couple have been extremely close in later life and shared all their friends and interests, the partner who is dying not only feels griefstricken but worries endlessly about the survivor's capacity to cope once they are gone. Similarly, a widow or widower whose grown-up child or children have been unable to stand on their own two feet and still depend on them emotionally can brood a great deal.

Sometimes the close bond may be between the person who is dying and a pet. Anguish about the fate of the pet can be just as great as if it were a human being left behind.

Those people who looked forward eagerly to retirement but now accept that they will not live long enough to enjoy it can feel especially bitter about dying.

I'm just choked . . . the one thing that kept me going the last few years at work was the idea that I'd be able to spend my time the way I wanted . . . on my allotment . . . now it's all going to ruin.

Nature of terminal illness

Many who realize that they are dying will be much affected by any previous experience of death. When they have witnessed a close relative or friend dying in an unpleasant and protracted way from a similar disease, they will find it hard to accept that their experience will be any different, despite reassurances to the contrary.

It's only 6 years since my dad died of cancer . . . of his throat. I used to be so proud of him . . . such a big strong man. It was awful to see him go like that – all skin and bones. His eyes seemed to be asking us to give him something to end it all. They wouldn't allow an animal to suffer like he did . . . they'd have it put down. They keep telling me they'll make sure I'm comfortable. I'd be a bloody fool if I believed them.

When the predominant effect of the illness is physical weakness this can be humiliating and intolerable to those who prided themselves on how active and independent they were. Similarly, patients who hold high standards of cleanliness and like to be in control can find becoming incontinent shameful and most distressing.

Breathlessness appears especially likely to cause mental distress (Hinton, 1963). Patients dying from diseases of the respiratory system including cancer of the lung or cancers which impede the airways through mechanical obstruction are, therefore, at particular risk.

Many patients are terrified that they will suffer pain and not be able to withstand it. Cancers are most likely to cause such pain and adequate early pain control will do a great deal to lessen emotional distress and fearfulness. Vomiting and nausea may also heighten any distress especially in younger patients. While some degree of confusion is common and may distress patients, especially those who were proud of their intellectual abilities, it may also protect others from realizing what is happening to them and thus lessen the level of concern.

The suffering will be intensified if treatments are used in a last-ditch attempt to save the patient and cause unpleasant side-effects. This is most likely in patients with advanced cancer. Instead of being allowed to prepare for death, they are given treatments which are usually most unpleasant.

I lie here thinking why, oh why did I have to go through all that hell. I told them I didn't think it would make a difference. The cancer had spread too far – even I knew that. I let them persuade me. I could kick myself. All those days lost – probably very few left.

Communication of awareness of dying

Patients who are aware that they are dying, and are looked after by staff who encourage them to disclose that they know and enable them to discuss their concerns, are significantly less likely to experience anxiety, depression or anger than patients who are discouraged from indicating their awareness (Hinton, 1979).

Patients who realize that they are dying but discover that their loved ones, as well as medical and nursing staff, have been holding out on them often become very sad, angry and frustrated. They can become increasingly withdrawn and lose interest in what is going on around them. They usually assume that their loved one has not told them in order to protect them from the bad news and inevitable upset. They tend to avoid broaching this for fear it will intensify the strain that they perceive their loved ones are already experiencing. This means that patients are then unable to share their real concerns with their loved ones and may lead to their feeling increasingly upset and isolated. Most importantly it can prevent them from dealing with any unfinished business; this will heighten their anxiety about their own death and the welfare of those that survive them.

Those who considered that they had a very good (73 per cent) or good relationship (59 per cent) with their spouse were less inclined to disclose their awareness that they were dying than those who admitted to having an average or poor (92 per cent) relationship (Hinton, 1980). Thus, paradoxically, patients who have a good marriage find it more difficult to 'hurt' their loved ones by admitting that they are dying and are at risk of being more distressed than those with poorer relationships.

Patients who think it likely that they are dying but are made uncertain because of contradictory information that they have been given by relatives, medical or nursing staff can become very anxious and depressed.

I feel I haven't got much longer. I'm so weak I'm no use to anyone. When the doctors come round they say I've responded a little. Who are they trying to kid? I'm so fed up with it all I wish I could go to sleep and not wake up.

Such uncertainty is heightened when the doctors and nurses behave in a way which conflicts with what they have told the patient.

They insist I'm getting better and keep telling me this. Yet they don't all come in my room like they used to. They stay outside and talk about me. When they do come in they all look so serious, not a smile between them. Why don't they admit I'll not get better.

The patient is most likely to be bewildered about what is happening when the doctors pursue active treatments right up to the last minute, which suggests that they still have a chance of surviving. When the doctors cease treatment death is usually very imminent and the patients have had very little opportunity to prepare themselves adequately for it.

Place of death

Over half of those who die do so in hospital, usually while being cared for in an acute ward. Many will have been in hospital for some weeks before death. The design of these wards and the different stages and kinds of illness treated within them makes them far from ideal for the care of the dying.

Many patients are in such wards because they are under investigation or being treated for potentially life-threatening acute illnesses. This creates a real conflict for most of the medical and nursing staff. Should they devote their time and energy to helping those with at least some chance of survival or spend it comforting the dying? Since they often lack experience and expertise in terminal care they usually find it easier to help the acutely ill patients and then justify this on the grounds that something positive can be done for them.

The discomfort that they experience when in the presence of dying patients may lead them to avoid these patients whenever possible. If the patients are in bed in the open ward they pass them by. When the patients are in a side room they visit much less frequently than when they were receiving 'active' treatments.

Most patients realize that they are being passed by and feel increasingly lonely, miserable and resentful, especially if they have no relatives or friends visiting them. Many consider that they are no longer regarded as human beings and feel hurt and angry or become apathetic. They are often most sensitive to the drop in the number of visits made by medical staff, both during ward rounds and at other times. This may also make them reluctant to burden such obviously busy and harassed staff with any complaints about pain or other distressing symptoms. Consequently, the staff are reinforced in their belief that these patients who are dying have relatively few needs compared with the other patients and so may neglect them even more.

Even when dying patients complain that they are experiencing distressing symptoms, these are often not accepted at face value by the staff. 'When I told her (the ward sister) that I felt the pain however I tried to lie in bed she said "oh come off it – it can't be as bad as all that".'

Consequently, attempts to relieve the symptoms are often inadequate and too late. This increases the chance that patients will become increasingly anxious and depressed.

Problems experienced in hospital by dying patients are frequently compensated for by the continued visits and support they receive from their loved ones and friends. Some patients wish their loved ones to be there as much as possible but others find too much contact very painful. It reminds them of what they are about to lose and fills them with sadness and anguish. They would prefer more time on their own and the chance to begin to separate from their loved ones.

The percentage of patients who die at home is 40 per cent. While being in familiar surroundings with loved ones can reduce the fear and distress it may also lead to difficulties. Complaints about pain, sickness and breathlessness may not be acted on by relatives because they wrongly believe that they are an inevitable consequence of the terminal illness and that nothing can be done to relieve them. Some patients are especially worried that being cared for at home will place too great a strain on those involved.

I'm so weak and useless now ... can't do a thing for myself ... not a thing ... I hate being like this. It's so hard on him ... he can't take much more ... he'll have a breakdown if it goes on much longer. Why doesn't God just take me away. It would be so much kinder all round.

They may also wish to protect their relatives from the pain of seeing them suffer and waste away. 'He used to tell me what a lovely figure I used to have ... look at me now ... just skin and bones. I can't bear him to see me like this.'

Patients' worries about the strain on their relatives can be considerably lessened by the provision of adequate support to the family. This may take the form of nusing help, help around the home, and the provision of practical aids.

Less than one in 100 patients who die end their days in a hospice or other unit devoted to the care of the dying. Admission into a hospice has the advantage that it clearly signals to those patients who are ready and able to acknowledge it that death is imminent. It is also clear that paying proper attention to the concerns and needs of the dying considerably reduces the level of physical suffering and mental distress (Hinton, 1979).

Attitudes and beliefs

Only a minority of patients still believe in an afterlife, rebirth or reincarnation but this may enable them to view death calmly. Patients with strong religious beliefs or no beliefs at all are usually much less apprehensive than those with only weakly held beliefs (Hinton, 1963). However, some of those with strong beliefs may be terrified of being punished by their God because of past misdeeds. Others with an equally strong faith begin to question what it all means and where it has led them. They wonder how and why God could have allowed them to contract a fatal illness and inflict such suffering at that point in their lives. They feel especially bitter towards God or his earthly representatives when they believe that they led obedient and blameless lives before their illness.

Strong feelings of betrayal and bitterness may also be evident in patients who had a profound belief in the ability of modern medicine to cure disease and prevent death. Rather than re-evaluate this belief, they may look for evidence of negligence on the part of the doctors and nurses who have cared for them. They can spend much of the time insisting that they would not be in this position if the illness had been diagnosed earlier or treated more energetically.

Some patients will have had more faith in other systems of medicine, for example, homeopathy or faith-healing. They may also have beliefs which preclude the use of treatments which could alleviate their suffering. To challenge these deep and long-held convictions in the name of scientific medicine can cause enormous distress. Demonstrating a respect for these views and reassuring patients that nothing will be done against their wishes may markedly reduce their suffering.

Denial

A few patients who are dying manage to continue to firmly deny the possibility despite strong cues to the contrary. They speak consistently as though they have a future and this can be discomforting for others to hear. Yet, providing that they seem in reasonable psychological balance and have no areas of 'unfinished business' which could cause serious problems to the surviving relatives if they are not attended to, the denial should be accepted and no attempt made to broach it.

Everyone keeps going on about this being a cancer hospital but I know it doesn't just deal with that. I've got this inflammation [lung cancer] in my lungs ... I'm sure I caught it in the tropics a couple of years ago – they haven't found a cure yet but I'm sure they will.

CLOSE RELATIVES AND FRIENDS OF THE DYING

Nature of death

Sudden death which occurs without any prior warning is extremely hard for most relatives and friends to accept especially when it occurs away from home. There is no transition period between a state of health and death. Telling relatives and friends that a person is dying allows them an opportunity to prepare for it, even though they may find it difficult to accept and be reluctant to use the transition period constructively.

They will usually feel shocked, very sad and concerned about how they will manage during this time. However, their main concern will usually be how to ensure that the patient suffers as little as possible and dies peacefully. A death accompanied by much physical and mental distress can cause relatives and friends to feel considerable anguish and strain. They may also become very bitter and angry, especially if they believe that the person who is dying is not being given sufficient help by the caring professions.

How could they let her come home like that . . . she's been in terrible pain ever since – nothing shifts it – I'm at my wits' end – there's nothing I can do for her . . . and what's worse, no one else seems interested.

The witnessing of such suffering can prove an almost intolerable strain for some close relatives and friends. Yet, they will usually try to pretend that they are coping with the burden because they believe strongly that they owe it to the dying person to keep going for their sake.

I don't think I can take any more . . . I feel I'm going to have a breakdown . . . I'm just strung up all the time. . . . It breaks me up to see her suffering like this, but I can't give in, I mustn't.

The awareness that the person is likely to die prompts many relatives and friends to reorganize their daily lives to cope with frequent visits to hospital or looking after the patient at home. They often find that they are spending most or all of their time with the dying patient and have to neglect other responsibilities and relationships, including their jobs, other family members, friends, social and leisure activities. When death occurs quickly, this may not matter but if it happens much later than was predicted by the doctors serious problems can arise.

The relative or friend who becomes this involved with the dying patient is likely to become separated from important sources of emotional support. They may become both physically and emotionally drained by the burden of continued visiting or care, yet feel they have to pretend that all is well for the sake of the dying patient. Nor do they usually feel able to take any time off lest this seems a desertion. Consequently, they may take 'on board' all the suffering experienced by the patient and find that they cannot stop thinking about it even when they are away from the patient. Such 'imprinting' can leave emotional scars which are difficult to heal.

I dreaded going to the hospital – I knew he'd be no better and would have lost even more weight – towards the end I felt I had to be with him all the time . . . just wasn't fair to leave him . . . he got so he couldn't breathe properly . . . he had to fight for every breath . . . I couldn't stand it . . . kept wanting to scream and get out of there . . . but I couldn't leave him.

Sometimes, relatives and friends are given no clear signal until death is very close. This may be inevitable because it was impossible to predict. At other times, it may happen because the doctors pursue active treatments until the last possible moment, even though it may seem clear to others that the patient is not going to respond. When they finally cease treatment there is little time before death and no time left for psychological preparation. Moreover, the patient is usually 'too ill' to complete any unfinished business.

The relatives and friends may accept this because they wanted every effort made to save the patient. However, they may feel bitter, frustrated and angry because they had realized the patient would not recover and did not wish them to be treated so energetically. Their feelings of anger may be even greater when the treatments used caused unpleasant side-effects and intensified the patient's distress. They may also feel guilty that they did not prevent such treatment being given.

I cannot get out of my mind what they did to him. All his hair fell out . . . he couldn't stop vomiting . . . he started bleeding from every orifice . . . I could strangle that doctor . . . I will if I ever get my hands on her . . . I'd told them I didn't want him to have any more treatment . . . I knew he was going to die . . . what really gets me is that I let them talk me into it. . . . I keep having nightmares . . . see his eyes pleading with me to help him out of his misery.

Doctors' predictions about when death will occur are often inaccurate and usually on the optimistic side. Occasionally, the patient lives much longer than anticipated. This may be difficult for relatives and friends to adapt to since they were prepared to put up with the strain when they believed death was imminent and geared themselves to it. They may find it impossible to make constructive use of such borrowed time.

Nature of relationship
The nature of the relationship that existed between the close relative or friend and the dying patient prior to the terminal illness is often a major determinant of how relatives or friends react when they realize the patient is dying.

When the relationship was mutually dependent and exclusive and neither partner pursued any independent friendships or interests the close relative or friend will commonly feel shocked and find it hard to believe. As realization dawns that they will soon be bereaved they may feel full of despair and consider that there will be little to live for. They anticipate that they will be desperately lonely when death occurs and wonder if they will be able to manage on their own. They cannot envisage any way in which the vacuum can be filled and may consider that it would be better if they were also to die soon. Even so, they will try to avoid worrying about the future in order to help their loved one or friend as much as they can.

Putting such worries to the back of their minds can be especially difficult if the relative or friend was too emotionally dependent on the dying patient. They cannot stop worrying about their future.

News that a friend or loved one is dying is also hard to accept when the relationship was very important because it compensated for inadequacies in other key relationships. For example, a mother may have found that her marriage fails to meet her needs and felt very unhappy. She finds consolation through a close relationship with her son whom she sees as the 'apple' of her eye. She puts considerable energy into ensuring that her son is happy and is given every opportunity to fulfil his hopes and ambitions. When the son then contracts a fatal disease this is experienced as a terrible blow, because the most important person in her life is to be taken from her. She may feel extremely bitter that he has been singled out rather than someone who was much less deserving and less important to her.

Why pick on him. What harm has he done to anybody. He's all that kept me going ... without him I can't see much point ... he was always so cheerful and cheeky. The others are so miserable ... don't do a thing to help ... why couldn't it have been one of them?

When the relationship between the parents and dying child was close but not excessively so, the parents may still be adversely affected. In particular, they may feel that they have failed the child since it was their duty to ensure that the child reached adulthood unscathed. This sense of failure also arises from the knowledge that death in childhood is rare. Parents may also feel helpless and try to compensate for this by spending too much time with the dying child.

Sometimes the relationship between the dying person, close relative or friend is characterized by strong feelings of ambivalence. There have usually been frequent serious arguments accompanied by expressions of anger and hate. On other occasions positive feelings of love and affection have been expressed. The close relative or friend will have very mixed feelings about the impending death and often feel guilty about things they have said or done. They may even feel they are responsible for the illness which leads to death.

I kept nagging him all the time about other women ... I couldn't help it ... couldn't leave it alone ... he got so mad with me ... I can't help wondering if this is what brought it all on?

When the relationship was bad before it was realized that the patient was dying, the close friend or relative may feel a great sense of relief that their own suffering will soon be over. However, they may find this difficult to admit to anyone. Relatives and friends may also wish that death would come quickly in order to prevent the patient and themselves suffering unduly, at the same time worrying that such feelings are selfish and shameful.

Communication with the patient
Worry about whether they are doing all they should for the patient is often heightened because they have elected to shield the patient from the truth. While on balance they continue to believe that this was the correct decision, they may have moments of serious doubt, especially if the dying person hints that he or she knows. This lack of openness makes it probable that the relatives or close friends will not have discussed where the patient would like to die and what the funeral arrangements should be. They may then experience considerable conflict in trying to decide these matters.

It is also likely that they will have been unable to discuss other important problems with the patient such as how they should dispose of their personal belongings, their own plans for the future, and any unresolved worries. Thus, a married woman may be agonizing about whether her husband would be pleased or hurt if she eventually remarried. A husband may be torturing himself about an affair he had and be desperate for forgiveness. A father may still feel deeply hurt after a serious row with his daughter during which she claimed to despise his lifestyle and beliefs. Now she is dying he is most anxious to clarify if she still feels this way and to try to sort it out. A son who acknowledges that he caused his father considerable worry during his adolescence and early adult life may wish to admit this to him and say how much he really appreciated him before his father dies.

When close relatives or friends are unable to discuss these concerns, usually because they do not want to distress or hurt the dying patient, they feel frustrated and upset. They find that they move further apart emotionally instead of together and this can cause much sadness and despair. The sense of frustration can be acute when the relatives or friends try to communicate openly but the patient will not respond to their efforts.

He goes on as though all is well and he's getting better . . . he just won't discuss anything – what am I going to do . . . he's got a business to dispose of.

Availability of support

The stress of coping with a person who is dying is less likely to cause serious psychological problems if the close relative or friend is able to share their worries, feelings and concerns with someone else. Thus, those who have no such confiding tie are especially at risk.

Some close relatives or friends feel that there is no one they can turn to and much resent the lack of concern shown them by those involved in the care of the patient; yet they do not usually feel able to acknowledge their own needs. This appears especially true of mothers of dying children and single people whose parents are dying. They feel upset and ashamed that they are experiencing such strain. Their difficulty in admitting their need for help is often exacerbated by their feeling that medical, nursing and social work staff appear eager to let them take on the burden of care and leave them to it.

I had to bath him, feed him and sit with him . . . no one else seemed to do much for him. I got so that I couldn't stand being there with him . . . his breathing got so rough . . . I kept thinking he was going to die on me . . . I wanted to get out . . . get away. They wouldn't let me . . . said it was my job to be with him. I nearly went out of my mind.

Close relatives and friends can feel very resentful that other friends and neighbours also begin to avoid them when they most need comfort and support.

When I go into the shop, they [other customers] look the other way. . . . It's as though I'm contagious . . . I only wish that I could tell them she was getting better . . . but she's not . . . she's dying . . . they don't want to hear that do they?

A few close relatives or friends tell those who are concerned with the dying patient that they are finding it too much of a strain to spend so much time with the dying person. They are then told that they should stay with the patient because he or she may not have much time left. Their fear of not being there at the moment of death causes them to stay but they feel extremely bitter at not being allowed any time out.

Anticipatory mourning

When some close relatives and friends realize that the patient is dying they react as though they have already been bereaved. While it has been claimed that such anticipatory mourning is helpful in assisting the bereaved to resolve their grief this does not now appear to be so (Fulton and Gottesman, 1980). They fare no better or worse than those who do not exhibit any anticipatory mourning.

HELPING PATIENTS, RELATIVES AND CLOSE FRIENDS

Acknowledging the difficulties

If those in the caring professions are to establish properly the needs of dying patients, their relatives or close friends, they must be able to communicate effectively with them. This is only possible if the carers first honestly acknowledge the difficulties involved and their tendency to avoid them.

Discussing with patients, relatives or close friends how they are feeling about the impending death brings the carer into direct contact with physical suffering, despair and loss. This can cause considerable strain and upset, especially if the person who is dying reminds them of someone they care for, or of themselves. Thus, an experienced ward sister found it very difficult to cope with nursing a woman dying from cancer who reminded her of her mother.

She was so like my mother . . . it was horrible . . . like losing her all over again. . . . I got ever so down and tearful . . . I dreaded going on duty.

Similarly, a young doctor found he was trying to avoid visiting a young man who was dying of leukaemia because it reminded him forcibly that he too was mortal.

It all seemed so senseless . . . there was nothing we could do for him . . . I kept seeing myself in that room and wondering how I'd face up to it all.

Confronting the reality of dying is also difficult because it conflicts with the carers' belief that modern medicine is powerful and usually prevents death. To accept that the patient is dying is to admit that treatment has failed. Such an admission can be painful and leave the carers feeling that there is nothing they can say or do to remedy the situation. They may also take it personally and feel they have let the patient and family down. These feelings make it more difficult for the carers to talk freely with the patients or relatives, especially as they may be asked awkward questions about how long the patient has to live or why treatment has failed.

Hence, it is easy to understand why many doctors, nurses and social workers prefer to avoid the dying patients, their relatives or close friends whenever they can, and devote their energies to the care of those patients who are likely to recover.

Avoiding communication

When carers are in the presence of the dying patient they often unwittingly use techniques which keep them at an emotional distance. They may try to 'jolly the patient along' by telling him or her that there is no reason to be upset. 'Ooh, don't you look down in the mouth this morning ... come on, let's have a smile .. that's better. This conveys the clear message that only cheerful positive feelings are acceptable. It prompts those patients who are feeling upset or unhappy to pretend otherwise however difficult that might be.

If they realize that the patient is anxious or depressed they commonly try reassuring statements like 'There's no need to be so worried ... I'm sure you are going to be alright ...', or 'Everybody feels like that but you'll feel much better in a few days'. This method of reassurance usually fails because it is premature. The person talking with the dying patient has not first established what he or she is anxious or depressed about. So their attempted reassurance serves only to increase any anxiety or depression.

What do they mean ... there's nothing to worry about ... they told my mother she'd not suffer and look what happened. She had a terrible time. I've never seen anyone in such pain.

Who do they think they are kidding. I *know* I've not got much longer. Why do they have to pretend I'm getting better.

Sometimes, when patients or relatives try to discuss their worries, attempts are made to divert them into less difficult areas. The carers often do not realize that they have done this since it has become an automatic response, but the patient feels hurt and frustrated. The following examples of such blocking manoeuvres are taken from tape-recordings of conversations between dying patients and those concerned with their care.

Doctor   How are you today?
Patient   [a woman dying from cancer of the breast] Not very well. I feel so weak. Can hardly lift my head off the pillow. I don't feel I'm making any progress ... I'm beginning to think I'm not going to get better.

Doctor   Have you had any pain?

Patient   [dying from lung cancer] Am I going to have any more of that drug treatment? [cytotoxic therapy]

Nurse   No, I don't think so.

Patient   Does that mean there's nothing more they can do for me?

Nurse   Have you had your bowels open today?

An alternative and frequently used strategy when carers are asked such awkward questions is to explain to the patient or relative that they should ask someone else.

Patient   [after bone scan] I suppose it's now spread to my bones?

Nurse   I don't know. You'll have to ask the doctor.

This nurse already knew that the patient was suffering from advanced cancer, had not responded to treatment and had widespread bony metastases.

Consequently, anyone who wishes to talk more openly with dying patients, relatives or close friends may have to begin by unlearning these avoidance strategies. They will also need to realize that other factors prevent patients and relatives from disclosing their concerns and needs.

Non-disclosure
Patients, relatives and close friends correctly perceive doctors and nurses as being very busy and responsible for many other patients (Maguire, Tait, and Brooke, 1980), and feel that they are not entitled to take up too much of their time. They are also loath to burden them with their worries when they see them looking so cheerful and confident, especially as they may be unsympathetic since they are so strong and able to cope.

Many patients, relatives or close friends feel ashamed that they have not coped better. They fear that if they admit they are finding it too much of a strain those caring for them will regard them as 'weak', 'pathetic', or 'ungrateful'. Their reluctance to disclose how they really feel is often reinforced by their realization that the carer's prime concern is with their physical wellbeing. Few concerned with care seem directly interested in how they have reacted emotionally or how they are now feeling about their predicament. They often need considerable persuasion that the carers are really interested in these aspects of care.

Some patients and relatives keep their problems hidden because they doubt that there is any solution. There is little point in mentioning them because nothing can be done. Others are equally reluctant to disclose any difficulties because they feel that they will not be believed. 'When I told him (the doctor) that I was having all this pain in my hip he wouldn't believe me . . . said I must be exaggerating it.'

What to ask

Since patients, relatives and close friends do not usually disclose their problems it is important to talk with them in a way which will make them more likely to do so. Enquiry about how the patient is getting on should, therefore, include questions concerning both likely physical and psychological problems. Questions about physical health should concern whether or not the patient has been experiencing any pain, nausea, vomiting, breathlessness, constipation, bedsores, incontinence, anorexia, sleeplessness or unpleasant smells.

Questions about psychological adjustment should cover how the patients, relatives and close friends have reacted so far, their current attitudes about the illness and treatment, mood, sleep pattern and the presence or absence of confusion. If problems become evident it is helpful to establish if the patient, relative or close friend has been able to confide them to anyone.

When the person indicates that the problems arise out of an awareness that the patient is dying it is worth determining the nature and extent of any previous experience that individual has had of dying in others. It is also important to discuss if they are worried about any 'unfinished business' and whether or not they have attempted to resolve it. Enquiry should be made to establish if they have any religious beliefs, how these have been affected and whether they need any spiritual help.

How to ask

It is important to talk to the patient or relative alone when possible. Otherwise they may be loath to raise any personal concerns. It is also crucial to allow sufficient time and avoid unnecessary interruptions.

The key areas should be covered in an open-ended way that avoids biasing or restricting the answers. Questions should thus take the form 'have you had any pain?' rather than 'you haven't had any pain?' When the response indicates that the patient or relative has experienced the symptom or problem the interviewer's task is to establish its full nature, extent and impact, as well as any factors which precipitate or relieve it.

During the course of such enquiry the patient or relative will usually give frequent and helpful cues about key problems. These may be in a verbal or non-verbal form. Thus, a patient may respond to a question about how she is feeling in herself by saying that she has been feeling very low because she is suffering constant pain, feels sick and is worrying about how her family are managing about her. She has given cues to four problem areas: pain, feeling sick, worry about her family, and feeling very low. The task of the interviewer is to be alert to such cues and to acknowledge and clarify each one in the following way: 'you say you've been feeling very low – can you tell me about it?' 'You mentioned you've been worrying about your family ... what exactly have you been worrying about?' Such acknowledgement and clarification of cues indicates to the patient or relative that the interviewer really is genuinely concerned to help them and to understand what is going on.

Non-verbal cues usually take the form of the patient or relative looking obviously worried, weepy, sad or in physical discomfort. The interviewer should try to convey that he or she has noticed the cue and would like to talk about it if the patient or relative wishes: 'You look very worried. Would you like to tell me about it?' or 'I can't help noticing that you keep catching your breath. Are you finding it difficult to breathe properly?'

When cues are not picked up by the interviewer, they are usually repeated several times. Should the interviewer still fail to respond the patient or relative ceases to offer any more cues. These techniques enable the interviewer to establish if the patient, relative or close friend is experiencing any problems, how they feel about their predicament and why. It is most important that what is disclosed is accepted at face value unless there are strong and valid reasons to do otherwise. The good interviewer is able to tune in to the patients', or relatives', or close friend's real world and does not try to distort it or fit it into some preconceived mould that accords with a notion of how people usually react.

Dealing with awkward questions

When assessing, in this way, how dying patients and their relatives are adapting it often becomes clear that they fully realize that death is imminent. They make this explicit during the conversation and no guesswork is needed. A few patients or relatives indicate equally clearly that they believe that the disease will be cured despite obvious cues to the contrary.

Sometimes, no clear indication of the patient's awareness is given. Instead the patient asks a question about the illness and its prognosis which indicates that he or she has some suspicion that all is not well. The interviewer has to gauge what kind of answer is really wanted, and should begin by reflecting the question back in the following kind of way: 'I'd be happy to answer your question but first I'd like to know why you asked me that'. In the answer the patient usually indicates that he or she has picked up clear cues that he or she is dying.

Well, they've stopped giving me the treatment. I only had two courses. Obviously I wasn't responding as they hoped. I know there's nothing more they can do now. That's right isn't it?

As in this example, they often also ask for confirmation that their perception is correct. The interviewer should respond honestly but make it clear that efforts can still be made to ensure that the patient does not suffer unduly. Sometimes, reflecting the question back results in the patient producing firm arguments that the illness will not be fatal. These should not be challenged unless serious problems are evident from the assessment. On a few occasions, the replies to the reflected question leave the interviewer no clearer as to what the patient knows or wants to know. The interviewer should then avoid being drawn into giving a firm answer.

Thus, it is not a matter of deciding whether to tell or not to tell a patient or relative. Instead, it involves confirming what they have already realized or prefer to think.

The problem of collusion

Occasionally, doctors and relatives and close friends agree to withhold the truth from the dying patient. They want to avoid distressing the patient or causing him or her to 'go to pieces'. Unfortunately, this makes communication between the patient, and relatives, and friends and between the patient and carers much more difficult and intensifies any difficulties the patient is experiencing. Since many patients realize that they are dying through the cues they are given, this collusion represents a humiliating vote of no confidence in their ability to cope with bad news. It can cause great unhappiness and result in the patient drifting apart from key relatives or friends. Most importantly, it prevents them from dealing with unfinished business.

Irrespective of whether or not patients are the victims of such collusion they should be dealt with in the way already discussed if they ask awkward questions. When such questions indicate that patients have realized they are dying they should be answered honestly, and their awareness communicated to the doctor and relative. The relatives may initially react with anger, but more often they experience considerable relief that it is out in the open, although they may then need help in coming to terms with their own anguish.

NEED FOR SUPPORT

The approach which has been advocated here exposes the health care professional to considerable physical and emotional suffering. Care must be taken to ensure that the carer is not overexposed and adversely affected by this work. One method of doing this is to hold regular meetings for all the staff involved. At these meetings they are encouraged to discuss their experiences of and feelings about particular dying patients, their relatives and friends, with their colleagues. This provides much needed support and continued guidance.

Some framework of support is essential if doctors and other health care workers are to remain effective and survive emotionally in this demanding area.

CONCLUSION

The more accurate determination of the needs of the dying, their close relatives and friends, should enable much more appropriate and effective care to be given. This should lessen considerably the suffering involved and make the subsequent grief-work for the relatives easier.

Acknowledgement

I am grateful to all the dying patients and their relatives who were so willing to discuss their experiences with me.

References

Adams, D. W. (1979). *Childhood Malignancy: The Psychosocial Care of the Child and his Family.* (Springfield, Ill.: Charles C. Thomas)

Brown, G. W. and Harris, T. (1978). *Social Origins of Depression.* (London: Tavistock Publications)

Cartwright, A., Hockey, L. and Anderson, J. L. (1973). *Life before Death.* (London: Routledge and Kegan Paul)

Fulton, R. and Gottesman, D. J. (1980). Anticipatory grief: a psychosocial concept reconsidered. *Br. J. Psychiat.*, **137**, 45

Hinton, J. M. (1963). The physical and mental distress of the dying, *Q. J. Med.*, **32**, 1

Hinton, J. M. (1979). Comparison of places and policies for terminal care. *Lancet*, **1**, 29

Hinton, J. M. (1980). Whom do dying patients tell? *Br. Med. J.*, **281**, 2, 1328

Maguire, P., Tait, A. and Brooke, M. (1980). Mastectomy: a conspiracy of pretence. *Nurs. Mir.*, **150**, 2, 17

Parkes, C. M. (1964). Recent bereavement as a cause of mental illness. *Br. J. Psychiat.*, **110**, 198

13

Therapeutic uses of truth

Michael A. Simpson

Communications, like tumours, may be benign or malignant. They may also be invasive, and the effects of bad communication with a patient may metastasize to the family. Communication may induce effects not unlike the immune responses induced by other foreign stimuli – including irritation and inflammation, resistance, and even (on occasion) shock. Like lymphocytes, 'caregivers' show differentiation into killers, helpers, and suppressors of response.

I believe that the supposed therapeutic benefits of lying or attempting to deceive the seriously ill patient have been greatly exaggerated. Much of the literature has been unhelpful because it has persistently asked and answered the wrong questions. Truth is one of the most powerful therapeutic agents available to us, but we still need to develop a proper understanding of its clinical pharmacology, and to recognize optimum timing and dosage in its uses. Similarly, we need to understand the closely related metabolisms of hope and denial.

Historically, differing views have been expressed. That keen observer of the human condition, Emily Dickinson, in her verse 'Tell all the truth but tell it slant' suggests that 'success in circuit lies', and that we should let the truth 'dazzle gradually'. The somewhat pompous old humbug, Oliver Wendell Holmes, advocated that the physician keep an impenetrable face and a stock of handy phrases 'for patients that will insist on knowing the pathology of their complaints without the slightest capacity of understanding the scientific explanation'. 'I have known the term "spinal irritation" serve well on such occasions', he added, 'but I think nothing on the whole has covered so much ground, and meant so little, and given such profound satisfaction to all parties, as the magnificent phrase 'congestion of the portal system'.'

Freud commented on how the analyst 'finds himself at a loss altogether for the lies and the guilt which are otherwise so indispensable to a physician'; adding most cogently that 'since we demand strict truthfulness from our patients, we jeopardize our whole authority if we let ourselves be caught by them in a departure from the truth'.

One of the distinct disadvantages of clinical lying is that we have no effective antidote. It is very hard to un-lie. By lying, you invalidate yourself as a source of further credible information, and lose the capacity to give later, better news; to comfort or to console.

In no situation are the problems of communication about a diagnosis and its implications more clear or more misunderstood than in the case of cancer. For cancer, as Susan Sontag (1978) has eloquently described, is in our age a diagnosis especially encumbered by layers of lurid metaphor. It is treated as a particularly dirty and morally contagious disease. 'Treatment for cancer', curiously, is the only disease or treatment specifically exempted from the Federal Freedom of Information Act, as its disclosure, 'would be an unwarranted invasion of personal privacy'. The diagnosis, the disease's words and names, are treated as if they are as invasive and damaging as the disease itself. And it is not cancer's reputation as a life-threatening disease that earns this special abhorrence. Someone who has had a coronary thrombosis is at least as likely to die of a subsequent coronary within the following few years as are many cancer patients likely to die of their cancer. Yet people do not strive so zealously to hide the truth from a cardiac patient; for their disease, however life-threatening, is not felt to be equivalently obscene, nor is the diagnosis itself treated as if the very words were life-threatening.

Those of us who have been involved actively both in the comprehensive care of patients with cancer and other life-threatening illness and in research in these areas, have witnessed a shift in general attitudes in recent years. Many studies throughout the 1950s and 1960s (Simpson, 1979 a, b and c) showed that the majority of doctors preferred not to reveal diagnoses of cancer, and to withhold information from their patients. They believed that profound and damaging emotional reactions could result from 'telling', including an almost automatic loss of hope, severe depression or psychotic reactions, rapid decline with acceleration of the physical disease process, or suicide. They believed that most patients did not want to know, and bolstered this belief by a communicational double-bind – holding that the patient who doesn't ask, doesn't want to know, while the patient who *does* ask, doesn't want to know, either, but is simply seeking reassurance that all is well. Most doctors expressed the wish to be told if they themselves were a cancer patient, while believing in withholding the information from their own patients, and being little more likely to tell doctors with cancer than any other patient.

Every one of these beliefs and suppositions proved to be untrue when tested by perfectly simple research techniques. While an emotional response including depression and anxiety is hardly surprising in a patient learning that cancer has been diagnosed, the occurrence of serious or damaging reactions is extremely rare. The withholding of truth in these circumstances is very similar to the tragically commonplace withholding of morphine from cancer patients for fear of producing dangerous addiction and tolerance problems. Though unnecessary and easily relievable pain is very common in such circumstances, addiction and tolerance – the feared complications – are very rare indeed.

Study after study has shown that patients do indeed want to know about their diagnosis, prognosis and treatment (Simpson, 1979a). Interestingly, patients seem to share the physician's double standards, though to a lesser degree, as not all those who wanted themselves to know believed that everyone else would want to know or should know. Cancer patients who do know about their illness are in most cases pleased to have been told. As one patient in one of my studies said: 'The day after my specialist discussed my bone marrow cancer with me, I felt on top of the world! I had guessed over a year previously, from my treatments, but I wanted to *know*. I am so much happier than when I lived in the "guessing and wondering" state.'

Further, our studies show that patients who ask about their condition do want to hear genuine and truthful answers; and that many of those who do not ask complain of not having been given enough information about their diagnosis, prognosis, treatment and progress. But they find it hard to ask for many reasons. They are diffident, do not want to be a nuisance or to seem ignorant about medical matters; or they see the staff as being too busy and too important to stop to talk to them. They usually try to raise the subject as subtly, obliquely and gently as they can, but usually this is not noticed, or ignored, or actively discouraged. More direct questions are often construed by doctors and nurses as being 'complaints', and this further discourages discussion. Patients often seek information from nurses, social workers, medical students, and other staff. But these people are still usually trained that it is the doctor's task and right to control what information the patient will receive, and at any rate are constrained in their freedom to respond by the local policy, and often the expressed wishes of the physician that no one else should meddle in these affairs.

More recent studies (Novack *et al.,* 1979) have shown a change in so far as a majority of physicians now tend to say that they favour telling patients who have cancer. This may not represent much change in what actually happens rather than in what we believe ourselves to be doing, which may not be the same thing at all. Although physicians often claim to judge each individual case on its merits, and to vary their approach according to the individual circumstances of each patient, observational studies show both a strong tendency towards stereotyping, using much the same response and even words to each patient; and also a heavy use of vague terms, euphemisms and circumlocutions, or on the other hand over-precise and incomprehensible technicalities.

Though marked psychological regression is little more common in cancer patients than tumour regression, common responses to the patient are not only often paternalist and patronizing, but also infantilizing. Only when treating children and cancer patients is it so common for the relatives to be told so much about what is going on, and the patient so little. This routine is rarely questioned, though it is far from being as benign as many would seem to believe. For example, not long ago I saw a couple in both of whom a serious cancer had developed within a short period. The husband had been told his wife's diagnosis and grave prognosis, and had been warned not to tell her. She had been told of her husband's diagnosis and poor prognosis, and had been warned not to tell him. The well-intentioned but mistaken physicians were surprised when both patients became seriously emotionally disturbed while trying to live out this macabre scenario.

One other source of problems rather than solutions has been the widespread and uncritical acceptance of the wholly fallacious but heavily promoted five-stage model popularised by Dr Elizabeth Kübler-Ross (1970)* who has been more the Aimée Semple McPherson of our discipline than the Madame Curie. The model was based on intuition rather than research, and has never yet been supported by any of the relevant subsequent research studies. In my model there are only two stages – the stage when you believe in the Kübler-Ross five (and other staging models) and the stage when you do not. Though each of the soi-disant 'stages' are among the repertoire of responses any seriously ill patient may show, none of the implicit assumptions of a staging model are true – the assumptions, for instance, that the stages are sequential or

*Her book described dying patients as experiencing the stages of Denial, Anger, Bargaining, Depression and Acceptance.

progressive (even if minor variations or regressions occur); that anyone is more than evanescently 'in' one or other 'stage'; that they are adaptive; or that 'acceptance', for example, is an appropriate goal for the patient to reach. None of these assumptions have been shown to hold true.

There has been, in this area, as in other areas of psychosocial inquiry, a sinister slide from *descriptive* to *prescriptive* models; from descriptions of what some people appear to do, to prescriptions of what everyone ought to do. This can lead to obscene practices, like the School of Nursing I encountered, where the junior nurses were given a half-hour lecture on the Kübler-Ross five, and were then sent out to the bedsides of terminally ill patients with the instruction to 'get them through to acceptance' in an hour. God protect us from crude amateur meddling – especially by professionals!

As I mentioned earlier, much of the discussion of these issues is devoted to answering the wrong questions, questions which presuppose a number of substantial and false assumptions about the situation. These also usually involve false dichotomous sortings of other people into discrete groups. You can divide the world into two types of people – those who divide the world into two types of people, and those who do not. One is often asked: 'Should you tell the patient?', or the slightly more realistic: 'What should you tell the patient?'. The following are some of the common false underlying assumptions. It is assumed that it is entirely or largely our choice whether we 'tell' or 'don't tell', and that in practice we are able to either 'tell' or 'not tell'. In fact while most of us realize that we can't 'tell' everything however hard we try to, we overlook the fact that we can't tell 'nothing' – total non-disclosure is simply not possible. It would be like trying not to tell a pregnant woman that she is pregnant.

If you are patently ill, feel bad, have investigations and treatments, and you are told nothing, or very little, or insufficient to account for what is happening, that tells you a lot, and it implies that what is unspoken is unspeakable. Saying 'nothing', says a lot. I have reviewed elsewhere (Simpson, 1979b) some of the many ways patients find out about their illness, both directly – by questioning different members of staff and comparing answers, or by reading their own charts or correspondence not meant for them, or by overhearing the private discussions doctors so often hold in public; and indirectly – by noticing the palpable decrease in quantity and intimacy of staff contacts after they have received a bad diagnosis or prognosis. As one patient remarked to me: 'I feel like a railway station that's been closed down – the ward round doesn't stop here anymore'.

It is therefore a mistake to assume, as many do, that people you haven't 'told', don't know. They may not have heard you; they may not have understood, for the basic communication skills of most caregivers are minimal; they may not comprehend the full meaning and implications of what they have understood; they may not recall all that they have previously understood; and they are likely to be using one of the many forms of that blessed and essential skill and defence – denial (Weisman, 1972, 1979). In one study, some 20 per cent of patients who were considered to have been 'told', claimed not to have been told anything at all.

It is assumed that people either 'know' or 'don't know', whereas there is not only a wide range of states of knowledge (knowing and comprehending how much about what) but free and frequent fluctuation between states of knowledge depending on changes in the communicational context. I urge you to explore the elegant and intricate variations and functions of that ubiquitous, helpful and essential mechanism of denial. As Hackett and Cassem, and myself, and especially Avery Weisman, have explored and demonstrated, denial has been negligently ignored by our profession and when not ignored has been inappropriately viewed as primitive and psychopathological. This denial of denial is unhelpful. What is crucial, however, is that the assessment of the patient's needs, and our attempts to meet them, must take account of and be prepared to support all healthy uses of denial they may make – but must not be governed by our own needs to deny aspects of reality that we find personally threatening. Most instances of denial shown by the cancer patient are healthy; most instances of denial shown in the professional context by the health professionals and by the caring systems themselves are unwholesome and unhelpful.

We should also remember that denial is an *inter*personal as well as an *intra*personal phenomenon and event. Denial varies not only with time, but also with whom. The patient will vary, with time, as to what he will deny in his relations with various others, including himself.

It is, then, also mistaken to assume, as so many do, that people either 'want to know' or 'don't want to know'. All the evidence and all one's clinical experience, suggests that people vary continuously as to what they want to know about what and from whom. People *don't* remain in a steady state of knowing. It is false to assume, as too many do, that there are some patients who 'should know' and others who 'shouldn't know'. Most people want to, need to, and should be able to learn more about their condition than their doctors believe, more often than their doctors believe; and yet many need to know less than their doctors may want to tell them, or not when their doctors want to tell them. Just as those of us who were pioneers in developing this field of clinical activity used to have to teach and remind clinicians that they should be more free to talk with patients about their illness, so now we have to remind some clinicians that many people do not want to know all about it all the time. The discussion should meet the *patient's* communication needs, not the *clinician's*.

Finally, there is the commonly held assumption that 'telling' people about their illness destroys 'hope' and leads to clinical and psychological decline. Hope (like its relative, denial) is far more flexible and strong than most people give it credit for, and is based on knowledge, not on ignorance. Hope, like denial, is rarely global and when it is, it cannot be sustained for long. Hope is the search for a future good of some kind, and depends on the knowledge and belief that there is an alternative, preferable, reachable situation or state. Several of these points were well shown in the recently published research study by Barrie Cassileth and others (1980) on information and participation preference among cancer patients.

They showed the variation in the degree to which cancer patients prefer to become informed about and to participate in their medical care, and that most patients prefer more information and participation than they are often offered. Patients who preferred more detailed information, compared to those who preferred less, were more likely to be younger, white, better educated, and to have had their disease diagnosed more recently; 80 per cent of patients wanted to know whether they had cancer, what body parts were involved, what exactly the treatment would do to them and what it would accomplish, what was the likelihood of cure, what were all the possible side-effects, and what their prognosis was.

Also, those who preferred active involvement in their own care were more hopeful than those who did not, and patients who wanted as much information as possible, good and bad, were more hopeful than those who preferred minimal or only good information. They concluded that, 'knowledge does not impede the application of selective denial as a protection against hopelessness', and that 'helping patients become well informed does not create depression but actually assists many patient in sustaining hopeful attitudes'.

What other conclusions can we draw? I would suggest that patients should be provided with the information they need and seek when they need and seek it, the process being determined by *their* needs and not *ours*. Health professionals need to become more adept at assessing these needs. We should attempt to assess and meet such needs by moving gracefully closer towards more direct and explicit *exchange* of information about the illness and its treatment rather than lunging in with a large bolus dose of data; to aim at a sort of mutual communicational seduction rather than rape. We should, above all, never expect our patients to move through a series of arbitrary and mythical stages, in a macabre terminal choreography. We must not constrain our capacity to comprehend the whole complex panoply of their responses by forcing it through a mean little conceptual sieve.

Previous policies and practices about communication with the terminal patient have served no-one well and have protected us all, not against dangers and disasters but against care and competence. Kalish has emphasized eloquently how impossible it is to have a warm personal relationship with the person with a life-threatening illness if one cannot relate to them in terms of their potential for dying as well as for living. He has described the 'horse on the dining room table syndrome': at a pleasant dinner party, a horse is sitting on the middle of the table; the guests talk as if it wasn't there, for to mention it might embarrass the host, and he doesn't mention it lest he embarrass the guests. Though it is studiously ignored in everyone's conversation, the horse still sits there, and it is the centre of everyone's thoughts all night.

References

Cassileth, B. R., Zupkis, R. U., Saffar-Smith, K., *et al.* (1980). Information and participation preferences among cancer patients. *Ann. Intern. Med.*, **92**, 832

Kübler-Ross E. (1970). *On Death and Dying.* (London: Macmillan)

Novack, D. H., Plumer, R., Smith, R. L., Ochitill, H., Morrow, G. R. and Bennett, J. M. (1979). Changes in physicians' attitudes toward telling the cancer patient. *J. Am. Med. Assoc.*, **241**, 897

Simpson, M. A. (1979a). Social and psychological aspects of dying. In Wass, H. (ed.) *Dying: Facing the Facts.* (New York: McGraw-Hill)

Simpson, M. A. (1979b). *The Facts of Death.* (Englewood Cliffs, NJ: Prentice-Hall)

Simpson, M. A. (1979c). *Dying, Death and Grief: A Critically Annotated Bibliography and Resource Guide.* (New York: Plenum Press)

Sontag, S. (1978). *Illness as Metaphor.* (New York: Farrar, Straus and Giroux)

Weisman, A. (1972). *On Dying and Denying.* (New York: Behavioral Publications)

Weisman, A. (1979). *Coping with Cancer.* (New York: McGraw-Hill)

14

At home and in the ward: the establishment of a support team in an acute general hospital

Thelma D. Bates

This chapter describes the origin and development of a Terminal Care Support Team designed to improve the standard of care of patients dying from cancer, in the setting and surrounding of an acute general hospital.

Any proposal concerned with patients dying from cancer in the care of an acute general hospital must take into account the needs and wishes of the patients and the problems specifically related to these hospitals.

The patients' views

There is no doubt that most patients prefer to die at home, in their own bed with their family near and under the care of their general practitioner. Some cannot do this because they have no-one to look after them, but many more could if the standard of medical care both in the hospital and in the community was improved. With help, many more families could cope with the considerable strains of death at home even if some could not face the prospect of the last day or two. These families need to know that rapid readmission of the patient to hospital is assured. In any event most of the 'dying time' is spent at home and it is here that help should be most readily available.

Patients who cannot die at home may well be content in a familiar hospital, in a ward they know and cared for by a ward sister and by doctors who have cared for them in the past. This is often the acute general hospital where they have had their previous treatment.

The problems of the acute general hospital

These hospitals have inherent difficulties in caring for dying patients as the wards are busy and geared primarily toward curative therapy. Understandably, dying patients tend to be regarded as medical failures and their prolonged stay in the ward will interfere with the admission of patients who *can* be cured. There is no lack of care in the acute general hospital, but care of the dying cannot be rushed and the tempo of these wards is fast.

In addition it is very often the junior hospital doctors who are responsible for the day-to-day care of dying patients, and regrettably medical students receive very little specific teaching related to the care of the dying. Junior doctors may not only lack experience in prescribing for the dying patient but, being young, they may well not have come to terms with death themselves, which will make communication with dying patients difficult. Nurses tend to have more understanding of their patients' needs. This is especially true of an experienced ward sister, but they are often far too busy and short of staff.

THE CONCEPT OF THE SUPPORT TEAM AT ST THOMAS' HOSPITAL

It was with these problems in mind that the idea of the St Thomas' Hospital Support Team was conceived in 1976, in the belief that if patients' symptoms were better controlled and if the family had more support, not only would more patients die in comfort, but more would be able to die at home with their family, if they wished to.

The original plan was to establish a team comprising two full-time senior specialist nursing sisters and a part-time social worker, backed up by a doctor already on the hospital staff and the hospital chaplain. The team was to act by giving advice and help at the request of a consultant with the patients remaining in their own wards under the care of their own doctors and nurses. Important aspects were: that the team would not take over the management of the patient completely, and, having no beds of its own, would provide not only expertise and additional time but the opportunity of teaching the skills of terminal care to a large number of different disciplines throughout the hospital.

PLANNING THE SUPPORT TEAM

As a radiotherapist and oncologist, used to working closely with fellow consultants of other disciplines, I felt that I was probably the person best equipped to put this concept into practice. I was aware that there might be problems in acceptance of an idea which implied a criticism of existing care and also contained an element of interference of a territorial nature for both doctors and nurses. It, therefore, seemed sensible to plan without a committee or working party and to seek no statistical data within the hospital formally to confirm that a need existed.

The planning took a year and began with a 4 month period of informal and individual discussion with consultant colleagues and ward sisters to discover their views of the existing standard of care and their opinion of the proposed Support Team. It was very soon clear that none of them was complacent about the standard of terminal care at St Thomas' Hospital. Most of the consultants volunteered that they had difficulty at times in controlling terminal symptoms, especially chronic pain. The response of the ward sisters ranged from total acceptance to total rejection. They were all concerned and aware of the need for improvement but some were anxious that another sister might cause confusion. With the wrong Support Team sister they could well have been right.

It was essential, at this early stage, to have the approval in principle of the district nursing officer and the head medical social worker and to locate possible initial funding from the St Thomas' Hospital Special Trustees in the event of formal approval. The dean of the medical school and the professor of general practice were put in the picture at a very early stage because of the relevance of the project to undergraduate teaching. Finally, the district administrator was briefed with a clear-cut, short project summary and a financial estimate for the first year. With his approval the second stage of planning – a phase of committees lasting 2 months – started.

The District Management Team gave the project a high-priority rating, but because of financial constraints urged a reduction in the number of sisters from two to one. The Medical and Surgical Officers' Committee of St Thomas' Hospital (comprising the Chairmen of the Specialty Sub-committees) gave their unanimous approval, which avoided the necessity of going through individual subcommittees. The hospital Special Trustees and the Samaritan Fund agreed to provide the necessary finance for the first 2 years.

There followed a 6 month period of detailed planning which included the job descriptions, advertising, interviewing and appointments of the sister and the social worker.

We acquired a centrally placed furnished office, a typewriter, a telephone and a hospital bleep. As the team was to keep its own typed notes for future research and self-assessment, specially designed history sheets and follow-up sheets were printed. The Patient Services Office was consulted, so that before starting we were aware of the statistics that we should be keeping. We also informed the Voluntary Services Bureau at St Thomas' Hospital, in anticipation of working with volunteers in the future, and the Friends of St Thomas'. Finally I attended a meeting of the local Community Health Council to tell them what we planned to do. In December 1977 we saw our first patient.

The original team in 1977 and early 1978 had one sister who fortunately had many talents, including considerable experience in geriatrics, terminal care (at St Christopher's Hospice) and teaching, which was important. In addition she was a good typist, which enabled us to keep typed notes from the start without a secretary. She was appointed with the status of a ward sister and thus wore the same uniform as the ward sisters, which may have helped integration in the wards. The first medical social worker had previously worked as the radiotherapy department social worker and was already well known in the hospital. My registrar in the radiotherapy department at this time had spent a year as medical officer at St Christopher's Hospice and his voluntary involvement in this team meant that we started with considerably more expertise than if I had been the only doctor.

MODE OF ACTION OF THE SUPPORT TEAM

The Support Team policy has not changed since its inception, in that it does not take over the management of patients but gives advice and family support when invited to do so by the patient's doctor. Sister and one of the doctors see a new patient on the day of referral, indicating to the patient that they have been sent by the consultant to help with a problem, such as pain. The problems are assessed and the solutions suggested are written in the hospital notes and discussed with the staff. The team then continues to work alongside the patient's own doctors, nurses and social worker, identifying problems as they arise and giving help without overlapping facilities. This requires a sensitive, tactful manner to ensure that there is no confusion in the minds of either patient or staff about who is responsible. Prescription of drugs is usually done by the junior hospital doctors under the guidance of the team, so that they will become familiar with these skills. The team visits inpatients early in the day every weekday, and at other times as necessary. The reason for visiting early is because this is when many clinicians do their ward rounds which provides an opportunity for meeting them and discussing problems. The team is available 24 hours a day, 7 days a week and because of its mode of action (leaving the patients primarily in the care of their own clinicians) most of the night and weekend problems can be solved over the telephone, although the sister or doctor on-call is always willing to go to the hospital if necessary. This availability has proved important, not only for the patients, but also for the acceptance of the Support Team by the hospital staff.

PROGRESS OF THE SUPPORT TEAM OVER THE FIRST 2 YEARS

Within the first month, the team had some success in controlling patients' symptoms and several very ill patients were able to go home. This unblocking of hospital beds stimulated further referrals and quite quickly there was a change in the pattern of work with the Support Team sister spending less time on the wards and more time visiting patients in their own homes. Within a few weeks, an outpatient clinic was started on one afternoon each week in the department of radiotherapy and oncology. In this clinic six patients and their families could be seen.

After 6 months, it became abundantly obvious that a second sister, to work in the community, and a part-time secretary were needed. Both of these appointments were approved without undue difficulty.

The community sister works in the same way as the hospital sister. She is involved with the patient only if the general practitioner is agreeable. She then works alongside the patient's own district nurse and general practitioner without taking over. The usual policy is for the general practitioner to be telephoned before a patient is discharged from hospital and, if he agrees, the community sister sees the patient in the ward and arranges to visit the patient at home. She is careful not to take over the district nurse's duties and is prepared to advise and do whatever is necessary to help.

A part-time secretary types the Support Team notes and makes sure that the general practitioner gets a letter at the first possible opportunity when his patient is about to be discharged from hospital or attends the outpatient clinic. The general practitioner is kept fully informed with a list of the patient's drugs and their present dosage and details of what the patient and family have been told about the illness. If, for some reason, a letter is not going to be quick enough, a Support Team doctor or sister will telephone the general practitioner.

There is a weekly meeting of all the team when patients' problems are discussed. The chaplain and social worker attend these meetings and are kept informed. If the patient already has a social worker, the original social worker usually retains responsibility but may hand over, or share care as seems appropriate. Similarly, if the patient is of another religious denomination the chaplain will make sure that the appropriate minister is informed. The weekly meetings are also a time for mutual support within the team, especially in times of particular stress.

During the first year 29 consultants and five general practitioners invited the team to help in the care of 207 patients. Most of these patients were in St Thomas' Hospital, in 26 different wards; 93 patients were able to go home for varying periods and 24 died at home (Table 1).

Table 1 Support Team statistics for the first 2 years

	1st year	2nd year
New patients	207	236
number of consultants referring patients	29	37
number of GPs referring patients	5	22
number of wards involved	26	31
Patients discharged home	93	139
Outpatients seen in the clinic	269	504
Home visits	301	1339
Patients dying at home	24	46
Patients dying in hospital	105	139
Patients dying in a hospice	22	25
Bereavement visits	7	135
Teaching sessions	59	76
Visitors	44	109

There was no change in the staffing of the team during the second year. By this time it was clear that the team was generally well accepted and well integrated within the hospital and patients were often being referred earlier in the course of their disease. There was a rapid increase in the home care service, so that by the end of the second year approximately 80 per cent of the patients cared for by the Support Team were outpatients. Not every general practitioner wished to work with the team, but the number who did increased, and during the second year 22 general practitioners referred their dying patients directly to the team. From the annual statistics (Table 1) it is obvious that the main change in the second year was the development of the home care service and the beginning of bereavement counselling.

ACCEPTANCE OF THE SUPPORT TEAM IN THE HOSPITAL

When the team first started there were anxieties in the hospital about it. Some doctors feared that the Support Team would take over the management of their patients, despite the fact that it was a well-defined policy not to do this. Others were concerned that their beds would be blocked by patients receiving terminal care, who would formerly have been transferred to a hospice. There were fears that the team might have a rigid policy of telling every patient the diagnosis or might upset patients and generally be too emotional. It was not difficult to overcome these fears in a short time. A more realistic fear was that of overlapping facilities which would cause confusion, particularly in regard to clinical responsibility. A few physicians felt that they wanted to look after their own dying patients without help and two ward sisters preferred not to work with the Support Team.

The likely reasons for this near-total acceptance within the hospital were that the team was very small to start with and that it has always worked in a quiet and tactful manner with little publicity. The personality of the team members was obviously extremely important. An aggressive or dogmatic attitude would not have been successful at this hospital. It was also probably easier to get acceptance in the hospital because I was already a member of the staff. Not least has been success in controlling patients' symptoms enabling unexpected discharge home.

ACCEPTANCE OF THE SUPPORT TEAM IN THE COMMUNITY

There has been much more difficulty in gaining acceptance in the community. It is still not uncommon for a general practitioner to decline Support Team help even though this has been given to his patient when in hospital. Sometimes this is because a group practice has its own nurse who specializes in terminal care and sometimes the general practitioner knows the patient and his family so well that he feels the Support Team to be unnecessary. Others find the Support Team an intrusion, especially since it is hospital-based. There is no doubt that there is a barrier between the hospital and the community despite the fact that this hospital has an academic department of general practice. It will take time for the Support Team to learn the differing views and needs of the local general practitioners.

It is a strict policy not to visit patients in their homes without first being in touch with the general practitioner. Whether he works with the Support Team or not, we feel that it is important to provide him with prompt letters about his patients and to offer to help rapid readmission to hospital should this be necessary. Local general practitioners have been informed about the Support Team's mode of action and given the names and telephone numbers of all the members of the team. The team has called on several of the larger group practices.

When the team works in the community the bulk of the routine cooperation is carried out by the community sister, but a medical member of the team will visit a patient in his home, preferably with the general practitioner, if this is requested. If the general practitioner refers a new patient, a Support Team doctor and the community sister will go to the patient's home to assess the problems and give advice in the normal way.

Liaison with the district nurses has been good from the start. The Support Team community sister was herself a district nurse for many years and therefore understands their problems. She had made it clear to them that she is there to help, and it is not unusual for a district nurse to encourage a general practitioner to call in the Support Team either for the control of symptoms or to give additional support to the family.

ROLES OF INDIVIDUAL MEMBERS OF THE SUPPORT TEAM

The hospital sister

The three most important attributes of the Support Team's hospital sister are, firstly, that she is able to get on well with other nurses, including not only the ward sister but also junior nurses and the sister tutors; secondly, that she had had experience and training in the care of the dying; and thirdly, that she can teach. In this particular pioneer team it has been very helpful that she was flexible, versatile, diplomatic and able to show initiative.

She starts her day by collecting the Support Team notes of the inpatients from the secretary and joining one of the team's doctors for the ward round. There are usually ten inpatients at any one time, although sometimes almost double this number. The round involves visiting several wards so that all inpatients are seen. She later goes back to the wards to be with any patients who need more time. She herself sees patients' relatives or arranges for the patient's own doctor or a Support Team doctor to see them. She acts as a link between the patient's doctors, nurses, social worker, physiotherapist, occupational therapist and any others concerned, making sure that everybody knows what is going on. In an acute general hospital such as St Thomas', the wards are often very busy and she is willing to carry out any nursing duties if the need arises. This *adaptability* and expert knowledge has made her particularly welcome on practically every ward that has cancer patients.

She also has a role within the team itself, to liaise and coordinate with the community sister, the team's social worker and the chaplain so that all are fully informed about any physical, social, or spiritual changes.

She attends the Support Team outpatient clinic and usually sees the patient and his family before they see the doctor. She accompanies the patient and his family into the consulting room and aids the patient's and family's communication with the doctor. Patients will often tell the sister important things that they do not tell the doctor. When necessary she helps the patient undress, collects prescribed medicines from the dispensary if no porter is available, and arranges the next appointment and possibly transport. If necessary she may telephone the patient's general practitioner or district nurse with new information.

The Support Team aims to see all new patients on the day of referral and has no waiting list. The hospital sister is often the first person to be spoken to about a new patient and she will accompany the team's doctor to see this patient. Being an acute observer she is able to make astute suggestions, and in the absence of a doctor she is perfectly capable of giving sensible advice. She is an experienced lecturer, trained as a clinical teacher, and her teaching duties range from ward tutorials with junior nurses to formal lectures at oncology conferences, attended by all relevant disciplines.

Sometimes she takes patients into the hospital garden or to concerts in the hospital. She may also drive patients and their families to see a hospice before transfer, which may make the change of location easier. When the community sister is on leave she combines her job with her own duties.

The community sister
Apart from accompanying a Support Team doctor when he visits patients in their homes, the community sister works largely on her own, acting as a link between the hospital and the home. Her present territory covers a 9 kilometre radius from St Thomas' Hospital but this is probably too large.

It is easy for her to create unnecessary dependency and she is selective in choosing which Support Team patient she visits and in deciding on the frequency of her visits. Some patients she may see only once a month, others she may see two or three times in a day. As previously stated, she works closely with the patient's district nurse and general practitioner. If the patient wishes to die at home, the efforts involved on the part of the family are often very considerable. It is an important role for both sisters repeatedly to help to assess whether the family can cope with this or whether the patients needs admission to a hospital or hospice, either permanently or in order to give the family a rest.

She makes sure that the patient and the family understand about the drugs which have been prescribed. She gives the patient a *drug card* on which is written the name of every drug, its description (such as a pink tablet or blue medicine), and when, how and why it is to be taken. One of the problems of patients cared for at home is occasionally a difficulty in obtaining an opiate mixture from local chemist shops, especially when the dose prescribed is high. The community sister makes a point of knowing exactly when a patient's medicine will run out and, if there is likely to be a problem, she will get it dispensed at the hospital. She keeps a record of all injectable opiates kept at the patient's home, abiding by the Dangerous Drugs Regulations. Any unused oral mixture is either formally disposed of by the family down the sink or returned to the pharmacy for their destruction according to law. Ampoules of injectable opiate are recorded on a special card and each time an ampoule is used it is stated on the card; any unused ampoules are returned to the hospital pharmacy. On two occasions only she has taught relatives how to give an intramuscular injection. This is not by any means always wise because of course the patient may die very soon after an injection, leaving the relative feeling responsible for death.

She and the district nurses between them ensure that the patient has all the aids he or she needs. For example, on occasions the community sister has gone to special trouble to obtain items not readily available in this area such as charcoal dressings for offensive fungating tumours. Between them they teach families how to care and encourage them to do so until the patient dies, if this is possible. In our district we are fortunate in having a night nurse and a twilight nursing service which can be called in to help when necessary.

The community sister carries a long-distance bleep and all her patients have both her bleep number and home telephone number. At weekends the team doctors and sisters take it in turn to carry the bleep so that the community sister can have some time off duty.

The community sister is usually at the hospital at the beginning of the day before the ward round, so that she can report her patients' progress to the Support Team doctors. She attends the Support Team outpatient clinic with her patients and is present at the team's weekly lunchtime meeting. Like the hospital sister she is flexible and adaptable and so helps the family and the district nurse in any way she can.

The social worker

The team's social worker gets in touch with the patient's social worker within the hospital if he has one, and between them they decide how best to deal with this aspect of the patient's care. It happens that the Support Team's present social worker has a special interest in bereavement counselling. If there is going to be this particular need when the patient dies, the Support Team social worker is the one most likely to be involved. This association with the patient and his family begins early so that by the time of death she will know them and their individual problems.

The social worker usually comes to understand all the detailed circumstances of the patient's family and home more fully than is ordinarily done by any other member of the team. Because of this knowledge she is able to give practical, even financial help by mobilizing the social services available – for example, families may need rehousing, improved heating, help with laundry or installation of a telephone.

She is in a position to help the patient and the family to cope with their stress and will spend time with them both in the hospital and at home. She is alert in particular to stress affecting any children of the family and she may discuss with parents the problem of talking with their children about the illness. When a patient is to be transferred to a hospice, there is much that she does to make this transition easier. Like the sisters, she encourages families to visit a hospice before the transfer and often continues to visit her patient when he has been admitted to the hospice so as to provide continuity of care. She encourages families to share their anxieties and sadness with each other. Accordingly, much of her work, in this time of impending inevitable death, is to some extent of prophylactic value in that it helps them toward normal grief.

If the family wish it, she usually makes her first bereavement visit on about the tenth day, by which time the funeral will have taken place and distant relatives and friends will have returned home. Thereafter she visits as often as she believes necessary while at the same time taking care not to create undue dependence. She encourages normal grief but is alert nevertheless to the signs of abnormal grief which may require medical help. At the time of writing, 25 bereaved families are being helped by her in this way. She is not the only member of the team to be involved in bereavement counselling but the whole team respects her expertise and values her guidance in this respect.

It is very important that the team's social worker cooperates closely with her fellow social workers and with the other members of the Support Team so that all are aware of the social circumstances affecting the patient and his family. By this means, she too receives support and is not working in isolation. She meets the rest of the team at the weekly meeting, and once a week she also has a formal meeting with me. On these occasions she keeps me informed, asks for advice and, when necessary, for money for special needs from the Support Team's fund, for instance, when the money cannot be readily obtained from other sources. The Support Team Fund is small and has been established by donations from grateful families. She has several opportunities during the week to have other discussions with team members, particularly with the two sisters.

The secretary

Her main role is to ensure quick communication with the general practitioner. She keeps the Support Team's own notes and types on the patient's card an entry every time the patient is seen whether in hospital, at home or in a hospice. Thus, the Support Team has its own clinical record of all the patient's problems and the manner of dealing with these (for example, the drugs used and their doses), so that this information can be kept and used for future reference or for research. If a patient is transferred to a hospice, a photocopy of the Support Team's own notes can be sent to the hospice so that the staff there will know what has been happening before.

The Support Team notes are kept separate from the hospital notes and thus do not get lost. The Support Team doctors write in the hospital notes in longhand and do not remove them from their proper place.

The chaplain

Like the doctors, he already has a full-time appointment at the hospital, being the principal chaplain at St Thomas' Hospital. From the start he has welcomed the opportunity to work as a member of the team.

He does more than attend to the purely religious needs of the patients, appreciating their emotional and physical fears. He is also alert to signs of stress in members of the team. He may establish a very close rapport with a family and continue to see them in their home during bereavement. At the team's weekly lunchtime meeting he learns which patients are likely to welcome a visit from a minister and, when appropriate, he will call in ministers from other denominations. Some patients at the outset may have rejected the idea of a minister's visit but their view in time may change, and in this event a member of the team will inform the chaplain that such a visit may now be welcome.

He prays not only for, but more importantly with, patients, always understanding that some people, unused to prayer, may be too shy to pray aloud. When asked to do so he gives communion, provides the laying on of hands, and will anoint patients.

He understands how a hospital patient may feel stripped of his status in life, with his clothes replaced by pyjamas, confined to a hospital bed. The chaplain spends time with patients, listening, responding but *never* lying to them. He allows them to express all their fears, whatever they may be, and not infrequently their anger, sometimes even anger directed against God Himself. Many patients at this time feel a sense of hopelessness and it is one of the chaplain's prime roles to allow a patient to discover for himself the uniqueness, wholeness and completeness of his life and to show him that his life is not a hopeless, useless, trivial thing, even though there may be little time left.

Two of our patients who were devout Christians experienced profound hopelessness, felt at least part of their lives to have been a sham and were deeply angry that God should deprive them of their fulfilment in life. It was particularly difficult for both patients to confide in members of their own church, but coming to know a new chaplain, who allowed this to be expressed and discussed, enabled them to be released from this severe strain and to accept themselves as they were.

The support team doctors
At the beginning there were two doctors, myself and my registrar who, as previously mentioned, had had a year's experience at St Christopher's Hospice. He is now a senior registrar and my present registrar has become the third doctor in the team. We are all employed full-time in the department of radiotherapy and our Support Team work is voluntary.

It is not easy to do this type of demanding work as well as a full-time job, but when establishing this pioneer team in a climate of economic difficulty it was important to start with doctors already on the hospital staff, who thus did not need extra salaries. In some ways the task has become easier with experience, but in other ways it has become more difficult because the success of the team has increased the work.

The doctor has four main roles: Firstly, he advises and constantly reviews the control of distressing symptoms – chronic pain being the most common; secondly, he helps the patient and his family by listening, responding appropriately and by being freely available; thirdly, he has a teaching role. By working alongside the patient's own medical attendants in the majority of wards in the hospital, and with an increasing number of general practitioners, broad-based, multidisciplinary teaching is achieved not only through the advice given but also by an *attitude to death and dying*. Teaching is considered to be one of the most important aspects of the Support Team's work. Up to now, most formal teaching sessions have been with nurses. Fourthly, the doctor has a research role, constantly to assess and improve methods of care.

The Support Team doctor is primarily a clinician with experience in terminal care and an understanding of malignant disease, extremely important in a team such as this which deals only with patients suffering from cancer. One patient who had previously been treated for a carcinoma of the cervix uteri was referred to the Support Team with an acute non-malignant abdominal condition. It is, therefore, vital that the doctor does not make the assumption because the patient has once had a cancer that she is still suffering from the cancerous condition in any later medical catastrophe. The team doctor therefore has to be able to diagnose the cause or causes of the patient's symptoms. In terminal care it is plainly preferable to do this by using clinical skills rather than by time-consuming and uncomfortable investigations.

A doctor with experience of cancers is in the best position to give a prognosis, though this must almost always be guarded. He is also in a good position to continue active, if only palliative, treatment of the disease while at the same time giving detailed attention to the control of symptoms. This skilful phasing in and out of active treatment is probably one of the things that can be done in an acute general hospital more easily than in a hospice where it may be assumed that no further active treatment is suitable. Ideally this type of terminal care could start much earlier than has previously been accepted as appropriate. Doubtless the majority of radio-therapists and oncologists will be in agreement with this. The presence of the other members of a team makes it possible for the doctor to achieve a very great deal more than he could possibly do on his own with his regular staff, however good they may be.

TEACHING

The root of the problem is that medical students, and to a lesser extent, nurses do not have enough training specifically related to the care of the dying. It is for this reason that our teaching role is considered to be extremely important.

At the beginning, the Support Team concentrated on teaching nurses. We did this because we were encouraged to do so both by the ward sisters and the Nursing School and we recognized that it is the nurses who are closest to the patients.

Medical students are not so far included in the team's teaching programme, but it is intended to introduce this teaching early in the medical course and to follow it up with further training during the clinical years. This will be with reference not only to hospital care but, we hope, working alongside the department of general practice, to teach students also how to care for people dying at home.

Teaching the nurses

The hospital sister talks to the nurses in the introductory block, again after about 18 months and finally in their third year. She always allows plenty of time for a free exchange of ideas and an opportunity for them to air their anxieties. The nurses can talk about their problems in the wards and the Support Team sister can try to do something to help them in this. For instance dying patients may ask very junior nurses about the diagnosis and prognosis and the Support Team sister can discuss this with them in the classroom. Junior nurses have been keen to have more discussion on the care of dying patients at ward report time and the Support Team sister has gone back to the ward sisters to tell them about this.

Informal teaching is given to small groups in the wards, perhaps on individual cases. More formal teaching is usually given by two or three members of the team. The usual policy is for each to give a short talk lasting 10–15 minutes in different but related subjects, with an opportunity for open discussion on each topic. This format has been used for nurses, both trained and in training. The hospital sister also talks to new staff on the orientation course so that they know about the Support Team from the start.

Trained nurses from St Thomas' and from other hospitals, even from other countries, frequently spend a day with the team, as do nurses on the joint board postgraduate course on terminal care.

Teaching the doctors

Of the doctors, it is the junior doctors who are motivated to learn most from the team because day-to-day prescribing for the dying patient is their responsibility. They are often uncertain about the choice of drugs and the need for flexibility of dosage, especially in the control of chronic pain. They learn far more by continuing to prescribe drugs than if the Support Team were to do it for them, and the day-to-day presence of the team on the ward ensures that changes are made as often as necessary. Of course if there is an urgent need for a prescription and the junior doctor is in the operating theatre the Support Team doctor will prescribe. By the end of their 6 month appointment as house officers, junior doctors should have gained confidence in prescribing for common symptoms such as pain, nausea and dyspnoea.

Teaching others
It is all very well to stand up in a lecture hall and talk about the care of the dying, but a much bigger and wider audience over a period of time can be reached by daily example in acute wards. The team is in great demand for study days for social workers, pharmacists, the clergy and others and it is usual to prefer short talks with plenty of discussion. Care of the dying is always incorporated in oncology study days, thus establishing it as a normal continuation of previous care, rather than a specialized or isolated topic.

PROBLEMS WITH THE CONTROL OF PAIN

Unrelieved chronic pain is still the commonest cause for referral and the main reasons for this fall into the following categories.

Clinical difficulties with the cause of pain
Without knowing the cause of a particular pain, it is of course difficult to know how to give the most appropriate treatment. A patient may have pain at several sites and not necessarily all of these are due to the malignant process. It is the usual practice of the team to begin by identifying each of the patient's pains, recording them on a body chart with the patient's help, deciding on the possible cause of each and noting the success or failure of previous treatment.

One of the features which we have seen is the assumption that strong analgesic drugs are the only method of treatment when death is close, forgetting that opiates can make some pains worse, in particular pain due to constipation, and headache due to raised intracranial pressure, conditions which might of course be better treated respectively by laxatives and by corticosteroids. In an acute general hospital, however, there is by contrast rarely a problem in arranging appropriate palliative radiotherapy, nerve blocks and internal fixation of pathological fractures, even in dying patients.

Difficulties in prescribing analgesic drugs

These difficulties stem primarily from carrying over into the management of chronic, persistent pain some of the attitudes adopted in the management of short-term (acute) pain. The principles for the prescribing of analgesic preparations in these totally different circumstances are almost antipolar. In managing acute pain it can confidently be expected that there will be less need for analgesics day by day, even, at times, hour by hour. In malignant disease, however, pain is usually continuous and often progressive.

Unfortunately, it therefore happens that many patients with cancer suffer pain even though there are very few in whom this cannot be prevented, provided that the necessary rules are understood and followed. The commonest cause of a pain becoming unrelievable has been failure to prevent it at an earlier stage. Some doctors are reluctant to use strong narcotic analgesics until death is very close. The following have been the main problems encountered.

Fears of addiction

Addiction is not to be feared in dying patients whose reason for taking the drug is relief of pain and not psychic dependence. This has been amply proven in the wards when, for example, the pain of a secondary deposit in bone has been relieved by palliative radiotherapy, and it has then been possible to discontinue the opiate without difficulty.

There is no reason why opiates should not be started even as long as a year before inevitable death. By recognizing and practising this, we have had several outpatients suffering from persistent rectal cancers whose pain has been well-controlled for long periods thus enabling them to lead surprisingly active lives. The alternative would have been long-term suffering from pelvic pain.

Fears of harmful side-effects

These may, for example, be respiratory depression, nausea, or dulling of consciousness.

In the terminally ill, some respiratory depression can be of advantage in relieving respiratory distress and this rarely shortens life. It is also true that opiates cause nausea, but this can almost always be controlled by an anti-emetic drug such as prochlorperazine (Stemetil). With the correct dose titrated skilfully according to the degree of pain, dulling of consciousness is usually a temporary problem. In carefully selected patients amphetamines may be of value to ambulatory patients on high doses.

The reluctance to acknowledge that a patient is dying
This is not uncommon on the part of doctors whose goal is cure, sometimes in collusion with a family who want to deny the seriousness of the prognosis.

Preference for giving opiates by injection
This is often done in the mistaken belief that it is more effective than giving opiates orally, but it not only leads to exhaustion of the injection sites but means that the patient has to stay in hospital. This was a common practice in our hospital and it doubtless stemmed from the routine postoperative prescription for pain.

Under prescription and prescription on demand
Another major error is the failure to appreciate that the chronic persistent pain of malignant disease requires careful adjustment of dosage and the giving of drugs at regular intervals to *prevent* pain rather than waiting for it to reappear. Prescription of drugs to be used as required (p.r.n.) was at one time a common practice but it is now much more widely accepted that this is inadequate treatment and often leads to unnecessary escalation of the dose required.

At the time of writing, morphine and diamorphine are the most useful drugs for the relief of severe pain. Though not available in all countries, diamorphine is available in Great Britain and has the advantage of being more soluble than morphine. Should injections become necessary this makes the subcutaneous route available at all levels of dosage. It is our practice to prescribe oral diamorphine alone in chloroform water so that the dose of diamorphine can be easily adjusted, no matter how often this becomes necessary. If cocaine is included in the mixture as in the Brompton mixture, this easy adjustment is impossible, because increasing the dose of diamorphine will then automatically also involve increasing the dose of cocaine and the cocaine may produce undesirable side-effects such as confusion.

This simple diamorphine mixture is usually mixed at the bedside with an antiemetic such as prochlorperazine syrup. This gives the mixture a more pleasant flavour and a distinctive blue colour, which makes it easy for the patient to say which medicine he is taking. When the patient is discharged home on a steady dose, the diamorphine and prochlorperazine can be dispensed together in the one bottle. When the patient is in need of a tranquillizer, chlorpromazine (Largactil) can be substituted for the prochlorperazine.

The usual dose is prescribed in 10 ml to be given 4 hourly, and a common failing is for the hospital to discharge a patient home with 300 ml, which will of course last only 5 days. Accordingly the patient may easily run out of his medicine perhaps over a weekend. If a patient is not to see a doctor for at least 2 weeks then he will need a litre of the mixture. As it is extremely difficult to pour 10 ml from such a large bottle, it is our policy to give two bottles, each containing 500 ml. Our Support Team sisters have a simple measuring device which they can apply to the outside of these bottles. This not only lets them know if the patient is taking the medicine as directed, but also predicts when a new bottle will be required.

Selection of an inappropriate analgesic drug
There is a simple practical scale of analgesic drugs ranging from the weak to the strong. Prescription has to be done on an individual basis according to need and will require constant review.

It was often not realized that pentazocine (Fortral) and oral pethidine are weak analgesics, that pethidine by injection, like oral dextromoramide (Palfium), has only a short period of action lasting from 1 to 2 hours, and that methadone (Physeptone), on the contrary, has a prolonged action and can lead to accumulation when given repeatedly, especially in the very debilitated patient.

One of the worst problems which we meet is pain which has not been controlled by high doses of Palfium due to its short period of action. It is often very difficult to wean such patients off Palfium while switching to an adequate dose of an oral opiate.

A very useful drug is oxycodone pectinate (Proladone), which is given as a rectal, or sometimes as a colostomy, suppository. As with most drugs given by the rectal route its period of effectiveness may vary, but it usually lasts for 8 hours and it is therefore of particular value for outpatients or for patients who are vomiting. Many general practitioners do not appreciate that Proladone is available on prescription from the chemist.

Failure to appreciate emotional aspects of pain
There is no doubt that fear and anxiety make pain worse. Sensitive medical and nursing care take this into account. The best way to deal with fear is to

let it come out into the open. The Support Team provides some of the time necessary for this care; time which is otherwise often difficult to provide in a busy ward. Anxiolytic and antidepressant agents sometimes have a part to play, but these can never overcome loneliness and the sadness of parting. Most doctors find this aspect of care very difficult to deal with, and we have often been told that a patient is 'too wide awake' when in fact sedation is not necessary.

Boredom also makes pain worse. Pain then, of course, tends to fill the patient's consciousness. It is therefore important not to isolate a dying patient unnecessarily but to make sure that he has people with whom he can talk, and to provide activities in which he can take part. We encourage inpatients to get dressed in their day-clothes, to walk in the garden when possible, and to leave the hospital for a few hours or even a weekend, assuring them that their bed will still be available for them upon their return.

SUPPORT TEAM POLICY ON WHAT TO TELL THE PATIENT AND HIS FAMILY

It is the policy of the Team to recognize that each patient is different and that therefore there can be no rigid rules on this subject. Some patients want to know the whole truth, some only part of the truth and others do not wish to hear anything of the diagnosis or prognosis. It is, however, our policy not to lie to patients or to their families. We do, however, take into account the obvious needs of the patient as well as the wishes of the patient's immediate family and of the doctors who are primarily responsible for his care.

A problem may arise when a patient's doctor has told him, erroneously, that he has not got cancer and that he is getting better. The Support Team may not feel that this is in the patient's best interests. In this event the team will respect the primary doctor's views and will avoid comment until they have had a chance to discuss this problem with the doctor. Usually a sensible compromise in the best interests of the patient and the family can be reached, but if there is disagreement the team would not disrupt a close liaison of trust between the primary physician and the patient. In this situation a hospital consultant will occasionally relinquish this responsibility to the Support Team.

In any event what the patient and family are told must be communicated to everyone who is caring for him. It must not be forgotten that the junior, as well as the senior, nurses and doctors need to be told what the patient and family know about the diagnosis and prognosis. It is also essential that before the patient is discharged from hospital, the same information is passed on to the general practitioner.

When the Support Team is given a free hand, the patient is usually asked 'What have your doctors told you?' The patient is always given every opportunity to ask questions, but information is never forced upon him. The team tries to incorporate in a sensitive manner the needs of the patient, the wishes of the family and the opinions of the family doctor and the nurses who care for him – combining any constructive facts with a degree of hope for the uncertain future.

The Support Team likes to see the patient and his family together and to encourage them to share their problems when this is appropriate, rather than collude with them in trying to protect each other with deception. The Team encourages opportunities for frank discussion.

It is not uncommon for a patient near the end of his life to sense a conspiracy between his spouse and his doctors if the truth has been largely withheld from him. A highly intelligent patient, with a loving wife, who insisted on concealing from him the seriousness of his condition, became so confused as to be paranoid. Despite a very highly disciplined background in life and a gentle nature, he eventually attacked nurses while trying to escape from the hospital in his pyjamas and even rejected his wife, believing her to be against him. The truth of the matter was that he could see for himself that his health was getting rapidly worse, and he felt trapped and isolated by the well-meaning collusion of his wife and doctors in showing an over-optimistic attitude. Sedation was the only answer for this patient because the collusion continued to the very end. The wife's subsequent grief was particularly severe. Had this loving couple been able to share these final problems together, he might have had a more peaceful death and she a more healthy grief.

The Support Team creates opportunities for the patient to discuss fears and anxieties about the illness, prognosis and even death itself. The team is well aware that patients and their relatives can either forget or deny what has been said in the past. The result is that information often has to be repeated. For example, a family may say that they have never been told that their relative has cancer, when as the patient's oncologist I know this to be untrue, but recognize why they must make this denial.

Very often a dying patient will establish a close relationship with one particular person. This may be a doctor whom he has known for many years or it may be a relatively junior nurse. This relationship is very important and it is well recognized by the Support Team that a one-to-one relationship of this sort may be hindered by a team approach. Accordingly the Team makes a point of preserving such relationships. A patient who has had a close relationship with his doctor and eventually discovers that this has been founded on lies may well feel betrayed and suffer because he feels he can then trust no-one. For this reason, the Team believes in a truthful approach.

DEATH IN THE HOSPITAL

The last few days of a person's life, especially the last few hours, should be anticipated, whether in the home or hospital. The hospital has the advantage of constant professional attention and facilities. Naturally to know this gives some patients and their families a feeling of comfort.

As previously said, the ideal place in a hospital, if death has to occur there rather than at home, is in a familiar ward with unrestricted visiting day or night. In this hospital, rooms are provided so that relatives can stay and sleep. The relatives can also get drinks of tea in the ward and obtain meals within the hospital.

The Support Team has a particular interest in the role of the family at this time and the degree to which they are involved in the patient's care. It is helpful for some families to be allowed to help with the nursing, but other families are in need of what they will regard as authoritative permission to return to their homes, knowing that the ward sister will telephone if the patient needs them. Some ward sisters have this sensitivity; others need to have it explained to them. One young girl found the constant presence of her devoted and distressed parents irritating even though she was equally devoted to them and thus had some relief when they were persuaded to leave the bedside to go away for their mealtimes. Other families do not want to be present at the moment of death and if this is so, a nurse at our hospital will usually stay with the patient to the end.

When a patient is likely to die in a hospital it is important to plan ahead, with a clear policy on when not to transfuse, treat infections or resuscitate after a collapse. It is plainly inappropriate to give intravenous or nasogastric feeding at such a time even for a patient who has intestinal obstruction. At this time good mouth care with sips of fluid and ice to suck are much more suitable. The clinician must anticipate that the patient may be unable to take his drugs by mouth and should therefore have prescribed injectable doses so as to forestall this difficulty, thus allowing the nurses to carry on the administration of the drug without interruption. It is usual to prescribe hyoscine in case it is necessary to prevent a death rattle which distresses the family more than the patient, even though we know at times that the hyoscine will not be necessary.

Some patients require rapid readmission, even in the last hours of their lives. It is important that this too is planned so that the patient can go straight to his old ward instead of taking a place in a queue in the casualty department. His drugs must be written up as soon as possible so that there is no interruption in their regularity. Although it is the general practitioner who arranges this readmission, the team can help by alerting the ward and the junior doctor before the patient arrives.

Some patients prefer to be in a side ward where they and their relatives can have privacy. Others find a side ward isolated and lonely. It need not be a general policy to draw the screens around the bed of every dying patient. On several occasions it has perhaps been helpful for other patients in the ward to see how peaceful death can be. When a patient dies, it is wise for the ward sister to let the neighbouring patients know rather than to keep silent.

The Support Team routinely visits a ward after a death, in order to find out if the death has been peaceful or not, and generally to give support if necessary to the ward staff. The death of a young patient, or one who has been in the ward for a long time, can be very distressing for them.

The Support Team also makes a point of letting the district nurses know when one of their patients has died in hospital. It is, of course, the routine for all hospitals to give this information to the general practitioner.

DEATH AT HOME

Even when previous terminal care has been good, the last few days of a patient's life at home can be a great strain on the family. If the patient's symptoms are well controlled it is often the family who need most care at this time. They will need clear guidance on how to nurse the patient and should, if possible, be told what to expect at the end. Anticipation of terminal events can be helpful. One patient with a fungating tumour in the groin died quickly and peacefully with a massive haemorrhage from the femoral artery. We had warned her husband that this might happen and advised him not to disturb the bedclothes but to sit and calmly hold her hand, which he did.

Particular problems arise when a patient is dying at home, during, for example, a weekend when his general practitioner is off duty and a completely strange emergency doctor has taken his place. At a time like this the family will turn to the Support Team. It has proved a great comfort for families to know that the team is always available and it is rare for them to telephone the team unnecessarily.

When a patient can no longer swallow his opiate mixture at 4 hourly intervals it is not easy to arrange for 4 hourly injections throughout a 24 hour period in the home, even with Support Team help. The rectal route is an alternative, but if this is not possible an increased dose of opiate at 6 hourly intervals is sometimes used in a semiconscious patient. An alternative is the use of a longer acting analgesic such as methadone at 8 hourly intervals. Even in the unconscious patient analgesic drugs must be continued.

Restlessness is a very distressing terminal symptom in the home. The district nurse and the team nurse can be alert to possible causes that they can rectify such as a distended bladder. Tranquillizers may also be necessary; chlorpromazine can be given as a rectal suppository or by injection and diazepam is a useful drug at this time.

Immediately after death a family may telephone the Support Team, especially the community sister, for comfort and for advice on what to do.

When a patient has died at home the Support Team will inform the ward nurses and anyone else in the hospital who has been involved with the patient's care.

FINANCING A SUPPORT TEAM

There is no great problem in raising charitable funds for a venture as worthy as improving the care of the dying, but there is sometimes a disadvantage with such funds in that they may lack permanence. Accordingly it is wiser to start with a small team with at least some of its members funded by the National Health Service in order to create stability and permanence. Our first sister's salary was, and still is, provided entirely from charitable funds and without their help the venture would never have got off the ground. From these funds the team became established, but since then a serious attempt was made to obtain funds for the salaries of new members from the National Health Service. The community sister, the social worker and the secretary now have their salaries provided from the national exchequer. The social worker's salary comes jointly from the hospital and the community and the secretary's salary is provided solely by the hospital. We are, however, at present in a time of serious economic difficulty in the Health Service and this particular team is unlikely to be offered any increase in staff if their salaries are to be paid by the Health Service. We need a third sister and her salary will have to be provided by charitable funds.

Fortunately, having no beds, there is no need to seek funds for running expenses or equipment. Some small items of specialized equipment which are often difficult to obtain in the National Health Service, such as triangular pillows, have been bought from funds given by grateful relatives.

GENERAL COMMENTS ON SUPPORT TEAMS

There are two main advantages of a terminal care team such as the one which I have described. Firstly, they are relatively inexpensive to run, even if they have their own beds, compared with a purpose-built hospice and, secondly, they have great teaching potential.

Terminal care teams have obvious disadvantages if not well run, not the least of these being the creation of confusion about responsibility for the care of the patient and even when the problems of acceptance in the hospital and in the community have been overcome, there remains the difficult nature of the work. It is very much easier to take over the total management of a patient in a hospice than it is to share care in either the ward of an acute general hospital or in the patient's home.

Terminal care teams should not be in competition with hospices and the ideal arrangement would be a good cooperative link between the two, recognizing each other's difficulties and advantages, and the ways in which the best choice of either can be made for the particular patient.

The St Thomas' Support Team was designed to fit our particular needs and I hope that its progress to date will help to encourage the formation of other teams. It is not suggested that all teams should be modelled on this one, but rather that their venue, staffing and mode of action should depend upon local circumstances.

From what we have learned, the bulk of the routine work can be done by experienced nurses but we would recommend that these nurses have the back-up of a doctor experienced in terminal care.

It may be necessary to start a team with a voluntary doctor who already has a full-time appointment, but this can only be attempted for a limited period because of the demanding nature of the work. Any doctor undertaking this work must have had special training, and if he has any doubts about his wish to do the work he should not do it. The ideal team, in my view, would be one staffed by a hospital doctor and a general practitioner in equal partnership.

Nurses, likewise, must have had training and because of the stresses of the work must be emotionally resilient. It is important for them to avoid excessive overtime or on-call duties. The rest of the team have to be alert to signs of stress. Sick leave without stigma needs to be taken early rather than late. This applies to all members of the team.

Despite the strains, the St Thomas' Support Team has had a lot of happiness from working together in this venture. We all recognize that the ultimate measure of the team's success will be when it is no longer required.

15

The role of the specialist or hospice unit

Eric Wilkes

INTRODUCTION

The realization that a specialist unit could handle more successfully some of the problems of terminal care has given rise to a movement operating in many countries and to well over 50 such units already at work in the United Kingdom, with more being planned. There is therefore a great variety of organization and interrelationship, of quality and emphasis, but there are certain general principles that are to be classed as characteristic of the movement.

First, such units are unique in that they are mainly geared to the problems of the dying patient. They may have other valuable activities, like the care of cases of motor neurone disease at St Christopher's Hospice, London, or the day unit of St Luke's, Sheffield with its special interest in the chronic disabled, but these activities are essentially parenthetical and subordinate. Most of the work is in dealing with the consequences of disseminated or inoperable malignant disease.

Secondly, the family unit is treated very much as the basic unit of care, so relatives are encouraged to be involved as much as possible, and bereavement is accorded a priority unknown in routine contemporary practice.

With much overlap there are three main phases to be traced in the development of this country's hospices. At first local initiatives and charities dominated the scene, as they are bound to do in any pioneering activity. The NHS was a supporter, by local prearrangement, advising and helping with the otherwise intolerable burden of revenue consequences, but not greatly influencing the design or policy of the project which remained basically a private enterprise.

As experience grew, however, and the value of such work became better substantiated, NHS units came onto the scene. Often the capital building costs would be provided in whole or in part from charitable organizations – here the National Society for Cancer Relief has played a vital role – but once built the unit was absorbed into the local structure and so far as policy, staffing and funding were concerned, these became specialized units of the NHS.

Inevitably NHS and private units have strong opinions about which is the better option, and usually identify what is most familiar as preferable. The NHS units point out the ease of access to other clinical resources, the financial security, the local voice in decision-making, the consultant status of those in clinical charge. They emphasize the dangers of the independent charity becoming outdated and complacent in its comparative isolation from the mainstream of clinical activity.

These may be valid criticisms but the independent unit is not slow in pointing to an inflexible and unimaginative NHS administration that may deprive the hospice unit of important resources because there is even greater need elsewhere; they remain unconvinced of the greater financial security of NHS units which may indeed have to work on a lower level of staffing; they deny complacency, claim valid specialist help is on hand for their patients too, and can point to a much more active volunteer input since they are safely away from the hostility of restrictive practices or the squalor of outdated buildings. And these volunteers on occasion can total several hundred, and combine a range of skills and a devotion that the NHS cannot possibly achieve.

Successful initiatives, predictably, are shared. Private units have opened up day-care and the role of the rehabilitation professionals, a NHS unit has the first consultant to be employed full-time in a domiciliary role, a private unit has the first training post in a vocational training scheme for general practice, and both are valuably involved in teaching and research. Probably here too Alexander Pope is right: whatever is best administered is best.

But such separate independent or NHS units are now no longer the only possible answers in the present third phase of development. The Royal Marsden Hospital has special wards for terminal care, and St Thomas' has, as Thelma Bates describes in Chapter 14 above, a support service without such special wards.

The hospice is no longer to be taken necessarily as a separate inpatient unit, with an outdated preoccupation with beds. In early plans the smallest viable inpatient unit was calculated to be at the level of 25 beds, and such units proliferated up and down the country; but this approach has now been broadened to include hospital-based or community-based support teams, with nurses supplemented by additional skills from the clinician, chaplain or social worker, in schemes which, whether carried out in association with a specialist unit or not, permit the upgrading of services without new expensive facilities.

Furthermore, because many of the patients are living difficult and narrow lives and so need a great deal more than a consultation yet less than full institutionalization, they are highly suitable candidates for day-care. We have now, therefore, got to the stage when specialist units can come into being with no beds, or with only a few beds, and through their domiciliary or day-care roles can have a genuine impact on the local situation.

The provision of a support service for the community involves almost as great an integration with the general practitioner and the attached district nurse as a hospital scheme does with ward sister and consultant. It is likely that such initiatives will dominate the needy 1980s; and integration and coordination of hospice and traditional skills will be increasingly achieved at both administrative and clinical levels. The day of the expensive 25-bed hospice unit is not quite over, but is usually to be justified only in big cities and in association with schools of medicine and nursing as a major teaching resource. What is required now is the willingness of the established services to exploit – if necessary on their own terms – the skills and the facilities made available by these new units. A further essential is that the detached or support nurses should be sensible professional colleagues who in their turn deserve and receive lasting and sensitive support in the emotionally demanding situations with which they are routinely faced. These nurses, it must be emphasized, complement and do not replace the responsibilities of those already involved.

Such nurses, although classed as specialists in their field, will often agree that with two exceptions they are no different from any other experienced high-quality nurse. One difference is that they are given time to deal more adequately with their dying patients than unhappily is often possible on the wards or in the community; and the other difference is their special experience and confidence in the art of communicating with these sick patients and their relatives.

Things have changed quickly over the last few years and it is no longer possible to guess at what percentage of experienced doctors now tend to share with their patients the true diagnosis or prognosis. What is certain is that it is much larger than a decade ago and is likely to be still increasing.

Novack and his colleagues (1979) have shown that whereas in 1961 in the USA 90 per cent of responding physicians did *not* tell cancer patients the diagnosis, in 1977 97 per cent did so – 'a complete reversal of opinion'. How relevant is this change in the United Kingdom has not yet been surveyed, for certain factors operating in the American scene are not so relevant here; the tendency, however, is likely to be in a similar direction.

Yet in a phase of rapid change one area that seems to have been modified slowly and in a very half-hearted way is the involvement of nursing staff in a counselling role. It is often to the nurse that, at certain times, patients reveal their knowledge and their fears, and too often on acute wards the nurse is forced gently – since this is the unit policy – to turn aside the question with 'you should really ask the doctor'; the doctors, of course, come comparatively infrequently in hurried groups that lend themselves more easily to evasions rather than to confidences. Perhaps this side of the doctor's work is less well taught now in the high technology era; perhaps with the expansion of the medical schools there is no longer repeated opportunity to see the consultant working up a relationship with the patient and telling the latter what is appropriate for that stage of their illness; perhaps the bright young doctors are too removed from the professional traditions of yesterday, or perhaps the seniors in present circumstances are able no longer to maintain those traditions so carefully. Certainly those who work in the specialist hospice-type units can be under no illusions about the difficulties of adjustment, the chances missed, and on occasion the resentment aroused, by our failure to inform, to share and to support.

History-telling is well taught in our medical schools and we can foray effectively into the past of the patient and attain our diagnosis; but counselling skills – the use of non-verbal communication, the asking of questions and the quiet exploration of answers so that the session is patient-dominated, these are skills not often to be shown in the turmoil of our outpatients or in the hubbub of our understaffed wards. They are skills far more characteristic of the hospice-type units, and are of course much easier to maintain in that less hectic environment.

The situation is easier also for the hospice units since they are coming in late in the patient's story. When a woman has had a mastectomy, radio-therapy, oophorectomy, various forms of hormonal therapy or chemo-therapy, and has recurrent problems, she needs quite different handling from the agonizing hopes of 3 or 4 or 15 years before. The woman with a lump or a discharge, no matter how formally ill-educated she may be, is already halfway to the truth. In one survey of patients admitted in the terminal phases of their illness to a specialist unit (Wilkes, 1977) only 9 per cent had no idea of their real situation. Even if the patient had no more than a vague suspicion, as soon as admission to the specialist unit is proposed there is little room for doubt or manoeuvre; so for such units a kind and optimistic openness is all we dare offer. We can promise to do our best, to control symptoms efficiently, always to be there, and hope, a day at a time, that they will have a lot of good living to do. We can get some 10 to 20 per cent of admissions home again, when we have controlled the symptoms or rested and briefed the family, and a far higher proportion can get home for a day out or for Sunday lunch. The impression is that once hope of cure is given up, more realistic hopes can be achieved with a more placid and genuine satisfaction. At this stage, hiding behind words and promises gains us no credit. However kindly it may be slanted, we must live in the world of truth. This means that outside doctors can get a wrong impression that hospice policy is invariably to tell all without delay. There is in hospice units so much knowledge of patients told too little and too late that we may on occasion overcompensate and tell too much too soon, and regret at leisure. The policy of most units is, however, to let patients tell us, in their own time and in their own way, to lead them to their own adjustment, and never to lie. At an earlier stage in the illness such a policy is compatible with many patients not being told their diagnosis if they show little sign of wanting to carry that burden; and although lines of communication must always be kept open and genuine trust maintained without falsehood, one accepts that sharing the truth with the patient in a caring skilled community is quite different from telling them early in their illness, when they are perhaps alone for long hours at home, and not yet ready for the situation that the great majority will face with courage and humour when nearer their time. One can perhaps put it another way, using the obstetric analogy of the premature, the postmature or the at-term baby, but with death instead of birth.

The premature death we fight, but if the battle is lost the patient may give up too quickly, and sit in front of the fire in his slippers wanting to die, eroding his own and the family's morale when months of limited but reasonable living could still be achieved. In contrast, there is the postmature death when life is debased by the patient striving desperately to maintain the business undertaking or the family responsibilities for which they no longer have the strength. It is the task of the family doctor or the specialist unit so to manage the patient and the family that the pre-death period avoids these extra pitfalls, and is as short and full as we can make it. Death when it comes should be a fitting and well-timed release with little of terror or suffering. Of course, we often fail; but the failures are usually only partial failures.

Doctors tend to underestimate the scant fear of death many of their patients have and yet this is often combined with a great and unjustified fear of the process of dying. Since most patients die by just a peaceful relaxation of their grip on life, we need to tell them of this or we risk missing the chance to comfort and reassure those who know they are soon to die, and also to neglect relatives watching at the bedside. This has perhaps been crowded out by the modern clinical climate but is part of the specialist unit's commitment.

The degree of success can be judged from a survey of 500 admissions to a specialist unit. The bedside nurses coded the quality of terminal life of those in their care for a week or longer before death. Their verdict was realized in an open meeting within, usually, 48 hours of the death. The nurses thought that 29 per cent of their patients had had an excellent quality of life, 70 per cent a satisfactory quality of life, and only 1 per cent a poor quality of life at the end (Wilkes, 1977). In the 1 per cent who had difficulties these were less likely to be problems of intractable symptoms than of psychiatric or personality difficulties superimposed on the physical illness. However, even patients with alcoholism, schizophrenia, even a Rampton or Broadmoor background, have achieved a peaceful final illness in the specialist unit, with respect both given and received.

THE INPATIENT UNIT

Despite all the variations in layout and personalities, the different terminal care units tend to have a surprisingly similar atmosphere: but they must be geared to problems as varied as the rural area around Christchurch, the retired at Worthing or the patients of a big industrial city. It was thought most useful to concentrate in this chapter on a description of St Luke's in Sheffield, as the unit best known to the author. It is the senior of the provincial units, opening its doors in 1971, and the first to have a purpose-built day unit. Furthermore, Sheffield likes, for all its 600 000 inhabitants, to call itself England's biggest village, and has a surprisingly stable population for such a major centre. It has, of course, all the problems of the big city but, despite the deprivation and detribalization of certain areas, these tend to be on a manageable scale.

Into the 25 beds of St Luke's are admitted some 350 to 400 patients each year – some 10 per cent of the local cancer deaths. The age of the patients varies from the late teens to the 90s but there are usually several patients under the age of 50 on the wards, making up 6 per cent of the total. It is, therefore, no geriatric unit, yet 13 per cent of patients are over 80. The average age is in the early to mid-60s for males and females, and the proportion of married to widowed to single patients is 5:3:1. Since the women look after their men, and then there is no-one to look after the women, usually three of the four five-bedded wards are for females (57 per cent of the total) and only one ward is for males. Flexibility is obtained through five single rooms, which tend to be allocated to those with offensive odours, or who are disfigured, or younger patients with children. We do not like admitting the very old to the single rooms, for the isolation encourages confusion. Occasionally when a couple is devoted and travel to the hospice is difficult, we admit both to a single room. This may be rather cramped but it does prevent the couple being parted in their last days.

This is in stark contrast to the routine in Sheffield – and indeed other towns – in which approximately two-thirds of all deaths occur in the acute hospital wards, yet over half of those patients have spent most of their last month in their own homes before being transferred to die among strangers (Ward, 1974).

The average duration of stay in St Luke's is something like 10 days for the men and 20 days for the women. Over a third will stay for between 1 and 6 weeks and 20 per cent for longer than 6 weeks. Typically, the men die quietly and speedily with lung cancer, the women much more slowly with breast cancers. These are the two commonest tumours, and with gastric and colorectal cancers they account for over half of the admissions. Although each year breast and lung primaries are admitted in roughly equal numbers, when compared with the lung cases, the breast cancers require two and a half times the bed-days for their care. The breast cases also provide a large proportion of the paraplegics (usually four or five among the 25 patients on the wards at any time) a large proportion of the 5 per cent of admissions who need to stay for several months, and also a large proportion of the 15 per cent or so of all admissions who can eventually, if temporarily, be discharged home. Of all breast cases 26 per cent go home, compared with 9 to 12 per cent of lung, colorectal or gastric tumours.

Some three-quarters of the admissions come, at the request of the general practitioner, straight from their homes, and the remaining quarter are transferred from acute hospital wards. The degree of local acceptance of the unit can be gauged by the fact that nearly 200 of the 280 principals in general practice in Sheffield applied over a period of 12 months for a patient to be admitted. Each year unfortunately over 150 cases die on our waiting list because we are unable to find them a bed. This figure is not helped by some 20 per cent of admissions coming from outside of Sheffield since we are classed as a supra-area specialty.

The pressures under which we work can be further demonstrated by the fact that nearly a quarter of our admissions are dead within 3 days: yet when a patient dies we always, at the request of the nursing staff, leave that bed empty for 24 hours so that both nurses and patients can mourn. Strange patients coming without delay into the newly empty bed were treated a little bit, despite our efforts, as intruders. Now that the nurses have time to explain and share the death with the others on the ward, it is clearly worth the small delay.

What sort of patients come to St Luke's? Although priests and nursing officers and professional colleagues have died with us, as the poorer social classes with fewer resources bear the strain of a terminal illness badly, we have more patients from social classes IV and V than on an ordinary ward. Of our patients 20 per cent are social isolates – quite often because they are aged and have outlived their close relatives and friends. Since at least 15 per cent of cancer cases dying at home in Sheffield are cared for by relatives themselves aged over 70, it is not surprising that the commonest single reason for admission is to give respite to exhausted families. We see little of rejection by relatives, especially if they can be given confidence and assured of constant support. What we do see much more frequently are exhausted wives who have not had their clothes off or a proper sleep for weeks and who cannot in any serious way be further involved in the care of their patient until they have had a period of rest. It may well be that pain or incontinence or confusion have added to the burden (see Table 1) of a lengthy illness and so led to admission. The resources of the family vary even more than those of the primary health care team; but we see exhausted families and unrelieved suffering often enough to agree with Isaacs' comment (Isaacs, Livingstone, and Neville, 1976) that if you are old and

Table 1   The ten major symptoms after admission in 296 cases of terminal cancer (per cent)*

Pain	58	Bedsores	15
Incontinence	38	Vomiting	13
Confusion	21	Open wounds	13
Dyspnoea	17	Cough	5
Nausea	16	Dysphagia	3

Note: Insomnia, anorexia, depression, anxiety and weakness are excluded since, although frequently noted, they were rarely complained of as the major problem requiring admission. Amended from Wilkes (1974) and published by permission.

dying at home, despite the massive resources of the NHS, what really counts is a good daughter and a good neighbour.

Yet we must always bear in mind that we only see a small spectrum of terminal care in the specialist units – rather less than 5 per cent of all deaths – and it is too easy to extrapolate our experience into an inaccurate picture.

When we look at the pattern of referrals, these will be controlled by the detailed family circumstances, by the degree of the general practitioner's commitment, and by the pressure on the beds of the consultant rather than by the problems of the individual patient. Yet having said that, the pattern of referral will not be totally meaningless and could be helpful.

For example, if we look at cancers of the urinary tract over 2 years in our half-million population we find that the average age of our bladder cancer patients (35 out of 700 or 5 per cent of admissions) was 71 years. The male to female distribution was 1:1. Three had second primary tumours confirmed, and their average duration of stay was 14 days; 16 had pain, six were incontinent, and five lived alone.

The prostatic cancers also had an average age of 71 years and made up (27 out of 700) 4 per cent of admissions. Their average duration of stay was 23 days and common problems were pain (11), paraplegia (four), cachexia (four) while four had elderly wives who could no longer deal with their needs.

The common symptoms of our eight renal cancers (with two patients in their 40s) were again pain (four) and cachexia (two), but other complicated problems included paraplegia, pathological fracture, dyspnoea, urinary retention, haematuria, confusion, hiccoughs, and living alone.

When we look at the gynaecological cancers who needed our care over a year, we can expect some 20 cases of terminal cancer of cervix, 20 of ovary

Table 2

Symptom	Cervix (19)	Uterine body (9)	Ovary (20)	Total
Pain	11	6	14	31
Nausea/vomiting	3	2	11	14
Ascites	–	–	6	6
Other oedema	1	2	3	6
Incontinent with fistula	6	–	1	7
Confusion	3	–	2	5
Cachexia	2	3	5	10
Dyspnoea	2	–	3	5
Pressure sores	3	–	1	4
Urinary diversion	4	–	–	4

and ten of uterine body. They will, in their final admission, stay for an average period of 3 weeks, and have an average age in the mid-60s. We can expect a steady trickle of young cases of cervical cancer in their 20s, 30s and 40s and older patients, from all three primary sites, in their 80s.

Of our actual major gynaecological cancers the numbers and main symptoms were as shown in Table 2.

These patients stayed with us for a total of 890 days. Nearly two-thirds had pain and over a quarter were nauseated. Indeed the ovarian cancers vomited more than the gastric cases in our series. So far as the ascites was concerned we were more impressed by the value of spironolactone in preventing or delaying the reaccumulation of fluid than by the local instillation of cytotoxics. We found the opiates controlled the pain well but that in difficult cases of sciatic pain intrathecal phenol injections gave good results. When opiates gave effective analgesia, there was little need to keep increasing the dose, yet some patients had suffered pain for 1 or even 2 years.

Cases needing admission for longer than a month were uterine body – two, cervix – four, and ovary – seven. The occasional case may need admission for many months, usually because of a combination of pain, weakness, poor home circumstances and incontinence associated with a cervical carcinoma. The excretion of an uncontrollable mixture of urine and faeces is a ghastly problem for the patient, but we achieved a late palliative colostomy more often with colorectal than with cervical cancers. The diversion of the urinary tract, for all it had usually been carried out months before, was not associated with a very high quality of life, and yet a less exacting procedure such as nephrostomy can lead to rather difficult nursing procedures. There are no easy answers.

We also admitted four vulval primaries over this period. All were old (70–89 years), and they tended to present late, with offensive lesions, in pain, confused or comatose. Two had a major recurrence of tumour in the groin. They all died fairly quickly after admission, but no matter how keen they were to keep their privacy and stay independent, one can imagine the smelly desperation that must have dominated their last months.

For such patients we could achieve little more than clean, dry sheets, and a sense of privilege in caring for them. Yet for many others we can attain genuine and rapid symptom-control. This too can produce its own complications.

If patients have lived for weeks with pain they may, when they lose it, feel lost and insecure. They need to work at something useful and relevant to them, or morale will get worse. Mobilization and partial independence can often be achieved. Thus if a patient survives 2 weeks in our unit the incidence of bedfastness – initially on admission at some 58 per cent – will be greatly reduced (even halved) depending on a combination of physiotherapy, confidence and pain-control.

Again, if a patient's life is taken up with physical symptoms, they may be living almost at an animal level; but once the symptoms are controlled they will be worrying about their future, and needing some proper occupation. The days of the dying patient are so often few and yet empty. Work under the supervision of an experienced occupational therapist can transform the aimless atmosphere on the wards, make enough money for the charity to pay for all the raw materials needed, give simple heirlooms for the family and dignity back to the patient.

It is perhaps helpful to summarize the staff of St Luke's. We have two part-time physiotherapists and some six volunteer aides, two occupational therapists and some 25 volunteer aides. These of course, are also involved in the day unit. We have a nurse : patient ratio of 1:1, but this includes so many part-time married nurses that the 25 full-time equivalents are made up of some 65 nurses. The medical care, permitting each patient to be seen by a doctor every day, is from three part-time general practitioners, of whom the author is one, plus the SHO, in training. We have a part-time chaplain, two chaplain's assistants, and two qualified social workers. We also have general administrative support of the highest calibre. This level of clinical staffing, however, does not permit us routinely to assess the suitability of patients prior to admission, but the general practitioners only rarely mislead us. We have difficulty keeping up with the needs of inservice training or an adequate programme of research.

We do, however, take regular social work students, we run several JCBNS courses a year – booked at the time of writing for some 2 years ahead, and are involved in regular teaching with local schools of nursing and medical students, as well as with a constant stream of professional colleagues, both local and overseas.

One of the questions often raised by our visitors is how we deal with requests for euthanasia. We get such requests with surprising rarity, especially when we remember that some 2 or 3 per cent of our stable middle-aged patients have attempted suicide, and very reasonably may have been referred to us in consequence.

Although on occasion we get patients who have had enough, who turn their faces to the wall and withdraw from life, those who talk of seeking a quick end are almost invariably admissions who have been with us a very short time. We often succeed in establishing good relationships very quickly but not always in a matter of hours. This naturally takes time to develop and sometimes time is short.

Usually these patients who express a wish to die quickly have resented their dependence, have hated being a nuisance and have, even in their own homes, been lonely and poorly supported, with the world already passing them by. Home is where the pain is and in the little bedroom they can scarcely hear the real world going on downstairs.

Once these factors have been palliated, although it may well have its bitter and sardonic moments, life usually is still sweet. This is no paradox in a place whose end-product is dying well and with dignity. For the terminal care unit, in the midst of death we are in life.

THE DAY UNIT

We were anxious about the patients we discharged home, although we weaned them gradually from full-time care, letting them home at first for a day, then perhaps for one or two weekends and then for a longer stay, so they and their family were properly trained for their return. But they often missed the company and the support even when the home circumstances were good.

We were even more anxious about those for whom we could not find a bed, or who needed help but not yet admission.

We appreciated that a small unit must have limited goals but we felt a day unit must surely be the right answer, especially as no more beds could be funded. After 3 years, we are convinced that this day unit was the right decision, and we are glad that we have been able to raise the £40 000 needed each year to run it.

There are now three parts to St Luke's – the inpatient unit, the day unit, and two Macmillan support nurses, both experienced community nursing sisters, based on our unit and funded by the National Society for Cancer Relief. These are the nursing sisters who arrange the details about the discharge of patients with their community nursing colleagues and the general practitioners. They also assess the suitability of cases referred for the day unit, and even with experienced assessment in the early days nearly a fifth of our day patients were only well enough to attend once. Finally these nurses offer support and advice to terminal cases in their own home, as an extra resource to the primary care team, without such cases necessarily having any contact with St Luke's. It is perhaps this close contact with the community that leads to almost all the day unit referrals being from general practitioners (Table 3).

Table 3   St Luke's day unit: referral source by major problem; 300 episodes involving 273
patients

Patient referral by	Pain	Family or carer stress	Nursing needs	Social problems	Needs a day out	Total of patient episodes
General practitioner	67	19	15	7	104	123
Hospital	12	4	3	2	21	25
Social worker	18	4	6	5	25	30
Community services including district nurse	24	7	11	3	35	46
On discharge from St Luke's inpatient unit	19	2	3	1	24	28
On return for further episode (mainly chronic disabled)	18	5	5	1	44	48
Total	158	41	43	19	253	300

These support nurses cooperate so closely with the day unit staff that it is
difficult to see how it could function effectively without them. They are
especially vital in visiting at home our day-patients in August and
December when the day unit closes, or when the patients are too ill to
attend.

Nurses actually employed in the day unit are the sister-in-charge, a state
registered nurse who always works on a particular day each week and so
knows the patients and their problems well, a nursing auxiliary rotating in
turn from the inpatient unit, and either a second auxiliary or a nurse in
training.

This rotation of inpatient nurses to the day unit is of especial help to day-
patients when they need admission. They settle in quickly when they see
one or two familiar and friendly faces on the wards. As well as this,
however, basic nursing care is important in the day unit. The patients may
not be able to be clean and well cared-for at home, and a weekly bath may be
a great luxury.

Bowels are always a problem. Toilet facilities may be so primitive that
diuretics can only be taken on day-unit days. As well as this we have
swollen post-mastectomy arms to be massaged in a mechanically inflated
arm splint, stoma care to be supervised, catheters changed, dressings
reapplied and medication checked.

The physiotherapist teaches them how to retain mobility with exercises,
and the use of gadgets that may vary from a walking tripod to an electric
wheelchair. The occupational therapists can offer them pottery, with the

fully glazed articles back from the kiln a week after they were made, painting, mosaic trays or tiles, and simple repetitive work that is speedily recognizable as a fruit bowl, plantpot holder or lampshade. A chaplain and social worker are available, the doctor's day-unit round is a significant if brief event (although we must accept a lower standard of symptom-control than would be required on the wards), the hairdressing and beauty salon is an integral part of the day unit although it serves inpatients also, and after a good lunch the most popular activity is bingo.

With this variety of activities available, a day from 10 am to 3 pm is as much as most of these patients can deal with. Some 85 per cent of them attend only once weekly, and this day becomes a club with relationships important enough for those who have had to become inpatients determinedly joining their old friends even, if need be, in their bed.

When we surveyed the patients and asked what they enjoyed least, we were not surprised that taking medicines was fairly unpopular. Neither were we surprised that even a brief and superficial contact with the doctor was very important. We were, however, taken aback when, despite the variety of talent waiting to greet them, our patients said that they enjoyed most of all their drive to and from the unit. It was for many the only time they could leave their home and they were driven by a volunteer driver who was punctual and reassuring. As relationships developed, the driver would alter the route so that the patients could see new developments and changes in their area that they had heard or read about. The journey became literally a lifeline. Despite this, we may soon have to carry more patients by our own ambulance for the younger pensioner-volunteers are finding the upkeep of their cars increasingly costly and two-car families may become rarer.

We were also surprised by the tremendous relief experienced by the family at having a day of respite not only from the work but also from the responsibility of caring. 'At last I felt supported', wrote one, and a quite independent visiting research worker was told the following by a 63-year old widow who had been admitted after a spell in the day unit:

Before the day centre I tried to commit suicide. I didn't know what to expect here, I thought I'd be out in a box, I said I don't want to be shut away, I thought it would be geriatrics. But it's given me a new lease of life, it's given me a life, I wait for my day here to come. On Tuesday we do modelling, it's given me something to live for and nothing is too much trouble for them. I was going to drown myself, that is all over now. Working for this place is the most important thing we can do. I'd do anything for this place. I made progress in my health, I've gone from wheelchair to calipers to a stick. The services here are lovely, they encourage you and give you hope. I was telling a nurse I was frightened of dying and they were really reassuring. I've seen three people die here and it's nothing, they just go to sleep: that was very comforting.

The work of the day unit has been greatly enriched by including a one in five proportion of chronic disabled – mostly old strokes, Parkinson's disease, longstanding rheumatoid or multiple sclerosis cases, for whom the NHS has so little to offer. Such cases attend once a week for 8 weeks or they may be taking up a place for many years; they then go on to a waiting list for another 8 week programme some 12 months later. It is clear that these cases benefit not only from their enjoyment of the social stimulus but also by their improved physical performance. Of course we realize that we are only scraping the surface of this area of unmet need.

Cases of malignant disease who attend the day unit can attend indefinitely. Younger cases with primary brain tumours have been long-term attenders and we need to give much support to the patient and spouse as their difficulties grow. Prostatic and bladder cases also can come over a long period (Table 4) but the typical long-term day-case is again the primary of breast. So long drawnout can their problems be that the day unit could be worthwhile for them alone.

Table 4 St Luke's day unit: average duration of final episode (weeks) by primary site

Tongue	18 weeks
Lower third oesophagus	6 weeks
Gastric carcinoma (unspecified)	3 weeks
Sigmoid colon	16 weeks
Rectum	3 weeks
Lung	14 weeks
Breast	12 weeks
Ovary	16 weeks
Bladder	23 weeks

It is important that men attending the day unit should not feel swamped in a crowd of women. Although the numbers of men and women are reasonably equal, since the women tend to attend for longer periods, men can become embarrassed and unhappy if there are no kindred spirits to keep them company.

It is interesting to note the great preponderance of husbands as the chief carers of these day-patients. They made up no less than 56 per cent of the chief carers (Table 5), with the wife taking the main responsibility in only 12 per cent and sibling or child in 21 per cent of cases.

The Dying Patient

Table 5 St Luke's day unit: relationship and age of carers at home*

	20–29	30–39	40–49	50–59	60–69	70–79	80+	Total
Husband	0	1	8	39	38	51	16	153
Wife	3	10	10	9	1	0	0	33
Daughter	3	3	11	11	1	0	0	29
Son	0	1	1	10	7	6	3	28
Brother/sister neighbour or other	2	3	7	7	3	3	0	25
All	8	18	37	76	50	60	19	268

Note: five had no carer

Table 6 St Luke's day unit: activity 1 January 1978 to 30 April 1980 (273 patients)

	Patient-episodes*	Attendances
Chronic sick	79	575
Malignant disease	221	2016
Total	300	2591

Note: An episode here means a fairly regular sequence of attendances; if the sequence is interrupted by admission, other treatment, or holiday, for example, subsequent return to the day unit is classed as a separate episode.

The pattern of transfers is for a gradual, and therefore tolerable, change in the monthly pattern of roughly 200 attendances. Each month we can expect about eight new recruits to day care, with two or three being transferred from inpatient to day unit and also a similar number going from day unit to inpatient care, where they may well die.

The pressing need for a change of environment was noted in no less than 228 out of the 273 patients, 144 needed help with pain or other symptoms, and family stress or nursing needs were of roughly equal frequency (38 and 43 respectively) in the chronic disabled and malignant disease patients. Major social problems were noted in only 5 per cent of the chronic disabled and in 6 per cent of the cases of malignant disease. The different needs of the two categories of patients are as might have been expected (Table 7)

Table 7 St Luke's day unit: assessment of major needs

	Total	Pain (per cent)	Family or carer stress (per cent)	Nursing needs (per cent)	Social problem (per cent)	Needs a day out (per cent)
Chronic sick	68	22	14	10	5	98
Malignant disease	205	65	14	17	6	82

and their common problems often led to a good mutual support system being developed between patients that was perhaps as important as the relief afforded to the relatives (Wilkes, Crowther, and Greaves, 1978).

Of the total of 11 per cent of inpatients discharged in 1979, 4 per cent attended the day unit following discharge, but 7 per cent did not. Although many of these not attending lived at a distance, it does mean that a small proportion of very ill patients can achieve a further genuine period of independence. Improvement in their quality of life, however, remains the main objective and, we hope, achievement of day-care.

Further details can be gleaned from Tables 3 to 11.

Table 8 St Luke's day unit: main problems by primary site (some had several main problems)*

Primary site	Pain	Family or carer stress	Nursing needs	Social problem	Needs a day out	Total
Tongue, mouth, oropharynx, tonsil, larynx	3	3	3	2	9	20
Oesophagus, stomach, small bowel	11	2	4	1	11	29
Large bowel	15	1	3	0	19	38
Lung	33	5	3	4	48	93
Breast	30	5	13	3	34	85
Ovary	7	0	3	0	7	17
Bladder	4	1	0	0	4	9

*Note: data on 165 of 205 patients with malignant disease

BEREAVEMENT

In an ideal world, the general practitioner would not be so besieged by stuffy noses and grazed knees or by people who had such cogent yet inalterable reasons for their anxiety and discontent. The doctor would have the knowledge of the families that comes with time while retaining the alert clinical watchfulness of youth.

One could watch the young marriages that tend to have difficulties in surviving, and the old partnerships that do not share roles, and try to equip them, years before, for their inevitable bereavement. Then we would never be faced with the intelligent woman who knows nothing of her financial state or how to mend a fuse, and all the widowers could cook a good meal and deal with the laundry.

Table 9 St Luke's day unit: pattern of attendance in commoner tumours

Primary site	Total weeks of attendance						Total patient episodes	Total patient attendances	Average number of attendances
	1–3	4–6	7–12	13–24	25–48	49–100			
Tongue, oropharynx, tonsil, mouth and larynx	6	3	0	0	1	0	11	47	4
Oesophagus, stomach and small bowel	9	3	3	0	0	0	17	68	4
Colorectal cancers	13	4	2	3	0	1	25	175	7
Lung and bronchus	25	8	9	7	3	2	57	505	9
Breast	16	7	7	9	4	3	52	625	12
Uterus	3	0	1	0	0	0	4	9	2
Ovary	2	2	0	4	2	0	11	137	12
Bladder and kidney	0	2	0	4	4	0	12	219	18
Prostate	3	2	0	0	0	0	5	20	4

Table 10 St Luke's day unit: episodes of 25 weeks duration or longer

Primary site	Duration (weeks)
Tongue	35
Sigmoid colon	27
Lung	67, 76, 25, 39
Breast	58, 27, 79, 41, 36, 30
Ovary	38, 46
Brain	26
Multiple myeloma	80, 32

Table 11 St Luke's day unit: outcome and main problems

	Admitted St Luke's inpatients	Admitted to other hospital	Kept at home	Died at home	Died elsewhere	Total
Pain	87	9	38	20	3	157
Family or carer stress	13	8	13	5	2	41
Nursing needs	21	4	12	5	1	43
Social problems	8	2	0	4	1	15
Needs a day out	95	25	98	30	4	252
Total	224	48	161	64	11	

In an ideal world, the hospital consultant would somehow find time to interview the patient in quiet privacy and relatives would have the truth explained in detail and then, as the students are taught they should do, given another appointment to come with a close friend or relative some 24 or 48 hours later, when the relatives can hear the truth again, and will have had time to prepare questions. Also this time, so as to confirm their understanding, relatives would be asked to repeat back the salient points of what they have been told.

But in the real world, the family doctor hardly ever meets the family, for home visits have declined by 60 per cent over the last 20 years, and patients come and go. They need referral to a hospital where they will often be dealt with by the variable talents of junior staff; operation notes are reliable but what patient or relatives have been told is not necessarily even entered up.

For example, after conscientious and detailed briefing, diabetics who were thought suitable for general practice care were discharged from a hospital clinic, yet at a later interview 20 per cent of the patients thought they had been discharged because they were cured. If this inability to comprehend is so great in a diabetic clinic, how much greater is it likely to be with the more distressing news of incurable illness? And such inability to take in bad news accurately is not restricted to ill-educated or elderly relatives.

By the time relatives come to visit at a specialist hospice unit, one would have expected that there is little left to be told. In fact, staff often have to spend more time briefing and consoling the relatives than the patients. And just as the grief reaction is likely to be more severe and long-lasting if the relative's death is sudden, it may be so in more chronic and long-term illness if the relatives have not been well briefed and supported.

Dying patients who have adjusted well to their situation still like to make impossible plans for the future; they can live with the truth, but not all the time. Relatives, similarly, like to come back to the future occasionally and when it suits them. It may be that dealing with this will be one of the important areas of responsibility suitable for delegation to the hospital terminal care support-nurse, a post in which experimental studies are proceeding and in which increasing interest is being shown.

The writings of Murray Parkes (especially 1972, 1976) have taught us the main points about bereavement: the numbness preceding the loneliness and the pining, the guilt and anger and resentment, before the months of gradual adjustment. We know that to some their grief is a superb opportunity for exploitation and manipulation, and for some others it marks the end to normal living. We must offer special help and solace to those at special risk: those left with young children, the survivor of the close childless couple, the frail elderly widower, or, in more general terms, those who showed a greater than usual sense of loss, and those who have poor community links or unreliable or indifferent family support.

Family doctors are showing an increasing awareness of this problem and relatives, in a small local survey, found their general practitioner more help in bereavement than any other of the health professionals, with ward sister and community nurse close behind and well ahead of clergyman or social worker. Some doctors now put the date of the bereavement on the front of the survivor's medical record, so that if they attend with a headache or a backache near that anniversary date, a more appropriate consultation may ensue.

But one must be impressed also by the high incidence of physical illness among the recently bereaved. In another small survey of some 34 relatives 6–12 months after bereavement 15 thought their health not good and only 11 thought it reasonably good; 12 were on psychotropic medication, 14 had attended hospital outpatients, and ten had been admitted to hospital.

Despite the temptation to prescribe tranquillizers and hypnotics, one is increasingly conscious of their very limited helpfulness. Indeed frequently they will delay adjustment rather than facilitate it; and this was one of the reasons why we felt it necessary to include a bereavement visiting service as part of the hospice unit's role.

The service is under the general supervision of the senior social worker but is not to be classed as a sophisticated counselling service. It provides more in the nature of a good neighbour's visit, and it usually takes place some 6 weeks after the patient's death. It is carried out by volunteers who may be nurses or who help in some other capacity at St Luke's.

The visitors are usually made most welcome, but it is not long before tears and questions, often easily shared and answered, come to the fore. If there is serious emotional disturbance, the case is reported back to the social worker and may be referred by her to the general practitioner. In most cases, and we contact 30 to 40 per cent of relatives of the cases dying at St Luke's, one to three visits are enough and the worst is over.

Indeed, the relatives feel such visits are so helpful that one is tempted to ask all family doctors to visit a few weeks after each death in their practice, to sit down and say to the relative 'Well, I suppose you don't think much of doctors now', and then to listen. On the other hand, our visitors too do not always get the full picture, since the unit they represent was involved in the case, and relatives handle us perhaps with diplomacy and tact just as they would their family doctor.

It is for that reason that an independent research worker performed some late bereavement visits for us, and a few selected case reports can be found in Appendix I (page 311). It needs emphasizing here again that such reports may not represent anything like 'the truth' and imply no condemnation of any colleagues; they are what the relatives remembered and felt, and as such they have, it was thought, some valuable lessons to teach.

Finally, the concept of grieving has been broadened somewhat. The mother has to mourn for the normal child she has not had before she can begin to cope with the handicapped child she must rear. One can mourn as much for one's lost leg as for one's lost spouse.

Prominent in this area of hardship stands the stoma case, often elderly and humiliated, bewildered and bereft. We are fortunate in having stoma nurses in the city now and since the small survey and the interviews in Appendix II (page 323) was recorded things are probably better. But it is always worth listening to the patient, and the teaching of professionals or students by the patient is very much in the hospice unit tradition. It gives patients status and a chance to air their views, and for the professionals to review their performance.

In these reports, however, the patients, no matter how distorted their recollections may be, could perhaps have received more than was on offer, at any rate in the art of communication.

References

Isaacs, B., Livingstone, M. and Neville, Y. (1972). *Survival of the Unfittest.* (London: Routledge and Kegan Paul)

Novack, D. H., Plumer, R., Smith, R. L., Ochitill, H., Morrow, G. R. and Bennett, J. M. (1979). Changes in physicians' attitudes toward telling the cancer patient. *Am. Med. Assoc.*, **241**, 897

Parkes, C. M. (1972). *Bereavement: Studies of Grief in Adult Life.* (London: Tavistock and Pelican)

Parkes, C. M. (1976). *Omega*, **6**, 303

Ward, A. M. W. (1974). *Soc. Sc. Med.*, **8**, 413

Wilkes, E., (1974). *Proc. R. Soc. Med.*, **67**, 1001

Wilkes, E., (1977). *Nursing Times*, **73**, 1506

Wilkes, E., Crowther, A. G. O. and Greaves, C. W. K. H. (1978). *Br. Med. J.*, **2**, 1053

Appendix I:
Ten bereavement interviews

Linda Liddamant

Note: Much bitterness was exposed to the research interviewer and only the details have been falsified to preserve anonymity: but the histories permit us a brief glimpse into the relatives' world. It is to be emphasized that here we are not necessarily concerned with the truth, for this has been distorted and disguised by eccentric ideas, by all kinds of misunderstandings, and by the guilt and resentment of grief. What they tell us is not how it happened. It is, damagingly enough, how it is remembered.

CASE 1

Note: Wife had wanted the husband admitted, but the patient had been reluctant – he was a hospital worker in his 50s; he had one son aged 10.

Mrs Plummer welcomed me into her comfortable flat, and we chatted over a cup of coffee. She would prefer to be at work, but cannot find a job where she could be at home when her son returned from school. Geoffrey had a very bad grief reaction to his father's death. He felt very insecure and kept his grief to himself until he became quite ill. Mrs Plummer's general practitioner advised her to give up work and give Geoffrey all the attention she could, and so she is now at home all day and very bored. She feels that the ideal answer is either a part-time job, or to do some home typing.

However, being at home all day gives her too much time to brood. This is slowing her progress to some extent, as became clear during our conversation. She tends to dwell on little details until they assume huge significance. For example, she is very bitter about the surgeon at the district general hospital. For 4 years her husband went to have a regular checkup and in all that time nothing was discovered. However, when an exploratory operation was performed at the end of that time, a large, inoperable tumour was found. Mrs Plummer believes that the cancer was there all the time but the specialists were too incompetent to find it and her husband could have been saved but for them.

Since her husband's death, Mrs Plummer has been under considerable strain. Her sister left her 'to paddle my own canoe', and her mother has been less than friendly since Mrs Plummer refused to have her to live in the flat. This has left her to be mother and father to Geoffrey and to help him through his grief as well as coping with her own.

In these circumstances the bereavement visitor was really welcome. It gave her a link with her husband and a chance to talk. She found the visits distressing, but felt that they did her good to let out her feelings. She was also helped by the thought that Mr Plummer had died in peace and with dignity, and (she thinks) with no idea of how ill he really was. The knowledge that the end can be faced without fear has been a help to Mrs Plummer in facing her own death, and her main worry about that is leaving Geoffrey.

The strain of coping after her bereavement has meant that she has been taking tranquillizers and sleeping pills. She smokes more too, and would be a compulsive eater if she did not keep herself in check.

She has had to subdue her own reactions to cope with her son's grief. She also worries about money, and feels she cannot make her son see that the funds are not limitless, but also feels sad she cannot give him everything the other boys have. Her health also worries her for Geoffrey's sake, especially since she feels estranged from her closest relatives. She was Mr Plummer's second wife, and so has stepchildren to whom she is not very close. Actual loneliness does not worry her very much as she describes herself as a 'bit of a loner'.

Her life has settled into a routine of caring for her boy, shopping and housework. She does not consider this sufficient to occupy her mind. She would really like to work, but the way social security and rent offices work would mean her being out of pocket unless she did not declare her earnings. As a result she broods. She admits to taking things too much to heart. (This is the cause of her estrangement from her mother who told Geoffrey to forget his father or he would have nightmares.) She even finds herself worrying about the hereafter. She thinks Mr Plummer, once reunited with his first wife, will forget her.

I think her adjustment is reasonable. She is lucky in a way to have her son to take up most of her time. She worries about him growing up wild, and what to do for the best, but it is the thing that keeps her going. It is something she can deal with and she does not feel as helpless as she did whilst nursing her husband. I think when Geoffrey is a little older and starts to think of himself as the man of the house, many of Mrs Plummer's worries will resolve themselves and she will be able to relax.

CASE 2

Note: Colostomy, discharge, pain and anxiety were the dead husband's problems.

This visit was doomed from the beginning. It should never have been made, since Mr Fox only attended the day hospital and did not die in the unit but at home. However, for some reason it was on my list of possible visits. I had difficulty finding the place, and was not expected because the letter had gone astray.

I hit Mrs Fox at a low-spirited time. She was just sitting in an untidy room full of dogs and cats, with a kitten on her lap. These are her only consolation since Mr Fox died. Mrs Fox was tearful, but asked me not to worry because she cried very easily. She was depressed and apathetic. She said she had no energy to clean the house, but was depressed because she knew it was dirty.

In a way I think my visit may have done her some good. During the 2½ hours I was there she got a lot off her chest, about hospitals, life in general and middle-class bitches in particular. Her main source of grief and bitterness are as follows in the next few paragraphs.

Grief is by far the largest problem. She cried as she told me she was married at 16 and had loved her husband deeply. She showed me photographs of him and talked for three-quarters of an hour about him and what a good, kind man he was. She still misses him, and has lost interest in herself and her appearance since he died. She knows she is overweight, but has no incentive to diet. I got the impression that she feels it would be disloyal to her husband to even attempt to make herself look attractive.

Mrs Fox told me that she is haunted by the memory of her husband's death. Although she would not go into details, it was clear that she regarded it as horrible, something she 'wouldn't wish on a dog'.

Mr Fox had been to the day unit and refused to go back after a few visits. The reason for his refusal lies at the root of Mrs Fox's antagonism towards the terminal care unit.

She was angry at the way the nursing sister had put Mr Fox off by *cheerfully* telling him of patients who had died since Mr Fox last saw them. She thinks Mr Fox did not appreciate the full truth about his illness, and therefore found these constant references to death very frightening.

Also Mr Fox had never been overenthusiastic about the day unit because of the attitude of some of the volunteers. Mrs Fox felt that ordinary working men like her husband did not like being patted on the head and patronized. She complained that it made her husband feel 'less than a man'.

Mrs Fox has been unable to find a job since Mr Fox died and so has too much time to brood. Therefore, she has a clear unalterable picture of the day unit (although she has never seen the place) and of the people who work there. Obviously it is not an unbiased view, since she got the details secondhand from her husband, and her grief and bitterness have coloured her interpretation.

Her health has not suffered, but her general morale is low. She just sits and worries, without the drive to do anything. Her main preoccupation is with money. The rent tribunal made her pay back a rent rebate when they discovered Mr Fox's son was living with her. She feels very bitter about this, since nobody had asked her if she was on her own, and then they treated her as if she had deliberately deceived the council. She objected to being addressed as 'my lass' by the 'lah-di-dah lady', whom, she suspects, does voluntary work in her spare time.

Taken as a whole the visit was not a success from my point of view. Mrs Fox is angry with the special unit for upsetting her husband. She has not adjusted at all well. She has lapsed into a state of alternating depression and violent bitterness against the terminal care unit for neglecting her when Mr Fox died. This makes life rather tiring for her relatives who have to deal with these moods.

Despite her avowal that she is seeking a job and could do with stimulation, I feel she has not yet shaken herself out of her apathy. She seems almost to enjoy thinking herself mistreated and snubbed by the world. She defends her inactivity by saying that she has no chance to succeed because everyone is against her.

CASE 3

I felt that Mr Higgins was rather suspicious at first. He told me quite abruptly that he had been trying to contact the social worker to see who I was and what I wanted. I tried to suggest that he could have refused to see me, but was ignored. He kept asking me if I knew this or that about his wife, as if checking up to see that I had done my homework. I was not too sure how much of this attitude was his usual manner or how much was a defensive measure.

However, after a cup of coffee the atmosphere thawed a little.

After Ethel died, Mr Higgins was greatly supported by the bereavement visitor and his local church. He did not mention his son. However, the estate on which he lives is large and has no facilities for social contact apart from the pub and the library. As a result, he spent days without seeing anyone, often just walking about the estate. The bereavement visitor was a great comfort to him, since the visits gave him a chance to talk and broke up the days. He got really depressed and restless after his bereavement, and had trouble settling down.

The amount he smoked increased, and for a while he took sleeping pills and tranquillizers. His weight did not alter, and he is not worried about his health. His main worries after Ethel died appear to have been financial, but he has now sorted these out.

Life has been transformed by the arrival of his new 'young lady', whom he met at the library. Since then, long days alone have ceased to be a problem. They go out together using their bus passes, and spend the afternoon at one flat and the evenings at the others. Marriage was not mentioned, and this informal arrangement seems to suit them both.

On the whole I would say that Mr Higgins' adjustment is fair. He has accepted Ethel's death, but has not come to terms with coping on his own. As a result he has found a lady who is said to resemble Ethel quite closely, and is now enjoying the sort of companionable retirement he was unable to share with his wife. I think he found this lady before he had completely resolved his grief, and may be putting off really coming to terms with it.

By the time I had heard all about the 'young lady' and how isolated people in the flats were on a 'rowdy' estate, Mr Higgins had shown me around the flat and seemed more relaxed. However, he was waiting to be collected by a relative who was taking him and his lady to stay for a short holiday, and Mr Higgins was loath to let me settle. He told me there was a bus in 5 minutes and I took the hint.

CASE 4

Mr Worrall welcomed me into a beautifully tidy house, and brought tea and cakes he had made himself. His wife had known her diagnosis and so had taught Mr Worrall to cook and do other household tasks while she was well enough to sit downstairs. He was very proud of his domestic activities and his large, tidy garden.

However, he was rather depressed. He had grieved deeply for Doris but had eventually roused himself sufficiently to take up dancing. This was to get a little female company, as his other hobby, rambling, was more or less an exclusively male preserve. Through his dancing he had met a new lady and they had considered marriage. However, when the time came to decide, neither would give up their present home and eventually they decided to call the whole thing off. This has put Mr Worrall back to feeling as he did just after Doris died, totally alone, and he had added guilt feelings about even considering a new life with someone else. He blames himself for trying to replace Doris, but admits to feeling the physical need for cosy contact with a woman, and dancing is the only way to get such contact without risking arrest. He clearly found it painful to express these ideas, but said he needed somebody to talk to.

This brought him to the topic of his two sons. He gives them both money but feels that they value this more than him as a person. Mr Worrall feels rather bitter about this attitude, especially as he gave the cash to the boys rather than take Mrs Worrall on holidays, etc. while she was well. His family support seems minimal.

However, Mr Worrall is active, and has a very busy schedule. He lectures a lot and his timetable for the week struck me as compulsive, never time to sit down and work things out, no time to think at all.

Although practically he is coping very well, and keeping himself occupied, I wonder what will happen when he is ill and has to stop dashing about and starts remembering things. He was pleased with the treatment Doris got but hurried through the questionnaire so that he could tell his news about dancing, etc.

CASE 5

Mr Burrows lives in a nicely kept house, full of pot plants. Like me he had a cold and so put a 'drop' of brandy in our tea. I could smell this 'drop' 5 feet away. However, this soon warmed us up and the conversation thereafter was very relaxed!

He was keen to talk about his wife, although he wept some of the time. He felt she was always in the house with him 'just around'. He was grateful to the unit for all the care she had received and wished everybody well.

His greatest problem is loneliness. Mrs Burrows had a rare illness in her youth which stopped them having any children. He does go out with his brother and sister-in-law but now the foursome is incomplete and it occasionally makes him feel worse. He is very aware that now his sister-in-law has nobody to talk 'female talk' to and though the men try to include her in the conversation, it's not the same. He's never been a drinking man and so has no mates at the pub for casual company. He was always a little solitary, having driven a crane for 20-odd years, where you don't speak to many people.

He has arthritis but when this permits he does take himself out for a change, although generally he sits and reads, enjoying the feeling that his wife is near him. He is a great fan of murder and mystery stories.

He then went into a general discussion of all the neighbourhood, for example '14 children and only done 6 *weeks* work in 29 years, mind you with 14 kids he's not got the strength'. That brought back happy memories or his wife and him on holiday, etc.

As I left, my attention was drawn to the barbed wire which extends the length of Mr Burrows' front door to deter vandals and thieves.

CASE 6

Mrs Cox lives in a pleasant council flat with her son. She herself has had two tumours removed, which our notes have as cancer. This has left her with partial paralysis and a 'dropped' left eye of which she is very self-conscious. Thus she is unwilling to go out. The son goes out quite a lot, but is clearly very close to his mother. However, she feels that even he cannot combat the 'loneliness of heart' she feels.

She finds some compensation in her belief in spiritualism. She considers herself to be psychic and told me her husband often sits in the chair I was occupying, and that she doesn't worry about her health because Mr Cox on the 'Other Side' sends spirit doctors to tend her during the night. She knows because she has seen them.

She seemed a little confused as to the purpose of the terminal care unit. When told that Mr Cox was to be given painkillers, she assumed we meant drugs to kill cancer, and that he died because we'd accidentally killed him! However, he was ill, and she didn't think we did anything unkind so she did not intend to take action.

She feels she is coping quite well with everything, although her pills make her dizzy and so increase her reluctance to go out, even with dark glasses and a scarf. She is bitter about the state of her face, as she maintains that the surgeon has refused to acknowledge she had a growth at all until a medical student noticed it. He then claimed he'd known about it all the time and was just testing. So now Mrs Cox, although she still goes to see him, dislikes the surgeon as unfeeling, and places more faith in a spiritual healer and her ghostly doctors.

CASE 7

Mrs Haddon lives in a lovely home with a large garden and is very busy. Her son is at home at present. Her activity is part of a definite plan to wear herself out each day to be able to get to sleep.

When she received a visitor from the terminal care unit, she felt it was good, and a very welcome contrast to the treatment she received from the hospital. She has very bad memories of that place and did not expect any consideration or compassion from it. She kept stressing that her grief for Bill was secondary to her anger at the way her husband was treated at the hospital. This anger has unsettled her and her resentment boiled over as she told me about her experiences.

She was told by the consultant that 90 per cent of her husband's pain was him acting, and people at the golf club as well were told that he was 'putting it on'. On one occasion she went to fetch him from the hospital to find him rolling on the floor in pain (he has done this before at home because none of the painkillers did any good). The consultant told a nurse to tell her husband to get up, and that his pain was no more than that from a slipped disc. Mrs Haddon was horrified and stood up to the consultant but to no avail. She did, however, refuse to take her husband home, and made sure he was kept comfortable.

She feels that the way he was treated at the hospital robbed her husband of his dignity. The terminal care unit gave him back his dignity and allowed Mr Haddon to die in peace, and without pain.

Mrs Haddon had tranquillizers, on doctor's orders, while her husband was ill. She has not taken them since, preferring to be tired from activity rather than 'dopey'. She still get very angry when she thinks of the hospital, and will not go past the building if she can help it. She resents the fact that she, an intelligent woman married to an educated man, was not to be trusted with the truth about her husband's illness. She still shudders when she remembers the pain he suffered going to and from the hospital.

CASE 8

Miss Venables is living at her father's home at present. She is a lady in early middle age, but very well groomed and so I found it rather hard to guess her exact age.

She was pleased with the treatment her father received at the special unit. Her main grumble was with her general practitioner. For 2 years she had suspected that there was something more wrong with her father than the general practitioner had made out, and so was very angry to learn that cancer had gone untreated for this time. She realizes that she cannot assess the difference an earlier diagnosis would have made, but feels he didn't really have much of a chance.

She thought the idea of a bereavement visitor was a good one, although not really necessary in her case. She was coping well, and although sad to have lost her father was continuing her life as before.

CASE 9

Mrs Harkness lives in a nice house. She has two sons; one is getting married next year and the other is mentally handicapped. This is a source of great worry to her. When I arrived the house was quiet, for once. She was alone except for the corgi. Her handicapped son was away for the week at a residential school. Much as she disliked sending him away, she was glad of a week to herself to get the house straight and have a rest, since she finds caring for him very tiring, especially as he is incontinent and there is always loads of bedding to be washed.

Her attitude towards her son is two-sided. She feels the burden of caring for him alone and worries about his feeling rejected when she has to send him away. On the other hand, he is the driving force that makes her get out of bed in the morning and gives her other things to worry about. She is not well herself at the moment. She was very tense about this and miserable, and awaiting surgery.

She appreciated a visitor from the special unit because she felt she couldn't burden the elder son with all her worries, especially not while he is in the middle of planning the wedding. She worries about how she will cope when he moves quite a distance away.

She talked at length about her husband's illness. Her theory is that the cancer was brought on by a shock he had some years ago. After that Mr Harkness was never the same and his health deteriorated afterwards.

The general practitioner who looks after her son was not nearly so good with the father. Mrs Harkness subscribes to the theory that doctors don't like cancer cases, it messes up their batting averages. She has good neighbours and friends around, but is very worried about being isolated when her other son gets married, though she's very fond of his future wife.

She is worried about getting more personal contact, but is very limited by her son, who clings more now that his father is gone. At present she is just hoping that she will have the strength to cope with him after her operation.

CASE 10

Mrs Farrar lives in a beautiful house. She is sad when she looks at it because it took years to build and her husband never had the chance to enjoy it. She now lives there with her two younger sons, who are at school, and their little dog.

Mrs Farrar was very pleased at the treatment she had received at the special unit and all the kindness she was shown in the way that the doctors talked to her. She found this in bitter contrast to the way she was treated at hospital. She was very discontented with the doctors and specialists there. Mr Farrar was treated for over 2 years by one specialist who did nothing when he ought to have been giving different treatment altogether.

She doubts whether the change would have done Mr Farrar any good as far as saving or lengthening his life was concerned, but she resents that the chance was not made available. It might at least have improved the quality of the last part of his life. She is very bitter towards the doctors who said it was 90 per cent nerves and there was no reason for him not to be at work. On changing specialists, the new doctor took one look at him and fetched a wheelchair.

She was also angry that her husband, an intelligent man, should not have been told what was the matter with him. He would never have had any idea if they had not applied for a mortgage and her husband had seen a letter regarding his health left lying around on a desk at work. He didn't tell her, so when she realized how ill he was it came as a great shock.

Since her husband's death she has brooded about this, and feels her grief is not abating as quickly as it would if she were able to resign herself to her loss. She is aware of being overprotective towards her younger son. To prevent him growing up too closely attached to her she has sent him away to boarding school. This took a great amount of effort, but thanks to help and advice she received from Cruse (the society for bereaved spouses) it has been sorted out.

Her bereavement visitor was the same age as her and also had a family. Mrs Farrar feels that this is very important, since another widow would depress her too much and even without her husband she still has a family life to carry on. She felt that more thought ought to be given generally to selecting visitors to suit people, and that when women were left on their own a male social worker would be useful to give practical advice about plugs, etc.

My visit lasted 4 hours and we covered general topics as well, since she enjoyed the chance to chat to somebody new.

Appendix II:
Stoma patients interviewed

E. E. Lawton

In 1978, of 44 patients interviewed after stoma surgery 28 had great anxieties prior to discharge home, as these quotations demonstrate:

Mostly about the smell. It is difficult not to worry about it: of course I also worried about getting well again. I felt quite weak. I didn't dare think about having to learn how to live with the colostomy.

I did not know how I was going to do it at all. My daughter asked the nurses to show her how to do it and was told that I would *have* to do it myself. How could I when I was never shown what to do, or how to do it? My children just told me I was not to worry but I felt that I would rather be dead than have to live with it. Even though they told me it was only temporary. When I saw myself in the mirror, after a bath – my first – then I wished I had died instead of having the operation.

Frightened of going 'mental'. Weak, pain – thought I was imagining it – cried a lot. Body image. I had not seen the 'pretty little bags'. Did not know why I couldn't get any information about living with it for ever. I asked if I could see the Association visitor – a man we had heard of.

All I thought about was my determination to die. Everybody who had this operation had cancer, I thought to myself. I never thought it possible that I would go home.

The smell; because I was conscious of it all the time I thought the patients could smell it. I felt a bit odd but I did try not to let others see I was very worried about it. It worked so often – fluid – and I got very sore.

I wanted to ask so many questions which worried me about coping. Trivial to them I suppose – for instance, how would I know when to change the appliances – every week, every day? What to eat, etc. How to get rid of the bags and go out or back to work.

323

When they first saw their stoma 20 patients felt degraded and ill-prepared:

> I was very *shocked* to see it. I did not know about it at all before the operation. I think they look awful, but I have got used to it now.

> I was upset because I didn't understand what was going on.

> I didn't want to think about it. I just thought I was going to die anyway. I just cried and cried. It looked awful. The morning I left the hospital a junior nurse told sister there was still a clamp on it. It was removed 20 minutes before I left so I still hadn't seen it or I would have seen the black thing.

> It was so big. After seeing *the book* showing a small 1″ stoma, like a button, I was very shocked and upset. I did not know how to tell my husband about it – the sight of it would surely put him off. This was when I realized 'That's it' – I would just *have* to cope with it.

> Oh my God – what a mess. Heartbroken. Body image. I suppose I was selfish but it really did upset me. It was a very personal thing I felt – not for my husband's sake at all. Not then, anyway.

> I went wild in the post-op convalescent unit. I did not eat because I was the only man in the ward who had one. I could smell it all the time. How could I sit at the table with other patients? I wanted to die rather than live with the dirty thing. I thought I was going to die anyway, so why bother?

> I was very upset one day when a nurse with a student came to do my dressing. She took off the dirty one and the student said, 'Ugh, how dreadful, I don't know how you are going to live with this for the rest of your life. It is *horrible.*' I went to the bathroom, took a good look at it and cried – not because of the stoma itself but because I was so hurt by her thoughtlessness.

Out of the 44, 38 felt they needed more information and 18 felt incompetent and unable to cope properly with their stoma:

> About my diet and why it was not essential to continue my previous regime, i.e. low residue. I know what upsets me. I did not know about appliances (I still don't) but I know that perhaps another type might be more suitable for me.

> About getting supplies, and the disposal collection service. My daughter would have liked to know more about stomas and to be taught herself by the nurse how to do it. (The district nurse showed her later.)

> How to manage the stoma in general. What to expect. But most of all, how to cope with the GP, i.e. getting a prescription and then getting what we needed from *a chemist*. Our chemist did not have any but ordered for us. It was running backwards and forwards for 2 weeks.

Too many people are involved. If one person could talk to you about the whole thing, give advice and answer questions properly about what to do in any given situation, I think things would be much better.

The right answers to the queries I made on several occasions. I just wanted someone to tell me what to do, what to expect, perhaps too much. If I had just known *who* to ask for advice after I got home. It was all I wanted – someone to ask, who would advise me.

No. No-one ever showed me how. I had no idea where to start.

No, because I didn't know how to change the bags myself.

Not at all. I couldn't put the appliance on properly. It kept coming off when I did it.

Out of 44, 35 felt that they needed more information and extra help; and when asked for the most helpful advice they ought to have received, they replied thus:

Where to get practical help and support.

If I had known just how to avoid or how to cope with leakage from stoma *and* the possible accident, it would have saved us that anxiety.

A proper and realistic discussion about the operation *before* having it. To be actually told the truth about what to expect. The book I was given was out of date. One should *not* be told to *expect* sexual problems, or one does.

Someone to discuss the problems with. Our sons and their wives are no support to us at all.

Where to go for help, which I very badly needed. Looking back it could all have been avoided if I had been told about everything you have mentioned.

There were 17 who felt they had managed badly in their early days at home.

An emotional reaction is natural and inevitable in such circumstances, nor is it necessarily characteristic of stoma cases only. Maguire and his colleagues (1978) have shown a 25 per cent incidence a year after mastectomy of anxiety, depression or both and 33 per cent of these patients had sexual difficulties.

These comments are not to be taken as justifying criticism of colleagues but as emphasizing the loneliness of the badly briefed patient. This is vividly exemplified by the following case-history, which was written down immediately after the interview. The patient seems to have had speedy referral, accurate diagnosis, and uneventful surgery. There will be no litigation here and no complaints.

This male patient aged 53 years approached his general practitioner after a fairly long – more than 6 months' – history of loose stools and loss of weight. There had been no pain or discomfort and no rectal bleeding.

As he had been, and still was, working and feeling quite well at this time, he did not *know* his doctor because he had always kept well; he just thought 'a few tablets would clear it up'.

After rectal examination the patient was given a letter to take to hospital for an appointment to see a consultant, whom he did not know. He was not aware that the consultant was a surgeon.

Within a few days he had attended the outpatient clinic, taking his wife along with him.

> I left the consulting room *absolutely stunned* after being told that I had a large ulcer in my seat which would require major surgery [a meaningless term to him at the time]. Here I was a working man, feeling quite well and after seeing two strange men [general practitioner and surgeon] in less than a week being told that I must go into hospital for 'major surgery'. What did it mean, we asked ourselves and there was no answer. We went and had a cup of tea.
>
> I did not go back to my own doctor because I didn't know him, nor did I think of it at the time. I had a holiday booked 6 weeks ahead and had asked in clinic if I could have my holiday first, then go into hospital. They hesitated and I thought later, though they didn't actually say so, that it would be better for me to cancel it. I did this and wrote to the surgeon to say that I would go into hospital when they wanted me to and I was admitted a few days later.

At this stage, neither the patient nor his wife had ever heard of a stoma. It had not been mentioned in the outpatient department.

Two days before surgery, a doctor came to talk to him about his operation, accompanied by a staff nurse. He told the patient brusquely, 'If you have this operation you'll live 5 years – if you don't you won't live another 2'.

> I just didn't know what to think, it was such a shock – not just to be told that – but the arrogant manner in which it was said to me, a take-it-or-leave-it attitude. Staff nurse saw I was taken aback and explained a little but the doctor said I hadn't listened to what he said. I felt very upset. When I said to him 'I don't win either way do I?' he then explained that after 5 years I would *probably* be all right. I still don't know quite what he was *really* saying, and it worries me. I haven't seen my own doctor or asked anyone about it. The experiences I've had since the operation need some coping with and I can't seem to sort it all out in my mind [27 days after discharge]. That same day I was taken to theatre – no anaesthetic – for a 'test'. I was told by the same doctor that it was for a 'second opinion' and I felt that might mean '*no operation*'. I was quite pleased to hear

this. What I endured for the next 20 minutes I will never forget. I had my knees up and they were 'snipping away inside me' – no anaesthetic and it was agony, and it did something to my blood pressure because they all got worried about it and I was sent back to the ward.

The next day an ambulance driver came to me and said 'Are you ready?' I thought he had the wrong man. 'No,' he said, 'it's you, to go to . . . . That finished me. I knew that was the cancer place. Sister didn't know anything about it, but she thought I had better go as it was arranged by the doctor. I was left in reception there, frightened to death – all this in such a short space of time – I couldn't believe it was happening to me. I was taken into a room and the nurses marked my body, for X-rays I was told. Then I was told to wait outside. I did – *for 3 hours* – not even a cup of tea, much less anything to eat. I was scared stiff and no-one said anything to me.

Later, I was taken back to the ward, I got a cup of tea and went to bed for a while, thinking, 'This is a good time for all this – I'm supposed to have major surgery tomorrow and I know nothing about it really'. The ward staff nurse was a gem, she tried to explain about the operation later that day when she came to see me about the catheter put in before the operation. The preparation for theatre was very 'degrading'. I felt humiliated by the bowel washouts, the catheter and the shave, and I felt very upset about it all. Looking back – I just didn't understand the reason all this was being done at the time. The need for an operation only came to me later when I realized the true nature and extent of the operation I had had. Although I was told about the 'stoma', I didn't know what it meant really.

A medical student came to talk to me, he was so gentle, he was sorry he wasn't allowed to tell me anything. What you need is someone to talk to you like a human being.

When I came to after the operation I had a drip and tubes all over me [catheter – rectal drain] and I didn't feel too badly really. But on the night of the second day the bag [stoma] burst, all over the bed it was, and so late at night. I didn't know what had happened so I called the nurse over; she had never seen one before so she went to ask the other nurse, who told her to clean it up.

When she came back to me she said, 'She never did like me that one – telling me to clean you up and I don't know where to start'. She implied that because the other nurse didn't like her she could do the dirty job herself.

Then she told me to get out of bed – I hadn't been up (48 hours postop) and didn't know what to do with all my tubes. I stood by the bed and she fetched a bowl of water, cleaned me up, changed the bed and told me to get back in. Then neither of us knew how to put the bags on again, but we managed to see me through the night.

There wasn't another patient on the ward with a stoma, but a girl in our office had one 4 years ago – I didn't know that. She came to see me and told me all that would happen to me – about having to learn to live with it, not being able to get supplies because of the chemist and a lot of things I didn't believe. I thought she was exaggerating then, but I don't now. It's a good thing I have a sense of humour, I would have gone mad.

Staff nurse asked an ex-patient to come and talk to me, but he was a young man, very sporty and half my age. I couldn't relate to him in any way because I am old enough to be his dad. In any case, he didn't have the same surgery, so how could he know? I would willingly talk to men in my age group if only to help them, save them the anxieties I have gone through. A patient talking to me later said, 'Aren't we lucky mate – there's some fellow in here walking about with a shit bag on – glad I'm not him, aren't you?' I felt sure that everyone could smell me, though I was changing my bags all right. I was only shown once and after that I had to do it myself.

When I came home they gave me a few and told me to get some more from the clinic. As they were the drainer bags, I could keep washing them out so when I saw the surgeon I asked him, and he sent me to the sister. She gave me two and a prescription to take to the chemist.

I went to two chemists who did not have them, so when I went to the stoma clinic I told sister, who told me to go to a certain chemist in town and to get my next prescription from my doctor. Why wasn't I told this at first? Next time I went for my sick note I asked the receptionist, who said: 'There is a dispensary in this health centre, go and see them'. So now all I need to do is get my supplies from there.

No-one told me how to get rid of the used ones, and because I want to go on holiday for a week before the winter, please will you advise me?

Reference

Maguire, G. P., Lee, E. G., Bevington, D. L., Kuchemann, C. S., Crabtree, R. J. and Cornell, C. E. (1978). *Br. Med. J.*, **1**, 963

Index

acute aortic dissection 64
addiction 279
  analgesics, and 279
age
  death, at 234
  renal transplantation and 92
agitation 221
  management of, in terminal illness 221
Alzheimer's disease 20, 23
  Down's syndrome, and 42
  toxins in 42
  transmissable agent, and 42
anaemia 215
  cytotoxic chemotherapy, and 121
  management of 87, 215
  renal failure, in 87, 98
  terminally ill, in 215
  severe 91
analgesics 187
  addiction to 279
  co-analgesics, and 193
  cocaine 191
  diamorphine 190
  prescribing difficulties, and 279
  morphine 190
  non-narcotic 193
  non-steroidal anti-inflammatory 194
  rectal preparations 199
  side effects of 279

see also named drugs
anus 159
  squamous carcinoma of 159
anorexia
  cardiac disease, and 67
  constipation, and 166
  cytotoxic chemotherapy, and 121
  elderly, in the 8
  management of 222
antiemetics 213
  Brompton cocktail, in 189
  narcotic therapy, and 191
anxiety 210, 233
  awareness of dying, and 237
  cardiac disease, in 78
  drugs for 211
  elderly, in the 9
  pain threshold, effect on 201, 281
aortic coarction 68
  diagnosis 68
aortic dissection, acute 64
aortic stenosis 60
  sudden death, and 60
arteriovenous fistula 67
  heart failure, causing 67
ascites 224
  ovarian carcinoma, in 185
  peritoneal malignancy, management in
    164